Chronic Kidney Disease: Underlying Molecular Mechanisms

Chronic Kidney Disease: Underlying Molecular Mechanisms

Editors

Márcia Carvalho
Luís Belo

MDPI • Basel • Beijing • Wuhan • Barcelona • Belgrade • Manchester • Tokyo • Cluj • Tianjin

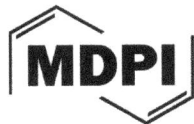

Editors
Márcia Carvalho
Faculty of Health Sciences
University Fernando Pessoa
Porto
Portugal

Luís Belo
Department of Biological
Sciences, Faculty of Pharmacy
University of Porto
Porto
Portugal

Editorial Office
MDPI
St. Alban-Anlage 66
4052 Basel, Switzerland

This is a reprint of articles from the Special Issue published online in the open access journal *International Journal of Molecular Sciences* (ISSN 1422-0067) (available at: www.mdpi.com/journal/ijms/special_issues/CKD_IJMS).

For citation purposes, cite each article independently as indicated on the article page online and as indicated below:

LastName, A.A.; LastName, B.B.; LastName, C.C. Article Title. *Journal Name* **Year**, *Volume Number*, Page Range.

ISBN 978-3-0365-8541-3 (Hbk)
ISBN 978-3-0365-8540-6 (PDF)

© 2023 by the authors. Articles in this book are Open Access and distributed under the Creative Commons Attribution (CC BY) license, which allows users to download, copy and build upon published articles, as long as the author and publisher are properly credited, which ensures maximum dissemination and a wider impact of our publications.

The book as a whole is distributed by MDPI under the terms and conditions of the Creative Commons license CC BY-NC-ND.

Contents

About the Editors vii

Luís Belo and Márcia Carvalho
Chronic Kidney Disease: Underlying Molecular Mechanisms—A Special Issue Overview
Reprinted from: *Int. J. Mol. Sci.* 2023, 24, 12363, doi:10.3390/ijms241512363 1

Manish Mishra, Larry Nichols, Aditi A. Dave, Elizabeth H Pittman, John P. Cheek and Anasalea J. V. Caroland et al.
Molecular Mechanisms of Cellular Injury and Role of Toxic Heavy Metals in Chronic Kidney Disease
Reprinted from: *Int. J. Mol. Sci.* 2022, 23, 11105, doi:10.3390/ijms231911105 5

Irina Lousa, Flávio Reis, Alice Santos-Silva and Luís Belo
The Signaling Pathway of TNF Receptors: Linking Animal Models of Renal Disease to Human CKD
Reprinted from: *Int. J. Mol. Sci.* 2022, 23, 3284, doi:10.3390/ijms23063284 29

Natalia V. Chebotareva, Anatoliy Vinogradov, Alexander G. Brzhozovskiy, Daria N. Kashirina, Maria I. Indeykina and Anna E. Bugrova et al.
Potential Urine Proteomic Biomarkers for Focal Segmental Glomerulosclerosis and Minimal Change Disease
Reprinted from: *Int. J. Mol. Sci.* 2022, 23, 12607, doi:10.3390/ijms232012607 55

Giorgia Magliocca, Pasquale Mone, Biagio Raffaele Di Iorio, August Heidland and Stefania Marzocco
Short-Chain Fatty Acids in Chronic Kidney Disease: Focus on Inflammation and Oxidative Stress Regulation
Reprinted from: *Int. J. Mol. Sci.* 2022, 23, 5354, doi:10.3390/ijms23105354 77

Chien-Ning Hsu and You-Lin Tain
Chronic Kidney Disease and Gut Microbiota: What Is Their Connection in Early Life?
Reprinted from: *Int. J. Mol. Sci.* 2022, 23, 3954, doi:10.3390/ijms23073954 101

Zhihuang Zheng, Yao Xu, Ute Krügel, Michael Schaefer, Tilman Grune and Bernd Nürnberg et al.
In Vivo Inhibition of TRPC6 by SH045 Attenuates Renal Fibrosis in a New Zealand Obese (NZO) Mouse Model of Metabolic Syndrome
Reprinted from: *Int. J. Mol. Sci.* 2022, 23, 6870, doi:10.3390/ijms23126870 119

Nazareno Carullo, Giuseppe Fabiano, Mario D'Agostino, Maria Teresa Zicarelli, Michela Musolino and Pierangela Presta et al.
New Insights on the Role of Marinobufagenin from Bench to Bedside in Cardiovascular and Kidney Diseases
Reprinted from: *Int. J. Mol. Sci.* 2023, 24, 11186, doi:10.3390/ijms241311186 133

Jing Liu, Elaine L. Shelton, Rachelle Crescenzi, Daniel C. Colvin, Annet Kirabo and Jianyong Zhong et al.
Kidney Injury Causes Accumulation of Renal Sodium That Modulates Renal Lymphatic Dynamics
Reprinted from: *Int. J. Mol. Sci.* 2022, 23, 1428, doi:10.3390/ijms23031428 155

Robert H. Mak, Sujana Gunta, Eduardo A. Oliveira and Wai W. Cheung
Growth Hormone Improves Adipose Tissue Browning and Muscle Wasting in Mice with Chronic Kidney Disease-Associated Cachexia
Reprinted from: *Int. J. Mol. Sci.* **2022**, 23, 15310, doi:10.3390/ijms232315310 . . . . **169**

Sara Mendes, Diogo V. Leal, Luke A. Baker, Aníbal Ferreira, Alice C. Smith and João L. Viana
The Potential Modulatory Effects of Exercise on Skeletal Muscle Redox Status in Chronic Kidney Disease
Reprinted from: *Int. J. Mol. Sci.* **2023**, 24, 6017, doi:10.3390/ijms24076017 . . . . **187**

About the Editors

Márcia Carvalho

Márcia Carvalho graduated in Pharmaceutical Sciences from the Faculty of Pharmacy, University of Porto (FFUP), Portugal. She holds a Master of Science degree in Quality Control—Scientific Area in Drug Substances and Medicinal Plants and a PhD degree in Toxicology from the same university. Marcia Carvalho is presently an Associate Professor of Toxicology at the Faculty of Health Sciences, University Fernando Pessoa (UFP, Porto, Portugal), a researcher at the I3ID/FP-BHS (UFP, Portugal), and an independent researcher in the Toxicology Group (FFUP, Portugal) of the Applied Molecular Biosciences Unit (UCIBIO, REQUIMTE). Her primary research interests are toxicological and toxicometabolomic studies to investigate the mechanisms of toxicity (particularly affecting the kidney and liver) of xenobiotics using in vivo and in vitro experimental model systems. She has published over 90 papers in international peer-reviewed journals, seven book chapters, and holds an h-index of 39 (Scopus).

Luís Belo

Luís Belo completed a Master's degree in Medicine in 2014 at the University of Porto (Faculty of Medicine), a PhD in Biochemistry in 2003 at the University of Porto (Faculty of Pharmacy), and a degree in Pharmaceutical Sciences in 1997 also at the University of Porto (Faculty of Pharmacy). He is currently an Assistant Professor with Habilitation at the University of Porto, a Medical Doctor in dialysis units, and a Researcher at REQUIMTE, the Applied Molecular Biosciences Unit (UCIBIO). His main areas of investigation are chronic kidney disease and obesity. He participated as a team member in several FCT-financed projects. He published more than 130 articles in international scientific journals and several sections of books. Since 2021, he has been a member of the Global Burden of Disease (GBD) Collaborator Network. He received 16 scientific awards and/or honors. His h-index is 31 (Scopus).

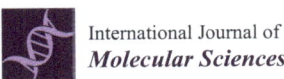

Editorial

Chronic Kidney Disease: Underlying Molecular Mechanisms—A Special Issue Overview

Luís Belo [1,2,*] and Márcia Carvalho [1,2,3,4]

1. Associate Laboratory i4HB—Institute for Health and Bioeconomy, Department of Biological Sciences, Faculty of Pharmacy, University of Porto, 4050-313 Porto, Portugal; mcarv@ufp.edu.pt
2. UCIBIO/REQUIMTE, Department of Biological Sciences, Faculty of Pharmacy, University of Porto, 4050-313 Porto, Portugal
3. FP-I3ID, FP-BHS, University Fernando Pessoa, 4200-150 Porto, Portugal
4. Faculty of Health Sciences, University Fernando Pessoa, 4200-150 Porto, Portugal
* Correspondence: luisbelo@ff.up.pt; Tel.: +351-220-428-562

Chronic kidney disease (CKD) is an epidemic health issue that requires global attention [1]. The worldwide increment of CKD incidence is related to an increase in traditional risk factors of the disease (e.g., diabetes, hypertension and human aging) that may be aggravated by other factors, such as environmental and occupational exposure to toxic heavy metals (e.g., cadmium and mercury) [2]. In this Special Issue, authors contributed with works that further the understanding of CKD's pathophysiology and its associated complications, highlighting the identification of potential new biomarkers of the disease and more effective therapeutic options.

Despite the etiology of CKD, inflammation is a common feature in the pathogenesis of the disease [3]. With this respect, the inflammation pathway driven by tumor necrosis factor (TNF)-α has received particular attention from the scientific community. Several studies in humans and involving animal models report an important role of the TNF system in renal disease [4]. The study of several plasma biomarkers—related to tubular injury, fibrosis and inflammation—revealed that a higher TNF receptor 2 (TNFR2) level was associated with the highest risk of progression of diabetic kidney disease [5]. Also, TNFR2 is distinguished amongst several circulating inflammatory variables because its levels present remarkable negative correlations with estimated glomerular filtration rate (eGFR) and increase with CKD progression [6]. TNF receptors (TNFR1 and TNFR2) might be useful not only for early CKD detection but also as biomarkers of CKD progression and prognosis [4].

New blood and urine biomarkers of CKD have been proposed, but many lack specificity and may only be detected in advanced phases of the disease [7]. Since there are various alternative pathways by which CKD can result, a panel monitoring multiple biomarkers may be a more reasonable method to better anticipate CKD development and access the disease's outcomes. Modern laboratory methods that enable the simultaneous analysis of several biomarkers are in use and have significantly impacted the identification of new biomarkers. Such is the case of omics technologies, despite being expensive and time-consuming [7]. For instance, Chebotareva and colleagues, by using proteomic analysis, identified potential profile urine biomarkers from patients with focal segmental glomerulosclerosis and minimal change disease, known as podocytopathies clinically manifested by the nephrotic syndrome [8]. Other investigators have used metabolomic studies and microRNA analysis [9].

Altered gut microbiota is involved in the pathogenesis of several pathologies, including kidney diseases [10]. Current knowledge supports the impact of the gut–kidney axis in CKD. A significant qualitative or quantitative alteration in the gut microbiota may lead to reduced production of beneficial bacterial metabolites, such as short-chain fatty acids (SCFAs). SCFAs are known to present important anti-inflammatory properties and their

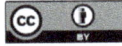

levels are reduced in CKD [11]. Thus, dysbiosis and microbiota metabolite changes may underlie CKD-associated inflammation, promoting disease progression and its associated complications. Recent data also suggest that gut microbiota dysbiosis is implicated in pediatric CKD and renal programming [12]. This programming increases the kidney's susceptibility to postnatal insults and increases the risk of developing CKD in the future.

The progression of CKD, which ultimately results in an irreversible state of renal fibrosis, is still not well controlled, despite the availability of general treatment methods. Recently, novel drug targets have been proposed: marinobufagenin (a cardiac glycoside) and transient receptor potential cation channel, subfamily C, and member 6 (TRPC6). According to Zheng et al. [13], pharmacological inhibition of TRPC6 may be a viable antifibrotic treatment approach for progressive tubulointerstitial fibrosis in hypertension and metabolic syndrome. Marinobufagenin has been suggested to be involved in profibrotic pathways and to have a relevant role in CKD [14]. Some patients could benefit from therapy with mineralocorticoid receptor antagonists (MRA) that have been shown to have a preventive effect on marinobufagenin-induced fibrosis.

Diuretics are widely used in CKD management, namely in treating edema and hypertension [15]. Diuretics may also affect renal lymphatic vessels, as they express the Na-K-2Cl cotransporter NKCC1, whose function is inhibited by furosemide. Liu and colleagues have demonstrated that lymphatic hyporesponsive to furosemide may occur in situations such as proteinuric kidney disease. Increased renal interstitial sodium after a proteinuric injury is associated with lymphatic vessel dysfunction [16].

Musculoskeletal disorders are moderately common complications in CKD patients [17]. CKD-associated cachexia (a syndrome that results in substantial loss of skeletal muscle mass and adipose tissue) has been linked to raised serum levels of pro-inflammatory cytokines, a redox imbalance and growth hormone (GH) resistance [18]. In CKD, some approaches have been proposed to improve muscular wasting, including pharmacological treatment and lifestyle changes. Using an animal model of CKD (mice model consisting of 5/6 nephrectomy), Mak et al. demonstrated that the administration of GH could increase food intake and weight growth, decrease uncoupling proteins and improve muscular mass and function [19]. GH also normalized myogenesis and muscle regeneration. This is in line with studies performed in hemodialysis patients, to whom the administration of GH increased muscle protein synthesis and muscle mass. Compelling evidence also suggests that exercise—a recognized pivotal factor in promoting skeletal muscle remodeling and metabolic adaptation—may help counteract muscle wasting in CKD [20]. Resistance exercise was shown to stimulate protein anabolism in patients under hemodialysis, and endurance exercise improved protein metabolism markers. Intradialytic regular exercise training was also shown to induce a reduction in inflammation and in various redox status parameters while improving physical performance in end-stage renal disease patients [21]. However, global exercise regimens must be implemented to better solidify the outcomes achieved thus far.

In synthesis, the molecular mechanisms involved in the pathophysiology of CKD and associated complications have been explored. The scientific community is also attempting to identify more sensitive and specific biomarkers of CKD but requires further study. Identifying and validating new and standardized therapeutical pharmacological and non-pharmacological options is also mandatory. As guest editors, we thank all the authors and reviewers for their valuable contributions to this issue.

Author Contributions: Conceptualization, L.B. and M.C.; writing—original draft preparation, L.B.; writing—review and editing, L.B. and M.C. All authors have read and agreed to the published version of the manuscript.

Funding: The authors acknowledge the support from FCT in the scope of the project UIDP/04378/2020 and UIDB/04378/2020 of UCIBIO and the project LA/P/0140/2020 of i4HB.

Conflicts of Interest: The authors declare no conflict of interest.

References

1. Lameire, N.H.; Levin, A.; Kellum, J.A.; Cheung, M.; Jadoul, M.; Winkelmayer, W.C.; Stevens, P.E. Harmonizing acute and chronic kidney disease definition and classification: Report of a Kidney Disease: Improving Global Outcomes (KDIGO) Consensus Conference. *Kidney Int.* **2021**, *100*, 516–526. [CrossRef] [PubMed]
2. Mishra, M.; Nichols, L.; Dave, A.A.; Pittman, E.H.; Cheek, J.P.; Caroland, A.J.V.; Lotwala, P.; Drummond, J.; Bridges, C.C. Molecular Mechanisms of Cellular Injury and Role of Toxic Heavy Metals in Chronic Kidney Disease. *Int. J. Mol. Sci.* **2022**, *23*, 11105. [CrossRef]
3. Yamaguchi, J.; Tanaka, T.; Nangaku, M. Recent advances in understanding of chronic kidney disease. *F1000Research* **2019**, *4*. [CrossRef] [PubMed]
4. Lousa, I.; Reis, F.; Santos-Silva, A.; Belo, L. The Signaling Pathway of TNF Receptors: Linking Animal Models of Renal Disease to Human CKD. *Int. J. Mol. Sci.* **2022**, *23*, 3284. [CrossRef] [PubMed]
5. Schrauben, S.J.; Shou, H.; Zhang, X.; Anderson, A.H.; Bonventre, J.V.; Chen, J.; Coca, S.; Furth, S.L.; Greenberg, J.H.; Gutierrez, O.M.; et al. Association of Multiple Plasma Biomarker Concentrations with Progression of Prevalent Diabetic Kidney Disease: Findings from the Chronic Renal Insufficiency Cohort (CRIC) Study. *J. Am. Soc. Nephrol.* **2021**, *32*, 115–126. [CrossRef]
6. Lousa, I.; Belo, L.; Valente, M.J.; Rocha, S.; Preguiça, I.; Rocha-Pereira, P.; Beirão, I.; Mira, F.; Alves, R.; Reis, F.; et al. Inflammatory biomarkers in staging of chronic kidney disease: Elevated TNFR2 levels accompanies renal function decline. *Inflamm. Res.* **2022**, *71*, 591–602. [CrossRef]
7. Lousa, I.; Reis, F.; Beirão, I.; Alves, R.; Belo, L.; Santos-Silva, A. New Potential Biomarkers for Chronic Kidney Disease Management-A Review of the Literature. *Int. J. Mol. Sci.* **2020**, *22*, 43. [CrossRef]
8. Chebotareva, N.V.; Vinogradov, A.; Brzhozovskiy, A.G.; Kashirina, D.N.; Indeykina, M.I.; Bugrova, A.E.; Lebedeva, M.; Moiseev, S.; Nikolaev, E.N.; Kononikhin, A.S. Potential Urine Proteomic Biomarkers for Focal Segmental Glomerulosclerosis and Minimal Change Disease. *Int. J. Mol. Sci.* **2022**, *23*, 12607. [CrossRef]
9. Shang, F.; Wang, S.C.; Hsu, C.Y.; Miao, Y.; Martin, M.; Yin, Y.; Wu, C.C.; Wang, Y.T.; Wu, G.; Chien, S.; et al. MicroRNA-92a Mediates Endothelial Dysfunction in CKD. *J. Am. Soc. Nephrol.* **2017**, *28*, 3251–3261. [CrossRef]
10. Li, L.; Ma, L.; Fu, P. Gut microbiota-derived short-chain fatty acids and kidney diseases. *Drug Des. Dev. Ther.* **2017**, *11*, 3531–3542. [CrossRef]
11. Magliocca, G.; Mone, P.; Di Iorio, B.R.; Heidland, A.; Marzocco, S. Short-Chain Fatty Acids in Chronic Kidney Disease: Focus on Inflammation and Oxidative Stress Regulation. *Int. J. Mol. Sci.* **2022**, *23*, 5354. [CrossRef] [PubMed]
12. Hsu, C.N.; Tain, Y.L. Chronic Kidney Disease and Gut Microbiota: What Is Their Connection in Early Life? *Int. J. Mol. Sci.* **2022**, *23*, 3954. [CrossRef] [PubMed]
13. Zheng, Z.; Xu, Y.; Krügel, U.; Schaefer, M.; Grune, T.; Nürnberg, B.; Köhler, M.B.; Gollasch, M.; Tsvetkov, D.; Markó, L. In Vivo Inhibition of TRPC6 by SH045 Attenuates Renal Fibrosis in a New Zealand Obese (NZO) Mouse Model of Metabolic Syndrome. *Int. J. Mol. Sci.* **2022**, *23*, 6870. [CrossRef] [PubMed]
14. Carullo, N.; Fabiano, G.; D'Agostino, M.; Zicarelli, M.T.; Musolino, M.; Presta, P.; Michael, A.; Andreucci, M.; Bolignano, D.; Coppolino, G. New Insights on the Role of Marinobufagenin from Bench to Bedside in Cardiovascular and Kidney Diseases. *Int. J. Mol. Sci.* **2023**, *24*, 11186. [CrossRef]
15. De Nicola, L.; Minutolo, R.; Bellizzi, V.; Zoccali, C.; Cianciaruso, B.; Andreucci, V.E.; Fuiano, G.; Conte, G. Achievement of target blood pressure levels in chronic kidney disease: A salty question? *Am. J. Kidney Dis.* **2004**, *43*, 782–795. [CrossRef]
16. Liu, J.; Shelton, E.L.; Crescenzi, R.; Colvin, D.C.; Kirabo, A.; Zhong, J.; Delpire, E.J.; Yang, H.C.; Kon, V. Kidney Injury Causes Accumulation of Renal Sodium That Modulates Renal Lymphatic Dynamics. *Int. J. Mol. Sci.* **2022**, *23*, 1428. [CrossRef]
17. Deme, S.; Fisseha, B.; Kahsay, G.; Melese, H.; Alamer, A.; Ayhualem, S. Musculoskeletal Disorders and Associated Factors Among Patients with Chronic Kidney Disease Attending at Saint Paul Hospital, Addis Ababa, Ethiopia. *Int. J. Nephrol. Renovasc. Dis.* **2021**, *14*, 291–300. [CrossRef]
18. Cheung, W.W.; Paik, K.H.; Mak, R.H. Inflammation and cachexia in chronic kidney disease. *Pediatr. Nephrol.* **2010**, *25*, 711–724. [CrossRef]
19. Mak, R.H.; Gunta, S.; Oliveira, E.A.; Cheung, W.W. Growth Hormone Improves Adipose Tissue Browning and Muscle Wasting in Mice with Chronic Kidney Disease-Associated Cachexia. *Int. J. Mol. Sci.* **2022**, *23*, 15310. [CrossRef]
20. Mendes, S.; Leal, D.V.; Baker, L.A.; Ferreira, A.; Smith, A.C.; Viana, J.L. The Potential Modulatory Effects of Exercise on Skeletal Muscle Redox Status in Chronic Kidney Disease. *Int. J. Mol. Sci.* **2023**, *24*, 6017. [CrossRef]
21. Sovatzidis, A.; Chatzinikolaou, A.; Fatouros, I.G.; Panagoutsos, S.; Draganidis, D.; Nikolaidou, E.; Avloniti, A.; Michailidis, Y.; Mantzouridis, I.; Batrakoulis, A.; et al. Intradialytic Cardiovascular Exercise Training Alters Redox Status, Reduces Inflammation and Improves Physical Performance in Patients with Chronic Kidney Disease. *Antioxidants* **2020**, *9*, 868. [CrossRef] [PubMed]

Disclaimer/Publisher's Note: The statements, opinions and data contained in all publications are solely those of the individual author(s) and contributor(s) and not of MDPI and/or the editor(s). MDPI and/or the editor(s) disclaim responsibility for any injury to people or property resulting from any ideas, methods, instructions or products referred to in the content.

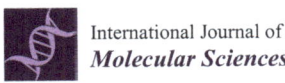

Review

Molecular Mechanisms of Cellular Injury and Role of Toxic Heavy Metals in Chronic Kidney Disease

Manish Mishra [1], Larry Nichols [2], Aditi A. Dave [1], Elizabeth H Pittman [1], John P. Cheek [1], Anasalea J. V. Caroland [1], Purva Lotwala [1], James Drummond [1] and Christy C. Bridges [1,*]

1. Department of Biomedical Sciences, Mercer University School of Medicine, Macon, GA 31207, USA
2. Department of Pathology and Clinical Sciences Education, Mercer University School of Medicine, Macon, GA 31207, USA
* Correspondence: bridges_cc@mercer.edu; Tel.: +1-(478)-301-2086

Abstract: Chronic kidney disease (CKD) is a progressive disease that affects millions of adults every year. Major risk factors include diabetes, hypertension, and obesity, which affect millions of adults worldwide. CKD is characterized by cellular injury followed by permanent loss of functional nephrons. As injured cells die and nephrons become sclerotic, remaining healthy nephrons attempt to compensate by undergoing various structural, molecular, and functional changes. While these changes are designed to maintain appropriate renal function, they may lead to additional cellular injury and progression of disease. As CKD progresses and filtration decreases, the ability to eliminate metabolic wastes and environmental toxicants declines. The inability to eliminate environmental toxicants such as arsenic, cadmium, and mercury may contribute to cellular injury and enhance the progression of CKD. The present review describes major molecular alterations that contribute to the pathogenesis of CKD and the effects of arsenic, cadmium, and mercury on the progression of CKD.

Keywords: chronic kidney disease; heavy metals; cadmium; mercury; arsenic; cellular injury

1. Introduction

Chronic kidney disease (CKD) is a major public health concern. According to the Centers for Disease Control and Prevention (CDC), about 15% of adults in the United States, or 37 million, are estimated to have some degree of CKD [1,2]. The Global Burden of Disease study from 2017 reported 697.5 million cases worldwide. It is clear that CKD is an important contributor to morbidity and mortality. More than 2.5 million patients are receiving renal replacement therapy and that number is expected to double to 5.4 million by 2030 [3,4].

CKD is a deteriorating, progressive, and irreversible loss of renal function. It is characterized by the presence of structural and/or functional abnormalities of the kidney with associated health implications that last more than three months. Individuals with CKD may have albuminuria, urine sediment abnormalities, abnormal renal imaging findings, serum electrolyte or acid-base derangements, and an estimated glomerular filtration rate (eGFR) of <60 mL/minute/1.73 m^2 [2,5]. CKD can progress silently to the advanced stages before the patient is aware of the disease; therefore, early detection and diagnosis are critical to slow or prevent progression [2,3]. There are different patterns of renal decline in patients with CKD. These patterns can be classified into very fast, fast, moderate, or slow decline, depending on the rate at which renal function declines. The differences in these patterns of decline reflect the heterogeneity of CKD origins and the related pathologies, adjunct comorbidities, and other harsh environmental exposures [6,7]. Diabetes mellitus, hypertension, obesity, and older age are the primary risk factors, while other risk factors include cardiovascular disease and a family history of CKD [2,3]. In addition, other factors such as human immunodeficiency virus (HIV) and exposure to toxicants or heavy metals have been shown to contribute to the development of CKD [8,9].

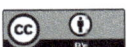

2. Pathophysiology of Chronic Kidney Disease

CKD can be due to various pathologic mechanisms, which can injure various components of the kidney, e.g., vasculature, tubular epithelial cells, interstitium, or the glomerulus. CKD is a consequence of two interrelated issues: an initial catalyst and a prolonging mechanism. The initial catalyst can be an intrinsic kidney defect, an inflammatory or immune-mediated cause, or exposure to nephrotoxicants [10]. The initial problem causes injury of affected glomeruli and leads to compensatory mechanisms in healthy nephrons, including glomerular hypertrophy and hyperfiltration. A continued cycle of hyperfiltration and consequent injury leads to sclerosis and nephron loss [11]. Although hyperfiltration initially compensates (partially) for the loss of functioning nephrons, the vicious cycle of nephron hypertrophy and sclerosis is a continuous process that results in CKD [12,13]. Atrophy and sclerosis of nephrons lead to further renal decline and alterations in normal fluid and solute homeostasis [10–12].

The purpose of this review is to describe some of the structural and molecular mechanisms that are involved in the pathogenesis of CKD (Figure 1). The pathogenic mechanisms may occur simultaneously, may be consequences of initial injury, or may be due to compensatory processes following injury. While this review covers a number of major cellular and molecular mechanisms that are involved in the pathogenesis of CKD, it should be recognized that there are numerous other factors that play a role in the pathogenesis and progression of CKD. Due to the complexity of the disease, is not possible to include all of the factors that contribute to its pathogenesis in one review.

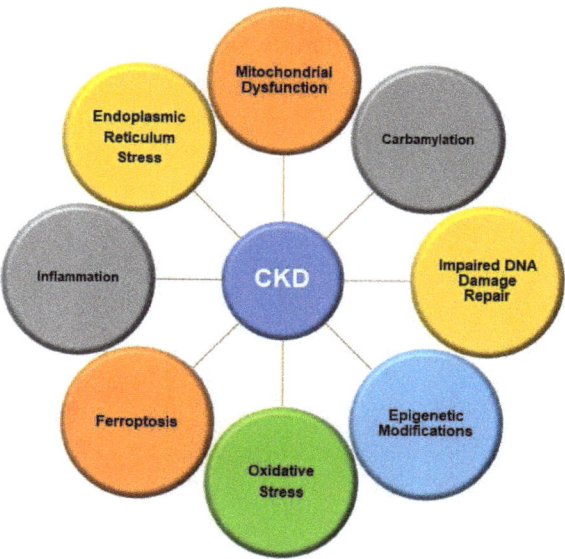

Figure 1. Molecular mechanisms involved in pathogenesis and progression of chronic kidney disease (CKD). CKD is a complex disease that involves dysregulation of multiple physiological processes. This diagram is meant to show the major molecular mechanisms that promote pathogenesis of CKD with the understanding that there are many other mechanisms that may also be involved in this process.

2.1. Structural Alterations within the Kidney

2.1.1. Podocytes

Podocytes are terminally differentiated cells that have three distinct compartments: the cell body, primary processes, and foot processes. Foot processes from adjacent podocytes are connected by a slit diaphragm, which forms the most selective component of the glomerular filtration barrier. Hyperfiltration causes foot processes and the slit diagram to be exposed to high tensile and fluid flow shear stress, which can cause stretching, injury, and loss of barrier function [14,15]. The changes in hemodynamic forces within the glomerulus modify the actin cytoskeleton of podocyte foot process, which can lead to effacement and disruption of the filtration barrier [16–20]. If hyperfiltration is not corrected, podocytes may detach, which leads to podocyturia, proteinuria, and decreases in GFR. Detachment is irreversible and often leads to glomerulosclerosis and CKD [21]. Studies in mice have found that vascular endothelial growth factor (VEGF)-A is required in developing podocytes to establish and maintain the glomerular filtration barrier [22]. In addition, the soluble VEGF receptor 1 (sFlt-1) appears to play a role in endothelial dysfunction observed in CKD [23]. Loss of VEGF-A can lead to dysregulation of podocytes, loss of endothelial cells, and collapse of glomerular capillaries [22].

2.1.2. Capillary Network

Peritubular capillary rarefaction (loss of capillary density) is a common feature of CKD. Interestingly, capillary rarefaction correlates strongly with CKD and has been used as a predictor of progression. Loss of peritubular capillaries is strongly associated with hypoxia and interstitial fibrosis, which lead to renal functional decline [24–26]. Alterations in the expression of endothelial cell-derived factors such as VEGF-A, angiopoietin, and thrombospondin-1 lead to an imbalance of proangiogenic and antiangiogenic factors. Thrombospondin-1 is reported to inhibit renal tubular epithelial cell proliferation, due to reperfusion injury, via the CD47 receptor [27]. Furthermore, inflammatory cytokines such as interleukin (IL)-1α and tumor necrosis factor-α (TNF-α) are secreted and block VEGF-A expression, a major proangiogenic factor [28]. It has been reported that small arterial changes might be crucial primary contributors to the development of glomerulosclerosis due to the decreased number of pericapillary pericytes, as pericytes are crucial for peritubular vessel function and capillary survival [29,30]. Thus, the alteration or disequilibrium of nitric oxide, endothelin-1, endostatin, throbospondin-1, and VEGF might be causative for a functional disruption in capillaries, leading to chronic hypoperfusion, ischemia, and nephron loss.

2.1.3. Tubular Epithelial Cells

The renal proximal tubule absorbs the majority of filtered solutes in an energy-consuming process. The reported contribution of acute kidney injury (AKI) to CKD has focused attention on the proximal tubule as the main target of injury in the progression of CKD Cells with high energy demand and slow proliferation, such as proximal renal tubules, are predisposed to oxidative damage and consequent injury [31]. Juvenile mice with a targeted deletion of endothelial nitric oxide synthase (eNOS) display renal cell death and renal cortical scars [32]. It is reported that patients with eNOS polymorphisms have increased susceptibility to the progression of CKD and thus, eNOS has been recognized as an important survival factor [33]. Tubular cells, which have a long life and high metabolic activity, rely heavily on proper mitochondrial function [34]. Mitochondrial density remains constant in hypertrophied renal tubular cells, but mitochondrial volume increases by over 50% [35]. Increased functionality may lead to additional mitochondrial oxidative stress, resulting in mitochondrial dysfunction. This dysfunction may lead to inflammation, additional alterations in intracellular homeostasis, and additional cellular injury [31,36,37].

2.2. Intracellular Alterations

2.2.1. Mitochondrial Function

Human kidneys comprise only 1% of body weight, but they utilize approximately 10% of total body oxygen. After loss of functional renal mass, nephrons become hypertrophic, which increases the oxygen consumption by up to 50% [38]. This level of energy expenditure cannot be maintained indefinitely and is limited by the capacity of mitochondria to match increased demands [34]. The means by which renal cells produce ATP varies among cell type. Proximal tubular cells produce ATP via oxidative phosphorylation, while podocytes, endothelial, and mesangial cells utilize glycolysis. These differences may determine the impact of mitochondrial dysfunction in renal cells and affect the progression of renal diseases [36]. It has been demonstrated that acute or chronic insults cause mitochondrial structural alterations, including mitochondrial DNA (mtDNA) damage and reduced matrix density [37]. The main mitochondrial dysfunction includes altered mitochondrial biogenesis, fusion/fission, mitophagy, and impaired homeostasis, which lead to a decrease in ATP production, alterations in calcium signaling, enhanced oxidative stress, and apoptosis [36,37].

Mitochondrial biogenesis is regulated primarily by peroxisome proliferator-activated receptor γ coactivator-1 (PGC-1α) [37]. PGC-1α activates many transcription factors such as nuclear respiratory factor-1 (NRF-1), NRF-2, and the estrogen-related receptors (ERR) [39], and together, these transcription factors regulate genes involved in mitochondrial biogenesis, lipid oxidation, glycolysis, and ATP biosynthesis. Reduced expression of PGC-1α along with decreased efficiency of mitochondrial biogenesis has been observed in CKD [36,40,41]. It is not clear if this reduced expression is a cause or an effect of CKD.

Alterations in mitophagy have been implicated in several kidney diseases, including CKD [42,43]. The expression of BNIP3 (Bcl2-interacting protein 3), a member of the Bcl2 (B cell lymphoma 2) family involved in mitophagy, is strongly reduced in renal tubular cells from diseased kidneys. This suggests that a disruption of mitochondrial quality control contributes to the pathogenesis of CKD [44]. Increased mitochondrial reactive oxygen species (ROS) causes inflammation and mitochondrial genome mutations, leading to mitochondrial dysfunction, which further increases ROS production and contributes to more mtDNA damage. This progressive damage in the mitochondrial genome has been implicated as a factor in the pathogenesis and acceleration of CKD [37,45].

2.2.2. Oxidative Stress

Oxidative stress occurs when there is a disruption in the balance of free radicals and antioxidants that degrade those free radicals [46]. ROS and reactive nitrogen species (RNS) are generated during oxidative phosphorylation [47]. Under normal conditions, moderate concentrations of ROS/RNS act as second messengers that regulate signal transduction pathways [48]. Mitochondrial dysregulation increases the production of ROS beyond the normal levels, which depletes antioxidants and leads to oxidative stress [46]. Increased ROS leads to lipid, DNA, and protein oxidation, which cause the formation of complex radical intermediates [46]. These highly reactive intermediates trigger the secretion of pro-inflammatory mediators during active inflammation [49]. Inflammatory cytokines, such as IL-6 and TNF-α, promote renal injury by perpetuating dysregulation in cellular processes [47]. Therefore, oxidative stress exacerbates cellular damage and enhances the progression of CKD [46].

2.2.3. Autophagy

Autophagy is a catabolic process that helps cells remove endogenous waste material and recycle cellular components [50]. Thus, autophagy is an essential pro-survival mechanism during cellular stress. Autophagy is initiated due to activation of major nutrient-sensing pathways, such as mammalian target of rapamycin complex-1 (mTOR1), adenosine monophosphate-activated protein kinase (AMPK), and sirtuin 1 [50]. Ischemic, toxic, immunological, and oxidative injury can enhance autophagy in proximal tubular cells and podocytes, modifying the course of renal diseases [50,51]. Dysregulation of autophagy can lead to progressive deterioration of renal function due to the accumulation of intracellular damaged proteins and enhanced oxidative stress [51]. Thus, autophagy is important in podocytes and proximal tubular cells to maintain proper homeostasis and prevent cellular injury [51,52]. Indeed, studies in mice and rats reported that a reduction in autophagy was associated with a buildup of dysfunctional mitochondria [53] and apoptosis [52,54].

2.2.4. Endoplasmic Reticulum Stress

There is experimental evidence that the accumulation of unfolded proteins in the endoplasmic reticulum of renal tubular epithelial cells may play a role in their death and associated interstitial fibrosis [55]. This accumulation causes endoplasmic reticulum stress, thereby activating the unfolded protein response, which is an evolutionarily conserved cellular response primarily regulated by the endoplasmic reticulum-resident chaperone glucose-regulated protein 78 (GRP78). Misfolded proteins cause GRP78 to dissociate from endoplasmic reticulum transmembrane proteins (PKR-like endoplasmic reticulum kinase, inositol-required enzyme 1, and activating transcription factor 6), thereby activating the cell survival unfolded protein response signaling pathways. This response attempts to maintain proteostasis by reducing general protein translation and increasing the production of molecular chaperones. Severe endoplasmic reticulum stress leads to apoptosis of renal epithelial cells. Endoplasmic reticulum stress also increases the expression of T-cell death-associated gene 51 (TDAG51), also known as pleckstrin homology-like domain, family A member 1. This increases the expression of TGF-β (transforming growth factor) receptor 1, which leads to the splicing of the *xbp1* (X box protein) gene. Spliced XBP1 protein leads to the activation of pro-fibrotic genes, and the development of renal interstitial fibrosis [55].

Acute kidney injury superimposed on CKD may accelerate the progression to kidney failure. One of the ways it may do this is by impairing nicotinamide adenine dinucleotide (NAD+) production, by repressing transcription of the gene for quinolinate phosphoribosyl transferase (QPRT, a bottleneck enzyme of de novo NAD+ biosynthesis), as part of the endoplasmic reticulum stress response [56]. A high urinary quinolinate-to-tryptophan ratio can serve as an indirect indicator of impaired QPRT activity and reduced de novo NAD+ biosynthesis in the kidney [56].

2.2.5. Carbamylation

The buildup of urea in CKD may drive the progression of disease via carbamylation [57]. Carbamylation is an irreversible nonenzymatic post-translational modification of proteins from the reaction between isocyanic acid and amino groups on lysine residues or the N-terminal extremity of proteins. Isocyanic acid derives mainly from spontaneous dissociation of urea into ammonia and cyanate (Figure 2). Cyanate is converted into its tautomer isocyanic acid, which is highly reactive and immediately binds to proteins and thus moves the equilibrium toward dissociation. The elevated levels of urea in CKD patients increases cyanate generation and therefore protein carbamylation. Isocyanic acid may also be formed from thiocyanate under the action of myeloperoxidase in the presence of hydrogen peroxide released by leukocytes in sites of inflammation. Carbamylated protein malfunction triggers unfavorable molecular and cellular responses and may accelerate the progression of kidney disease [57].

2.2.6. Ferroptosis

The process of ferroptosis may be important in the progression of CKD [58]. Ferroptosis is a form of regulated cell death driven by iron-dependent phospholipid peroxidation and oxidative stress. With CKD, iron accumulates in renal tubular cells. If lipid peroxide repair capacity by the phospholipid hydroperoxidase, glutathione peroxidase 4 (GPX4), is lost in the presence of this iron, ferroptosis may ensue. If the uptake of cystine via the cystine/glutamate antiporter, system x_c^- is lost, or glutathione synthesis is otherwise impaired in the presence of this iron, ferroptosis may occur. In animal models of CKD, an iron-restricted diet exerts a renal protective effect by inhibiting oxidative stress and aldosterone receptor signaling [58].

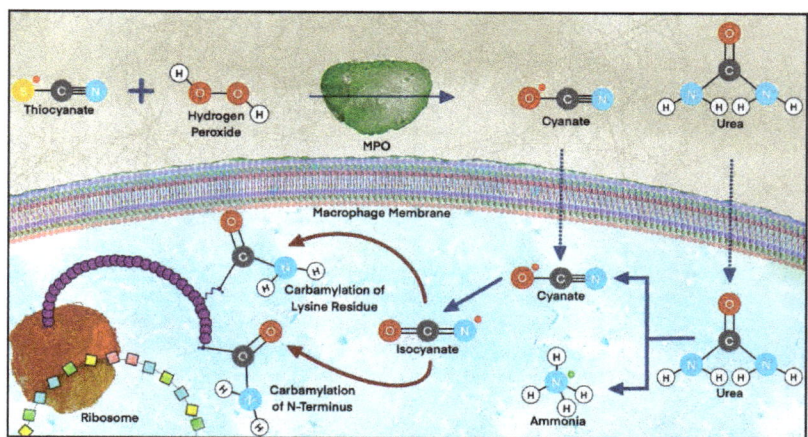

Figure 2. Process of carbamylation. Carbamylation occurs through two primary pathways that converge due to the spontaneous reactivity of isocyanate with lysine residues and the N-termini of nascent polypeptides. The first and predominant pathway is the spontaneous dissociation of urea to cyanate and ammonia. The second pathway is the conversion of thiocyanate and hydrogen peroxide to cyanate under the action of myeloperoxidase. Once cyanate is formed, it is converted into isocyanate, and the spontaneous and irreversible process of carbamylation commences. MPO, myeloperoxidase.

2.2.7. DNA Damage and Repair

Insufficient response to DNA damage leads to various insults that enhance apoptosis or result in a dysfunctional phenotype [59]. Several studies have shown a maladaptive response of renal tubular cells during AKI and suggest that an insufficient response to DNA damage could accelerate CKD [10,59,60]. Many studies have described DNA damage as a hallmark of various forms of renal damage characterized by dysfunctional cell cycle proteins of G1/S and G2/M checkpoints and subsequent cell cycle arrest through the activation of p53 or p21 signaling cascades [61,62]. These mutated cells become senescent and have a specific secretome-defined phenotype (senescence-associated secretory phenotype; SASP), which is accompanied by genomic damage and epigenetic abnormalities [63]. The synthesis and release of SASP factors is associated with the activation of the transcription factors, nuclear factor kappa B (NF-κB), and CCAAT enhancer binding protein β (C/EBPβ) [64]. Thus, both altered DNA damage response and NF-κB activation significantly contribute to establishing and maintaining SASP, which produces and releases more senescent secretomes, contributing to functional deterioration of neighboring cells and accelerating the process of cellular death.

2.2.8. Epigenetic Modifications

Several factors such as uremic toxins, oxidative stress, and inflammation increase the prevalence of epigenetic changes and enhance the progression to CKD [65,66]. Inflammation, a major factor in the pathogenesis of CKD, correlates with global DNA methylation [67]. Indeed, a significant association has been identified between DNA methylation and the prevalence and incidence of CKD [66]. Experimental studies observed that hypomethylation in the promoter region of the connective tissue growth factor (*ctgf*) gene is associated with reduced GFR and declined renal function [68]. Data from experimental studies in rats and mice indicate that altered DNA methylation is an important mechanism that initiates the transition from AKI to CKD [69]. In models of unilateral ureteral obstruction (UUO), it was observed that hypermethylation of the Klotho promoter by TGFβ decreased Klotho protein expression, which led to tubular and interstitial fibrosis. Similarly, hypermethylation of the *Vegfa* gene promoter led to reduced VEGF-A signaling, which can lead to capillary collapse and subsequent hypoxia and fibrosis [70]. In ischemic reperfusion rat models, aberrant methylation of the complement C3 promoter region in tubular epithelial cells activated the complement system. This is strongly associated with inflammation and accelerated renal decline [63,71]. Other studies showed that complement component, C5a, promotes DNA hypomethylation of several genes that have integral roles in the initiating cell cycle arrest and senescence [63]. Aberrant hypermethylation of laminin genes has been reported to cause the development of glomerulosclerosis and tubulointerstitial fibrosis in older kidneys, while aberrant methylation of the *rasal1* (Ras protein activator-like 1) gene induced the activation of the Ras–GTPase pathway in fibroblasts, leading to proliferation and fibrosis [72].

In addition to DNA methylation, numerous studies suggest that RNA interference via microRNA (miRNA) is a key factor involved in the pathogenesis and progression of CKD [73]. Several miRNAs, which are involved in post-transcriptional regulation of gene expression, have been linked to inflammation and fibrosis and may enhance the progression of CKD [66,74,75]. One of the most studied miRNAs is miR-192, which plays a role in the expression of profibrotic genes [75]. Upregulated expression of miR-192 leads to the activation of TGF-β and Smad3 signaling pathways, which lead to renal fibrosis through the deposition of collagen and fibronectin [75]. Similarly, the activation of TGF-β pathways increases histone methylation and increased expression of genes involved in deposition of extracellular matrix proteins [75].

2.2.9. Cellular Senescence

Cellular senescence appears to play an important role in the pathogenesis of CKD [76,77]. The accumulation of senescent cells may be responsible for insufficient repair capacity and functional loss. Senescent cells accumulate in the renal parenchyma, leading to tissue deterioration, fibrosis, and aberrant signaling in different types of cell populations [29,69,78]. Senescent cells of renal system express several markers, such as cell cycle arrest proteins of G1/S and G2/M checkpoints such as p16INK4A, p21WAF/CIP1, p27KIP1, and p53, but they do not express proliferation markers such as Ki67 [79–81]. Interestingly, selective ablation of senescent (p16INK4a-positive) cells in transgenic mice is linked to diminished expression of TNF-α, IL-6, and IL-1α in many tissues, including the kidney [79]. Cellular senescence has been linked to telomere shortening [82], which upregulates a DNA damage response and activates phosphatidylinositol 3 kinase-like kinases and Rad3-related kinases that lead to p53 activation. Active p53 upregulates transcription of pro-apoptotic genes and/or genes that inhibit cyclin-dependent kinase (i.e., $p21^{cip1/waf1}$). Activation of $p21^{cip1/waf1}$ may cause permanent cell cycle arrest [62,80].

Importantly, senescent cells have a specific secretome-defined, senescence-associated secretory phenotype (SASP), which includes a broad range of pro-inflammatory cytokines, chemokines, growth factors, and matrix-degrading factors (e.g., IL-6, IL-1α, IL-1β, chemokine ligand 1 (GROα; CXCL1), connective tissue growth factor (CTGF), plasminogen activator inhibitor 1 (PAI-1). C-C motif chemokine 2 (CCL2)) [79,80,83]. Recent studies report that the expression of integrin β3 increased significantly in senescent cells, which led to the activation of p53 and the secretion of TGF-β [84]. These molecules and others, such as TNF-α, IL-6, and monocyte chemoattractant protein 1 (MCP-1), can promote an inflammatory microenvironment and might be important drivers of inflammation-related injury and enhance progression of CKD [83,85].

2.2.10. Inflammation

Inflammation and fibrosis contribute to the progression of CKD via many pathways in glomeruli, tubules, and interstitium. In the final common pathway to end-stage renal disease, nephron loss causes hyperperfusion and high glomerular capillary hydrostatic pressure in remaining nephrons. This results in injury to the major cell types within glomeruli: endothelial cells, podocytes, and mesangial cells [86]. Injured endothelial cells detach from the basement membrane, express more leukocyte adhesion molecules, and secrete more proinflammatory cytokines. Injured podocytes also detach from the basement membrane, allowing proteinuria, associated with increased angiotensin II, aldosterone, and TGF-β. Injured mesangial cells proliferate and synthesize extracellular matrix constituents, MCP-1, CGTF, and TGF-β. Monocytes recruited to injured glomeruli become macrophages, and glomerular inflammation leads to glomerulosclerosis [87].

Interstitial inflammation and fibrosis also contribute to the progression of CKD. Lymphocytes and macrophages infiltrate the renal interstitium. Lymphocytes are recruited into the interstitium early. Monocytes are recruited into the interstitium, where they become macrophages. Macrophage infiltration after nephron loss is chiefly in tubulointerstitial regions. The CC chemokine receptor type 1 is important in interstitial but not glomerular recruitment of leukocytes. Dendritic cells appear in the interstitium, with peak concentration at one week after nephron loss. Mast cells are identifiable in areas of tubulointerstitial inflammation and fibrosis [88]. Myofibroblasts secrete the components of extracellular matrix, leading to fibrosis. The predominant source of these myofibroblasts is from pericytes around blood vessels and resident fibroblasts, with a minor contribution from de-differentiated proximal tubule cells [89].

In the progression of chronic kidney disease, the cell type probably most often central to the various processes involved is the macrophage [90]. The mononuclear cell chemokine, CCL2, mediates migration of monocytes to the injured kidney. CCL2 blockade attenuates glomerular and interstitial infiltration of pro-inflammatory macrophages, but other chemokines such as CX3CL1, CXCL16, and macrophage migration inhibitory factor (MIF), also contribute to macrophage recruitment in kidney disease [85]. Opposing this recruitment, the mononuclear cell chemokine C-C motif chemokine 5 (CCL5) constrains CCL2 expression, macrophage infiltration, and kidney damage and fibrosis in hypertension via blood pressure-independent mechanisms. This balance illustrates the complex network of overlapping chemokines working to maintain renal health [85].

Macrophages polarized to the M1 phenotype play a pathogenic role in inflammatory renal injury, and macrophages polarized to the M2 phenotype play a pathogenic role in the follow-on renal fibrosis. Recruited macrophages produce a range of cytokines, including TNF-α and interferon-γ (IFN-γ), which increase M1 polarization and the progression of CKD. Damage-associated molecular patterns (DAMPs) from renal parenchyma such as high-mobility group protein B1 (HMGB1) and C-reactive protein (CRP) also augment the renal accumulation of pro-inflammatory macrophages. Additionally, DAMPS released from damaged renal tubular epithelial cells (RTEC) have been shown to increase the expression of pattern recognition receptors (PRR) on healthy RTEC. This leads to the expression of pro-inflammatory cytokines, which leads to further recruitment of inflammatory monocytes and macrophages [91]. There is experimental evidence that macrophage polarization to a pro-inflammatory phenotype, associated in turn with increased pro-inflammatory cytokines and renal inflammation, is promoted by a high salt intake, suggesting that this is one of the mechanisms by which a low-salt diet ameliorates the progression of CKD [92].

Macrophage phenotype is partly determined by prostaglandins in the microenvironment. Arachidonic acid metabolism into prostaglandins plays a role in renal inflammation and fibrosis. The lipoxygenase family of enzymes convert polyunsaturated fatty acids into bioactive lipid eicosanoids such as hydroxyeicosatetraenoic acids, hydroxyeicosaoctadecaenoic acids, leukotrienes, lipoxins, and resolvins [93]. The enzyme 15-lipoxygenase worsens inflammation and fibrosis in a rodent model of chronic kidney disease. Silencing 15-lipoxygenase promotes an increase in M2c-like wound-healing macrophages in the kidney and alters kidney metabolism, protecting against anaerobic glycolysis after injury [93].

The presence of free fatty acids may drive some of the inflammation causing the progression of chronic kidney disease. Renal tubular injury from free fatty acids may be partly mediated by increased expression of the CD36 scavenger receptor due to increased expression of the peroxisome proliferator-activated receptor (PPAR)-γ nuclear transcription factor [94]. Renal tubular injury and inflammation due to increased circulating free fatty acids could partly explain the accelerated progression of CKD in patients with insulin resistance (type 2 diabetes mellitus) and obesity. The decelerated progression of CKD by sodium-glucose co-transporter 2 (SGLT2) channel inhibitors may be partly from attenuated CD36 expression from downregulated PPAR-γ [94]. IL-33 may be an important driver of progressive CKD [95]. IL-33 is a member of the IL-1 cytokine family and exerts pro-inflammatory and pro-fibrotic effects via the suppression of tumorigenicity 2 (ST2) receptor, which, in turn, activates other inflammatory pathways. Recent studies have shown that a sustained activation of the IL-33/ST2 pathway promotes the development of renal fibrosis [95]. This pathway is a potential target for therapeutic intervention.

Excess amino acids from the heavy nutritional load of a high-protein diet are thought to increase renal inflammation and fibrosis primarily indirectly by increasing glomerular hyperfiltration, but also partly by increasing proinflammatory gene expression. Later in the course of chronic kidney disease, excess amino acids promote fibrosis by increasing TGF-β. Whatever the mechanisms, a low-protein diet slows the progression of chronic kidney disease [96].

2.2.11. Fibrosis

Renal fibrosis is the end result of nearly all progressive renal diseases. Fibrosis is a maladaptive repair process associated with chronic inflammation. It is characterized by progressive remodeling and destruction of renal tissue in an attempt to replace injured cells. Although the initial stages of this repair process may be beneficial, prolonged activation of growth factors and cytokines leads to the replacement of normal renal parenchyma with collagen and other connective tissue fibers [97].

It is generally accepted that fibroblasts and myofibroblasts are key cells involved in renal fibrosis. Under normal conditions, fibroblasts synthesize many of the constituents of the extracellular matrix. It is well accepted that myofibroblasts are activated fibroblasts. Renal injury leads to numerous stimuli that may cause transformation of fibroblasts to myofibroblasts. These stimuli include the production of inflammatory cytokines (e.g., TGF-β, platelet-derived growth factor (PDGF), fibroblast growth factor 2 (FGF-2)), hypoxia, and cell contact with leukocytes and macrophages. Interestingly, renal fibroblasts maintain their activated phenotype in a setting of fibrosis even if the initial cause is no longer present [93].

Published evidence suggests that renal epithelial cells play an important role in renal fibrosis due to epithelial-to-mesenchymal transition [98–100]. This transition appears to be induced by interleukin-like epithelial mesenchymal transition inducer (ILEI) in response to TGF-β1 through Akt (protein kinase B) and ERK (extracellular signal-regulated kinase) pathways [101]. Following this transition, renal tubular epithelial cells lose their normal morphology, tight junctions, and epithelial cell markers (e.g., E-cadherin), and begin expressing mesenchymal markers such as α-smooth muscle actin (α-SMA) and vimentin. These alterations facilitate the progression of renal interstitial fibrosis and CKD [101].

PDGFs play an important role in the processes that lead to renal fibrosis [102]. PDGF receptor-β (PDGFR-β) is a tyrosine-kinase receptor for PDGF-B and PDGF-D. Upon activation, PDGFR-β induces downstream signaling that triggers cell proliferation, migration, and differentiation, leading to extracellular matrix deposition. There is experimental evidence that PDGFR-β activation alone is sufficient to induce progressive renal fibrosis and renal failure, key aspects of CKD [103]. PDGFR-β is a potential target for therapeutic intervention to slow the progression of kidney disease.

3. Molecular Effects of Environmental Toxicants on CKD Progression

As CKD progresses and GFR decreases, the ability of patients to eliminate metabolic wastes, xenobiotics, and toxicants declines significantly. Considering that the current environment is contaminated with numerous toxicants, it is important to understand how patients with a reduced ability to excrete toxicants are affected by environmental nephrotoxicants. Of particular concern is exposure to nephrotoxic heavy metals that are present throughout the environment. Today's environment is heavily contaminated by toxic metals such as arsenic, cadmium, and mercury; therefore, human exposure to one or more of these toxicants is nearly unavoidable. Indeed, the World Health Organization included these three metals on the list of top ten chemicals of public health concern [104]. A thorough understanding of the way in which these metals are handled by diseased kidneys is necessary to manage this important global health problem.

3.1. Arsenic

Arsenic (As) is a naturally occurring metalloid found in the Earth's crust [105]. As may exist in inorganic (arsenopyrite, pentavalent arsenate, trivalent arsenite) and organic (e.g., monomethylarsonic acid, dimethylarsonic acid, trimethylarsonic acid, arsenobetaine) forms [106]. Inorganic As seeps into groundwater reservoirs via environmental weathering of ores and contaminates underground aquifers. Inorganic As, in the form of arsenite ($As(OH)_3$) and arsenate (H_3AsO_4), is often found in water wells located in rocky terrain around the world [107,108]. Anthropogenic activity has also contributed to increased arsenic pollution through use of pesticides, handling of arsenate-containing wood preservatives, and semiconductor manufacturing [109]. While it can be inhaled or absorbed via dermal contact, human exposure occurs primarily via drinking water contaminated with inorganic arsenic [110].

Exposure to As is a serious global health concern that is associated with numerous health effects. Acute physiological effects of As exposure include various multiorgan symptoms ranging from colicky abdominal pain to encephalopathy [111]. Chronic exposure to arsenic is known to cause bladder, skin, and lung cancer. It is linked with kidney, liver, and prostate cancer and may cause numerous other health effects [112,113]. A meta-analysis of literature related to heavy metal exposure and CKD reported a link between exposure to As and risk of proteinuria, an early sign of CKD [114]. Similarly, it has been reported that exposure to heavy metals such as As may increase the risk of developing CKD [114]. Indeed, chronic exposure to As has been shown to result in glomerulonephritis, acute tubular necrosis, albuminuria, and renal papillae necrosis [115,116].

Exposure to As can lead to significant oxidative stress, which can exacerbate renal injury and enhance the progression of CKD (Figure 3). Studies in rats have shown that As increases production of ROS, which enhances the expression of inflammatory cytokines through the NF-κB pathway [117]. This induces apoptosis primarily by decreasing Bcl-2 and Bcl-xl (Bcl-2 associated protein) expression while concomitantly increasing expression of p53 and Bax in As-treated rats [117]. Recent studies in mice showed that exposure to As activates the MAPK/NF-κB and NRF2 pathways in kidney. While activation of these pathways may improve cell survival, exposure to As also led to increased activity of myeloperoxidase and increased expression of inflammatory cytokines, such as IL-1α, IL-6, IL-12, and TNF-α, which may lead to an inflammatory response [118,119]. Furthermore, elevated expression of inflammatory cytokines was shown to disrupt homeostasis of helper T cell populations (Th1/Th2/Th17/Treg). The balance among T cells populations is critical to maintain proper immune function. Exposure to As alters the balance and leads to inflammation and immunosuppression [118,120]. Use of newer immunotherapeutics and their impact on kidney function is a new and expanding area of research. Some immunotherapeutics have been reported to exacerbate or cause renal damage [121]. The complexity of renal function and inflammation makes this an interesting new area of research with great potential.

Studies using cultured myoblasts indicate that As exposure leads to apoptosis through pathways involving ROS, mitochondrial dysfunction, and endoplasmic reticulum stress [122]. A similar pathway may play a role in As-induced nephrotoxicity. Interestingly, trivalent forms of As have been shown to inhibit the production of glutathione, which may lead to unrestricted oxidative stress [123]. Arsenic can cause lipid peroxidation and damage mitochondrial membranes, leading to the formation of peroxyl radicals and dimethylarsenic radicals, and eventual cell death [123].

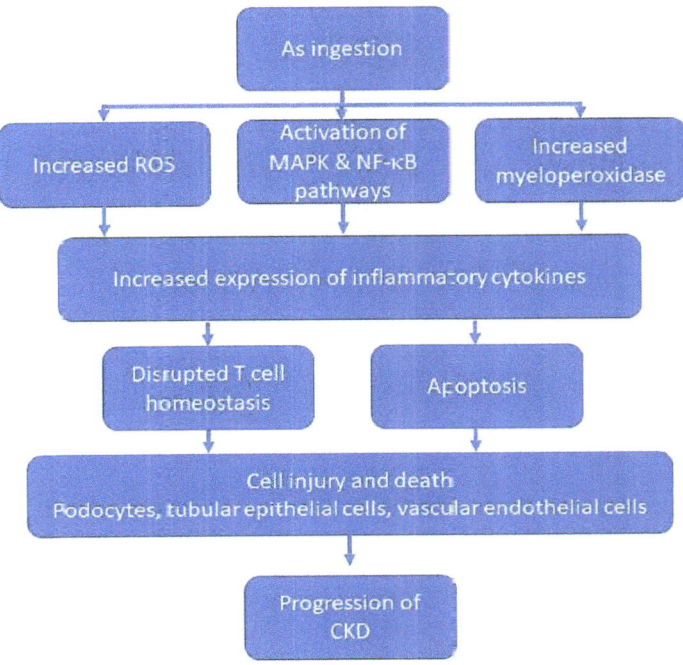

Figure 3. Flowchart summarizing major effects of arsenic (As) exposure in relation to the progression of CKD. As-induced injury is a complex, multifactorial process that cannot be summarized completely in a single figure. Thus, while this figure includes major pathways of As-induced injury, it does not cover all mechanisms and routes of injury.

3.2. Cadmium

Cadmium (Cd) naturally exists in zinc, lead, and copper ores as a divalent cation in the Earth's crust and marine environments at low concentrations and accumulates in air water and soil through volcanic activity and erosion [124]. While trace amounts of Cd in the environment are byproducts of these processes, the majority of environmental Cd is the result of industrial and agricultural use [124]. Soluble Cd ions from phosphate fertilizers can contaminate water and soil and subsequently accumulate in aquatic organisms or plants such as tobacco, grains, and root vegetables [125,126]. Because of accumulation in tobacco plants, individuals who smoke are exposed to significant levels of Cd through the inhalation of cigarette smoke. Cigarettes may contain 1.8–2.5 µg/g Cd [127], and data from the National Health and Nutrition Examination Study (NHANES) reported that smokers had average blood and urine Cd levels of 0.376 µg/L and 0.232 µg/L, respectively [128].

Following exposure, Cd is absorbed readily by epithelial cells in the gastrointestinal tract and lungs. Once ingested, ionized Cd^{2+} binds to albumin and the resulting complexes are then transported to target organs, including the kidney, bone, liver, and lung. Cd is taken up into hepatocytes via Ca^{2+} channels and membrane transporters [129]. Within the cell, Cd has been shown to impair electron transport chain complexes II and III, which impedes electron flow and generates ROS [112]. The generation of ROS promotes binding of the metal-regulated transcription factor 1 (MTF-1) to metal response elements (MRE), which subsequently activates transcription of metallothionein (MT) [110]. Intracellularly, MT binds to Cd to create a MT–Cd complex, and a fraction of the complex is exported into the circulation [130]. MT–Cd complexes are filtered freely by the glomerulus and are reabsorbed by proximal tubular epithelial cells via multiple mechanisms, including megalin and cubilin receptor-mediated endocytosis, ZIP8 and ZIP14, and the divalent metal transporter 1 (DMT1) [131,132].

Environmental and occupational exposure to low levels of Cd has been shown to cause renal tubular injury [133]. Owing to its toxic renal effects, chronic exposure to Cd increases the risk of developing CKD from 10% in the average population to 25% in exposed individuals [134]. Analyses of NHANES data showed that individuals with blood Cd levels over one mcg/L had a significantly higher association with CKD and albuminuria [135]. It is clear that exposure to Cd reduces GFR and impairs overall renal function. Here, we summarize the molecular mechanisms that underlie these pathologies and contribute to the development and/or progression of CKD (Figure 4).

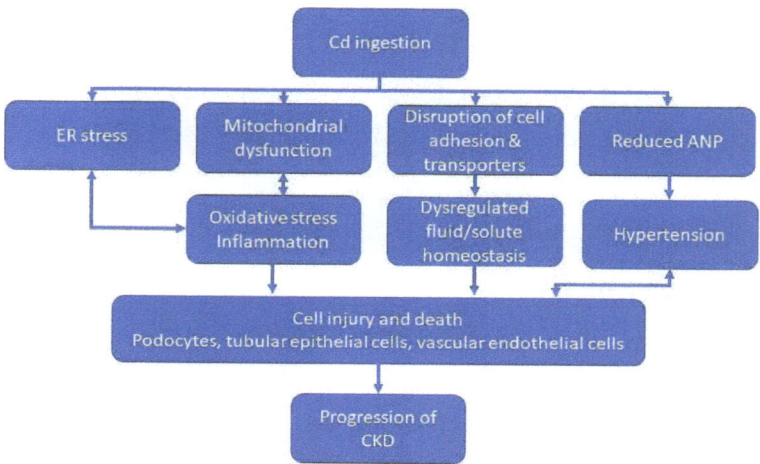

Figure 4. Schematic to summarize major factors that contribute to progression of CKD following exposure to cadmium (Cd). Additional factors not included here also contribute to Cd-induced progression of CKD.

As discussed in the previous sections, diabetes is a major risk factor for developing CKD. Exposure to Cd appears to increase the risk of developing diabetes in some individuals [136]. Diabetic mice (db/db) exposed to Cd were found to be hyperglycemic and exhibited an increase in white adipose tissue and weight gain [137]. Interestingly, exposure of these mice to Cd also decreased serum leptin levels, which may enhance appetite and lead to weight gain. In contrast to these findings, a recent study using streptozotocin-induced diabetic mice (C57BL/6) exposed to Cd showed that body weight decreased after exposure [138]. This variation could be due to differences in the frequency and dose of Cd exposure. This study, however, confirmed findings that exposure of hyperglycemic animals to Cd enhances the risk of renal injury [138]. Specifically, in vitro studies using cultured podocytes indicate that exposure to Cd under hyperglycemic conditions leads to mitochondrial dysfunction and ROS. Podocyte viability is reduced, leading to apoptosis, fibrosis, and decreased renal function [138]. These studies suggest that exposure of diabetic individuals to Cd may exacerbate renal injury and lead to CKD or enhance the progression of CKD by causing additional injury.

Hypertension is another major risk factor for the development of CKD. A meta-analysis study of published literature found a positive association between hypertension and Cd levels in blood and hair [139]. Indeed, Cd has been shown to decrease plasma levels of atrial natriuretic peptide (ANP) [140], an important regulator of blood pressure. Cd appears to reduce the affinity of the ANP receptor for ANP and also decreased the number of binding sites available [141]. Reduced levels of ANP and reduced sensitivity of the receptor may decrease the ability to regulate blood pressure, which may lead to hypertension and subsequent renal injury. The development of hypertension is characterized by low ANP plasma concentrations [142] and its suppressed ability to regulate blood pressure via inhibiting the renin–angiotensin–aldosterone system. In addition to causing vasodilation of the afferent arterioles, ANP binds to natriuretic peptide receptor-A, catalyzing the conversion of GTP to cGMP. cGMP phosphorylates and allosterically binds to basolateral sodium-potassium ATPase channels and apical cyclic nucleotide-gated, heterometric channels of transient receptor potential V4 and P2 [143]. While the mechanism remains entirely unclear, damage to the kidney's response to ANP may potentially be mediated by Cd-induced oxidative damage. In one study, increased production of thiobarbituric acid reactive substance after exposure to Cd was accompanied by decreased glomerular filtration rate and increased creatinine levels; upon bolus injection of ANP in compromised rats, high blood pressure and low glomerular filtration rate remained remarkably uncorrected. Without the counteraction of salt and fluid retention from ANP due to compromised receptor response, Cd may play a role in exacerbating hypertensive conditions precipitating kidney injury and eventual CKD [143].

In addition to the association with diabetes and hypertension, exposure to Cd has been shown to cause generalized cellular injury in renal epithelial cells. A major consequence of Cd exposure is intracellular oxidative stress. Studies using male Sprague Dawley rats found swelling, deformation, and vacuolation in mitochondria of renal tubular epithelial cells. In addition, expression of superoxide dismutase 2 (SOD2), found in mitochondria, decreased, indicating an inability to counteract the production of ROS. Indeed, increased cellular content of ROS was accompanied by increased expression of cytoplasmic superoxide dismutase 1 (SOD1). Interestingly, expression of catalase was reduced, which would prevent cells from responding appropriately to oxidative stress [144]. Other studies reveal the association of Cd exposure to substantial activity reduction in antioxidant enzymes, including superoxide dismutase, catalase, and glutathione reductase, that may amplify the progression of chronic kidney disease from oxidative species overwhelming antioxidants [145].

In addition to oxidative stress, Cd has been shown to induce ER stress and autophagy (via BNIP3) in HK2 cells and SD rats [146]. Studies in cultured rat pheochromocytoma cells (PC-12) showed that exposure to Cd enhanced autophagy [147]. In contrast, studies in mice exposed to Cd showed that protein components of autophagosomes (e.g., p62, Sirt6, and LC3-II) accumulated in the cytoplasm of renal tubular cells rather than participate in the formation of autophagosomes. This resulted in the inhibition of autophagy and the initiation of apoptosis [148]. Similarly, a study in cultured proximal tubular cells reported that treatment with Cd led to the accumulation of p62 in the cytoplasm and the inhibition of autophagy. Furthermore, it was reported that elevated levels of p62 led to increased nuclear translocation of Nrf2 [149]. Persistent activation of Nrf2 can lead to lysosomal dysfunction, which prevents fusion of lysosomes and autophagosomes [150]. Cd may also induce apoptosis in renal epithelial cells through p-53 mediated, DNA damage autophagy modulator (DRAM) and BAX signaling [151]. Cd has also been shown to activate inflammatory cytokines, such as NF-κb, TNF-α, and iNOS, and induce necroptosis [152,153].

Exposure to Cd has also been shown to disrupt cadherin-dependent cell adhesion in proximal tubular cells. Alterations in cellular adhesion have been shown to alter the membrane localization of the Na^+K^+-ATPase, which can lead to alterations in transport [154]. Similarly, other studies in proximal tubules showed that exposure to Cd decreased expression of SGLT1 and SGLT2. This decrease was attributed to the replacement of Zn in the Sp1 DNA binding domain, which reduced activation of SGLT1 and SGLT2 promoters [155].

Cd is a toxic metal to which humans continue to be exposed throughout their lives. Continued studies related to Cd-induced cellular injury in renal tubular epithelial cells are necessary to understand how exposure to this metal affects patients with renal disease.

3.3. Mercury

Mercury (Hg) is a toxic metal found in various environmental and occupational settings. It may exist in an elemental (metallic), inorganic, and/or organic form. Elemental mercury (Hg^0) is particularly unique because it exists as a liquid at room temperature. Inorganic mercury is usually found as mercurous (Hg^{1+}) or mercuric (Hg^{2+}) ions salts. Organic forms of mercury include phenylmercury, dimethylmercury, and monomethylmercury (MeHg), which is the most common form encountered by humans. The majority of human exposure is due to the ingestion of contaminated food. Upon ingestion, MeHg is absorbed readily by enterocytes along the gastrointestinal tract [1], after which they can enter systemic circulation and be delivered to target organs. Within biological systems, a fraction of MeHg is slowly transformed to Hg^{2+} [156–159].

Exposure to all forms of Hg has been shown to have significant renal effects (Figure 5). Experimental models (uninephrectomy) of early-stage CKD suggest that acute renal injury is more pronounced in uninephrectomized rats exposed to a nephrotoxic dose of $HgCl_2$ than in corresponding sham rats [160–162]. It was found that mercury-induced proximal tubular necrosis was more extensive in 50% nephrectomized animals than in sham animals. Additionally, the urinary excretion of cellular enzymes and plasma proteins, including lactate dehydrogenase, γ-glutamyltransferase, and albumin, was greater in uninephrectomized animals than in sham animals [162,163]. Interestingly, when 75% nephrectomized rats were used as models of late-stage CKD, it was found that the accumulation of mercury per g kidney is significantly greater in 75% nephrectomized rats than in sham rats, suggesting that cellular accumulation of Hg may be greater in the remnant renal mass from 75% nephrectomized animals than in kidneys of sham animals [164].

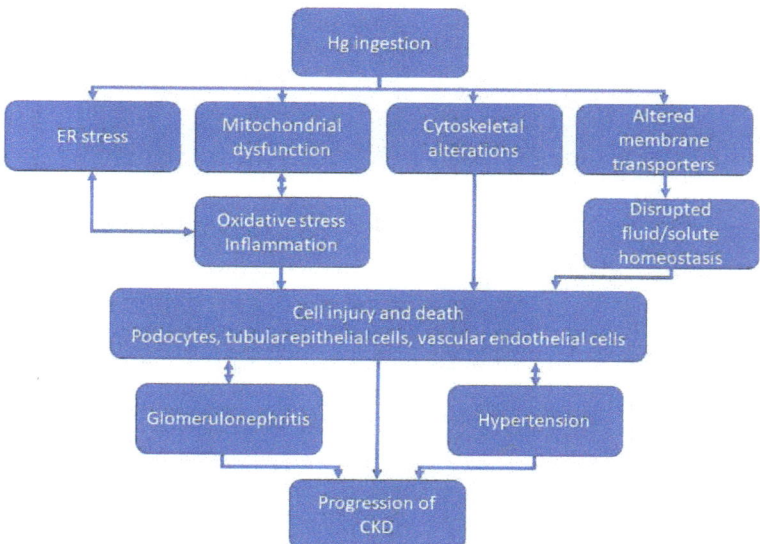

Figure 5. Flowchart outlining major mechanisms involved in mercury (Hg)-induced progression of CKD. Other factors not specified here also play a role in the progression of CKD induced by exposure to Hg.

In humans, chronic exposure to mercury has been associated with glomerulonephritis, particularly membranous nephropathy [165,166]. Membranous nephropathy is characterized by tissue damage due to activation of membrane attack complexes (MAC) by antigen–antibody complexes deposited on the glomerular basement membrane (GBM) [167]. This damage results in podocyte damage and disruption of the anionic charge barrier, leading to massive proteinuria [167]. Analyses of patient biopsies found that patients with Hg-induced membranous nephropathy exhibited more mesangial deposits and smaller podocyte foot processes than patients with idiopathic membranous nephropathy. Interestingly, podocyte effacement was less severe in Hg-induced cases than in idiopathic cases [168]. In vitro studies have shown that exposure to Hg leads to autoimmune disease characterized by anti-GBM antibodies, glomerular deposits of immunoglobin G (IgG), proteinuria, and acute tubulointerstitial nephritis [169–171]. Studies in Brown Norway rats have shown that exposure to $HgCl_2$ leads to a T-cell dependent autoimmune syndrome that leads to the production of anti-laminin antibodies that interact with the GBM [172,173]. Exposure to $HgCl_2$ leads to the appearance of non-antigen-specific CD8+ T-cells [174]. Additional studies in Brown Norway rats showed that RT6+ T cells decreased, which inversely corresponded with the autoimmune response to the GBM [175]. Escudero et al. showed that the HUTS-21 epitope of the beta-1 integrin on lymphocytes appears to be involved in Hg-induced nephritis by promoting lymphocyte infiltration into renal interstitium and deposition of anti-GBM antibodies [176].

Exposure to Hg may also play a role in the development of hypertension. A study of non-Hispanic Asians using NHANES data found that higher blood Hg levels were associated with hypertension [177]. Studies using spontaneously hypertensive rats (SHR) found that exposure to Hg accelerated the development of hypertension by increasing the production of nitric oxide and other ROS [178,179]. However, it appears that Hg also induces vasoprotective mechanisms such as increased plasma levels of nitric oxide and hydrogen peroxide to counteract other vasoconstrictive effects [179]. In addition, plasma levels of angiotensin-converting enzyme (ACE) were found to be increased in SHR rats following exposure to Hg [180], which can lead to vasoconstriction and hypertension. In a recent review, Hazeeb et al. outlined the molecular mechanisms by which Hg exposure leads to hypertension [181]. Hg has been shown to increase atherosclerosis as well as stimulate the proliferation of vascular smooth muscle cells, which would further increase the risk of hypertension.

The effects of Hg on renal tubule epithelial cells can be detrimental to total renal function. Studies in cultured proximal tubular cells have demonstrated that exposure to Hg induces significant cellular alterations [182,183]. Specifically, the most profound modifications were noted as increased oxidative stress, cytoskeletal rearrangements, increased intracellular calcium, and reduced cellular viability.

In the mitochondria, mercury-induced oxidative stress has been shown to disrupt the overall structure, leading to swelling, destruction of mitochondrial membrane potential, altered membrane, and increased release of Cytochrome C [184]. Exposure of human embryonic kidney epithelial (HEK-293T) cells to $HgCl_2$ revealed a decrease in cell viability due to a downregulation in the expression of the silent information regulator (Sirt1) and PGC-1α signaling pathway, a key mechanism in mitochondrial homeostasis [185].

Cytoskeletal alterations have been detected following exposure of normal rat kidney cells (NRK-52E) to MeHg [186]. These alterations are a result of epigenetic modulation of matrix metalloproteinase 9 (MMP9) via demethylation of its regulatory site. The subsequent increased expression of MMP9 led to loss of cell-to-cell adhesion and disturbances in cytoskeletal proteins such as F-actin, vimentin, and fibronectin [186]. Similarly, exposure of NRK-52E cells to $HgCl_2$ also led to loss of cytoskeleton integrity [182].

The ER is another cellular target in acute $HgCl_2$ toxicity. Experiments in NRK-52E cells showed that ER stress, as indicated by expression of GRP78 (78-kDa glucose regulated protein) and CHOP (C/EBP homologous protein), is a marker of renal cell injury [187]. GRP78 is an ER chaperone, which is upregulated upon stress; however, if the ER experiences prolonged stress, CHOP, a transcription factor specializing in regulation of apoptosis-related genes, will also be upregulated. Both of these proteins are positively correlated with renal damage. In addition, $HgCl_2$ has been shown to enhance the activity of Caspase 3 and the expression of $IRE1_a$ (inositol-requiring enzyme 1), GADD-153 (growth arrested and DNA damage-inducible gene 153), and Caspase 12, resulting in the death of tubular and glomerular cells [188].

Exposure to Hg also affects the activity of various transporters, which may lead to tubular injury and renal disease. Studies in Wistar rats exposed to a low dose of $HgCl_2$ showed that Hg inhibited the Na^+/H^+ exchanger (NHE3) in proximal tubular cells.

It was suggested that Hg enhanced phosphorylation of NHE3 and thereby reduced its activity [189]. NHE3 is the main isoform of the Na^+/H^+ exchanger in the proximal tubule and it plays a major role in the reabsorption of sodium from the lumen. Alterations in the activity of NHE3 could indirectly affect reabsorption and secretion of important molecules and fluid. In addition, $HgCl_2$ has been shown to inhibit Na-K-ATPase [190], which would alter solute gradients necessary for water reabsorption and lead to increased urinary output, a common sign of renal injury. Mercury has also been shown to bind to cysteine residues in aquaporin 1 (AQP1) [191], located in the proximal tubule and thin limbs in the loop of Henle [192], and inhibit its activity. AQP1 facilitates reabsorption of 70% of water from the ultrafiltrate entering the proximal tubule [193]. Therefore, the inhibition of AQP1 is also a likely cause of increased urinary output following Hg intoxication.

Collectively, the results of these studies suggest that kidneys of animals with reduced renal mass are more susceptible to the toxic effects of Hg. Similarly, individuals who have reduced renal function, due to CKD or other disease processes, may be more susceptible to renal injury following exposure to a nephrotoxicant such as Hg.

4. Summary

The pathogenesis and progression of CKD result from numerous physical and molecular changes that create a complex intracellular environment. Physical changes due to hypertrophy and hydrostatic forces may cause injury to cells and lead to an inability of the cells to manage small intracellular changes. Increased oxidative stress, ER stress, DNA modifications, mitochondrial dysfunction, and many other cellular and molecular changes lead to dysregulation of intracellular processes, cellular injury, and eventual cell death. Exposure to environmental toxicants such as heavy metals may lead to additional cellular injury and enhance the progression of CKD. Because of the complexity of the CKD, eliminating one path of pathogenesis may enhance pathogenesis via a different route. Stopping the progression of CKD will likely require a combination of multiple therapies, but each component of combination therapy will likely cause its own negative effects. The only reasonable and attainable goal may be slowing down the progression of this disease.

Author Contributions: Conceptualization, C.C.B.; investigation, M.M., L.N., A.A.D., J.P.C., E.H.P., P.L., A.J.V.C., J.D. and C.C.B.; writing—original draft preparation, M.M., L.N., A.A.D., J.P.C., E.H.P., P.L., A.J.V.C., J.D. and C.C.B.; writing—review and editing, M.M., L.N., A.A.D., J.P.C., E.H.P., P.L., A.J.V.C., J.D. and C.C.B.; funding acquisition, C.C.B. All authors have read and agreed to the published version of the manuscript.

Funding: This research was funded by NIH ES030867.

Institutional Review Board Statement: Not applicable.

Informed Consent Statement: Not applicable.

Data Availability Statement: Not applicable.

Conflicts of Interest: The authors declare no conflict of interest.

References

1. ATSDR. *Toxicological Profile for Mercury*; Public Health Service, Ed.; U.S. Department of Health and Human Services, Centers for Disease Control: Atlanta, GA, USA, 2008.
2. Gaitonde, D.Y.; Cook, D.L.; Rivera, I.M. Chronic Kidney Disease: Detection and Evaluation. *Am. Fam. Physician* **2017**, *96*, 776–783. [PubMed]
3. GBD Chronic Kidney Disease Collaboration. Global, regional, and national burden of chronic kidney disease, 1990-2017: A systematic analysis for the Global Burden of Disease Study 2017. *Lancet* **2020**, *395*, 709–733. [CrossRef]
4. Liyanage, T.; Ninomiya, T.; Jha, V.; Neal, B.; Patrice, H.M.; Okpechi, I.; Zhao, M.H.; Lv, J.; Garg, A.X.; Knight, J.; et al. Worldwide access to treatment for end-stage kidney disease: A systematic review. *Lancet* **2015**, *385*, 1975–1982. [CrossRef]
5. Levin, A.; Stevens, P.E. The authors reply. *Kidney Int.* **2013**, *84*, 623. [CrossRef]
6. Li, L.; Astor, B.C.; Lewis, J.; Hu, B.; Appel, L.J.; Lipkowitz, M.S.; Toto, R.D.; Wang, X.; Wright, J.T., Jr.; Greene, T.H. Longitudinal progression trajectory of GFR among patients with CKD. *Am. J. Kidney Dis.* **2012**, *59*, 504–512. [CrossRef]

7. Yan, M.T.; Chao, C.T.; Lin, S.H. Chronic Kidney Disease: Strategies to Retard Progression. *Int. J. Mol. Sci.* **2021**, *22*, 10084. [CrossRef]
8. Ekrikpo, U.E.; Kengne, A.P.; Bello, A.K.; Effa, E.E.; Noubiap, J.J.; Salako, B.L.; Rayner, B.L.; Remuzzi, G.; Okpechi, I.G. Chronic kidney disease in the global adult HIV-infected population: A systematic review and meta-analysis. *PLoS ONE* **2018**, *13*, e0195443. [CrossRef]
9. Jha, V.; Garcia-Garcia, G.; Iseki, K.; Li, Z.; Naicker, S.; Plattner, B.; Saran, R.; Wang, A.Y.; Yang, C.W. Chronic kidney disease: Global dimension and perspectives. *Lancet* **2013**, *382*, 260–272. [CrossRef]
10. Ferenbach, D.A.; Bonventre, J.V. Acute kidney injury and chronic kidney disease: From the laboratory to the clinic. *Nephrol. Ther.* **2015**, *12* (Suppl. 1), S41–S48. [CrossRef]
11. Charles, C.; Ferris, A.H. Chronic Kidney Disease. *Prim. Care* **2020**, *47*, 585–595. [CrossRef]
12. Chevalier, R.L. Evolution, kidney development, and chronic kidney disease. *Semin. Cell Dev. Biol.* **2019**, *91*, 119–131. [CrossRef] [PubMed]
13. Hostetter, T.H.; Olson, J.L.; Rennke, H.G.; Venkatachalam, M.A. Hyperfiltration in remnant nephrons: A potentially adverse response to renal ablation. *J. Am. Soc. Nephrol.* **2001**, *12*, 1315–1325. [CrossRef] [PubMed]
14. Srivastava, T.; Dai, H.; Heruth, D.P.; Alon, U.S.; Garola, R.E.; Zhou, J.; Duncan, R.S.; El-Meanawy, A.; McCarthy, E.T.; Sharma, R.; et al. Mechanotransduction signaling in podocytes from fluid flow shear stress. *Am. J. Physiol. Ren. Physiol.* **2018**, *314*, F22–F34. [CrossRef] [PubMed]
15. Kriz, W.; Lemley, K.V. A potential role for mechanical forces in the detachment of podocytes and the progression of CKD. *J. Am. Soc. Nephrol.* **2015**, *26*, 258–269. [CrossRef]
16. Blaine, J.; Dylewski, J. Regulation of the Actin Cytoskeleton in Podocytes. *Cells* **2020**, *9*, 1700. [CrossRef]
17. Kim, J.J.; Wilbon, S.S.; Fornoni, A. Podocyte Lipotoxicity in CKD. *Kidney360* **2021**, *2*, 755–762. [CrossRef]
18. Wanner, N.; Hartleben, B.; Herbach, N.; Goedel, M.; Stickel, N.; Zeiser, R.; Walz, G.; Moeller, M.J.; Grahammer, F.; Huber, T.B. Unraveling the role of podocyte turnover in glomerular aging and injury. *J. Am. Soc. Nephrol.* **2014**, *25*, 707–716. [CrossRef]
19. Hodgin, J.B.; Bitzer, M.; Wickman, L.; Afshinnia, F.; Wang, S.Q.; O'Connor, C.; Yang, Y.; Meadowbrooke, C.; Chowdhury, M.; Kikuchi, M.; et al. Glomerular Aging and Focal Global Glomerulosclerosis: A Podometric Perspective. *J. Am. Soc. Nephrol.* **2015**, *26*, 3162–3178. [CrossRef]
20. Wiggins, J.E.; Goyal, M.; Sanden, S.K.; Wharram, B.L.; Shedden, K.A.; Misek, D.E.; Kuick, R.D.; Wiggins, R.C. Podocyte hypertrophy, "adaptation," and "decompensation" associated with glomerular enlargement and glomerulosclerosis in the aging rat: Prevention by calorie restriction. *J. Am. Soc. Nephrol.* **2005**, *16*, 2953–2966. [CrossRef]
21. Trimarchi, H. Mechanisms of Podocyte Detachment, Podocyturia, and Risk of Progression of Glomerulopathies. *Kidney Dis.* **2020**, *6*, 324–329. [CrossRef]
22. Eremina, V.; Sood, M.; Haigh, J.; Nagy, A.; Lajoie, G.; Ferrara, N.; Gerber, H.P.; Kikkawa, Y.; Miner, J.H.; Quaggin, S.E. Glomerular-specific alterations of VEGF-A expression lead to distinct congenital and acquired renal diseases. *J. Clin. Investig.* **2003**, *111*, 707–716. [CrossRef] [PubMed]
23. Di Marco, G.S.; Reuter, S.; Hillebrand, U.; Amler, S.; Konig, M.; Larger, E.; Oberleithner, H.; Brand, E.; Pavenstadt, H.; Brand, M. The soluble VEGF receptor sFlt1 contributes to endothelial dysfunction in CKD. *J. Am. Soc. Nephrol.* **2009**, *20*, 2235–2245. [CrossRef] [PubMed]
24. Babickova, J.; Klinkhammer, B.M.; Buhl, E.M.; Djudjaj, S.; Hoss, M.; Heymann, F.; Tacke, F.; Floege, J.; Becker, J.U.; Boor, P. Regardless of etiology, progressive renal disease causes ultrastructural and functional alterations of peritubular capillaries. *Kidney Int.* **2017**, *91*, 70–85. [CrossRef]
25. Ehling, J.; Babickova, J.; Gremse, F.; Klinkhammer, B.M.; Baetke, S.; Knuechel, R.; Kiessling, F.; Floege, J.; Lammers, T.; Boor, P. Quantitative Micro-Computed Tomography Imaging of Vascular Dysfunction in Progressive Kidney Diseases. *J. Am. Soc. Nephrol.* **2016**, *27*, 520–532. [CrossRef] [PubMed]
26. Urbieta-Caceres, V.H.; Syed, F.A.; Lin, J.; Zhu, X.Y.; Jordan, K.L.; Bell, C.C.; Bentley, M.D.; Lerman, A.; Khosla, S.; Lerman, L.O. Age-dependent renal cortical microvascular loss in female mice. *Am. J. Physiol. Endocrinol. Metab.* **2012**, *302*, E979–E986. [CrossRef] [PubMed]
27. Rogers, N.M.; Zhang, Z.J.; Wang, J.J.; Thomson, A.W.; Isenberg, J.S. CD47 regulates renal tubular epithelial cell self-renewal and proliferation following renal ischemia reperfusion. *Kidney Int.* **2016**, *90*, 334–347. [CrossRef]
28. Kida, Y. Peritubular Capillary Rarefaction: An Underappreciated Regulator of CKD Progression. *Int. J. Mol. Sci.* **2020**, *21*, 8255. [CrossRef]
29. Schmitt, R.; Melk, A. Molecular mechanisms of renal aging. *Kidney Int.* **2017**, *92*, 569–579. [CrossRef]
30. Uesugi, N.; Shimazu, Y.; Kikuchi, K.; Nagata, M. Age-Related Renal Microvascular Changes: Evaluation by Three-Dimensional Digital Imaging of the Human Renal Microcirculation Using Virtual Microscopy. *Int. J. Mol. Sci.* **2016**, *17*, 1831. [CrossRef]
31. Berkenkamp, B.; Susnik, N.; Baisantry, A.; Kuznetsova, I.; Jacobi, C.; Sorensen-Zender, I.; Broecker, V.; Haller, H.; Melk, A.; Schmitt, R. In vivo and in vitro analysis of age-associated changes and somatic cellular senescence in renal epithelial cells. *PLoS ONE* **2014**, *9*, e88071. [CrossRef]
32. Forbes, M.S.; Thornhill, B.A.; Park, M.H.; Chevalier, R.L. Lack of endothelial nitric-oxide synthase leads to progressive focal renal injury. *Am. J. Pathol.* **2007**, *170*, 87–99. [CrossRef] [PubMed]

33. Noiri, E.; Satoh, H.; Taguchi, J.; Brodsky, S.V.; Nakao, A.; Ogawa, Y.; Nishijima, S.; Yokomizo, T.; Tokunaga, K.; Fujita, T. Association of eNOS Glu298Asp polymorphism with end-stage renal disease. *Hypertension* **2002**, *40*, 535–540. [CrossRef] [PubMed]
34. Weinberg, J.M. Mitochondrial biogenesis in kidney disease. *J. Am. Soc. Nephrol.* **2011**, *22*, 431–436. [CrossRef] [PubMed]
35. Hwang, S.; Bohman, R.; Navas, P.; Norman, J.T.; Bradley, T.; Fine, L.G. Hypertrophy of renal mitochondria. *J. Am. Soc. Nephrol.* **1990**, *1*, 822–827. [CrossRef]
36. Galvan, D.L.; Green, N.H.; Danesh, F.R. The hallmarks of mitochondrial dysfunction in chronic kidney disease. *Kidney Int.* **2017**, *92*, 1051–1057. [CrossRef]
37. Eirin, A.; Lerman, A.; Lerman, L.O. The Emerging Role of Mitochondrial Targeting in Kidney Disease. In *Handbook of Experimental Pharmacology*; Springer: New York, NY, USA, 2017; Volume 240, pp. 229–250.
38. Layton, A.T.; Edwards, A.; Vallon, V. Adaptive changes in GFR, tubular morphology, and transport in subtotal nephrectomized kidneys: Modeling and analysis. *Am. J. Physiol. Ren. Physiol.* **2017**, *313*, F199–F209. [CrossRef]
39. Baldelli, S.; Aquilano, K.; Ciriolo, M.R. Punctum on two different transcription factors regulated by PGC-1alpha: Nuclear factor erythroid-derived 2-like 2 and nuclear respiratory factor 2. *Biochim. Biophys. Acta* **2013**, *1830*, 4137–4146. [CrossRef]
40. Lynch, M.R.; Tran, M.T.; Parikh, S.M. PGC1alpha in the kidney. *Am. J. Physiol. Ren. Physiol.* **2018**, *314*, F1–F8. [CrossRef]
41. Chung, K.W.; Lee, E.K.; Lee, M.K.; Oh, G.T.; Yu, B.P.; Chung, H.Y. Impairment of PPARalpha and the Fatty Acid Oxidation Pathway Aggravates Renal Fibrosis during Aging. *J. Am. Soc. Nephrol.* **2018**, *29*, 1223–1237. [CrossRef]
42. Ishihara, M.; Urushido, M.; Hamada, K.; Matsumoto, T.; Shimamura, Y.; Ogata, K.; Inoue, K.; Taniguchi, Y.; Horino, T.; Fujieda, M.; et al. Sestrin-2 and BNIP3 regulate autophagy and mitophagy in renal tubular cells in acute kidney injury. *Am. J. Physiol. Ren. Physiol.* **2013**, *305*, F495–F509. [CrossRef]
43. Namba, T.; Takabatake, Y.; Kimura, T.; Takahashi, A.; Yamamoto, T.; Matsuda, J.; Kitamura, H.; Niimura, F.; Matsusaka, T.; Iwatani, H.; et al. Autophagic clearance of mitochondria in the kidney copes with metabolic acidosis. *J. Am. Soc. Nephrol.* **2014**, *25*, 2254–2266. [CrossRef] [PubMed]
44. Tang, C.; He, L.; Liu, J.; Dong, Z. Mitophagy: Basic Mechanism and Potential Role in Kidney Diseases. *Kidney Dis.* **2015**, *1*, 71–79. [CrossRef] [PubMed]
45. Sun, H.; Sun, Z.; Varghese, Z.; Guo, Y.; Moorhead, J.F.; Unwin, R.J.; Ruan, X.Z. Nonesterified free fatty acids enhance the inflammatory response in renal tubules by inducing extracellular ATP release. *Am. J. Physiol. Ren. Physiol.* **2020**, *319*, F292–F303. [CrossRef] [PubMed]
46. Daenen, K.; Andries, A.; Mekahli, D.; Van Schepdael, A.; Jouret, F.; Bammens, B. Oxidative stress in chronic kidney disease. *Pediatr. Nephrol.* **2019**, *34*, 975–991. [CrossRef]
47. Gyuraszova, M.; Gurecka, R.; Babickova, J.; Tothova, L. Oxidative Stress in the Pathophysiology of Kidney Disease: Implications for Noninvasive Monitoring and Identification of Biomarkers. *Oxidative Med. Cell. Longev.* **2020**, *2020*, 5478708. [CrossRef]
48. Sauer, H.; Wartenberg, M.; Hescheler, J. Reactive oxygen species as intracellular messengers during cell growth and differentiation. *Cell. Physiol. Biochem.* **2001**, *11*, 173–186. [CrossRef]
49. Rapa, S.F.; Di Iorio, B.R.; Campiglia, P.; Heidland, A.; Marzocco, S. Inflammation and Oxidative Stress in Chronic Kidney Disease-Potential Therapeutic Role of Minerals, Vitamins and Plant-Derived Metabolites. *Int. J. Mol. Sci.* **2019**, *21*, 263. [CrossRef]
50. Rubinsztein, D.C.; Marino, G.; Kroemer, G. Autophagy and aging. *Cell* **2011**, *146*, 682–695. [CrossRef]
51. Huber, T.B.; Edelstein, C.L.; Hartleben, B.; Inoki, K.; Jiang, M.; Koya, D.; Kume, S.; Lieberthal, W.; Pallet, N.; Quiroga, A.; et al. Emerging role of autophagy in kidney function, diseases and aging. *Autophagy* **2012**, *8*, 1009–1031. [CrossRef]
52. Kimura, T.; Takabatake, Y.; Takahashi, A.; Kaimori, J.Y.; Matsui, I.; Namba, T.; Kitamura, H.; Niimura, F.; Matsusaka, T.; Soga, T.; et al. Autophagy protects the proximal tubule from degeneration and acute ischemic injury. *J. Am. Soc. Nephrol.* **2011**, *22*, 902–913. [CrossRef]
53. Kume, S.; Uzu, T.; Horiike, K.; Chin-Kanasaki, M.; Isshiki, K.; Araki, S.; Sugimoto, T.; Haneda, M.; Kashiwagi, A.; Koya, D. Calorie restriction enhances cell adaptation to hypoxia through Sirt1-dependent mitochondrial autophagy in mouse aged kidney. *J. Clin. Investig.* **2010**, *120*, 1043–1055. [CrossRef] [PubMed]
54. Hartleben, B.; Godel, M.; Meyer-Schwesinger, C.; Liu, S.; Ulrich, T.; Kobler, S.; Wiech, T.; Grahammer, F.; Arnold, S.J.; Lindenmeyer, M.T.; et al. Autophagy influences glomerular disease susceptibility and maintains podocyte homeostasis in aging mice. *J. Clin. Investig.* **2010**, *120*, 1084–1096. [CrossRef] [PubMed]
55. Carlisle, R.E.; Mohammed-Ali, Z.; Lu, C.; Yousof, T.; Tat, V.; Nademi, S.; MacDonald, M.E.; Austin, R.C.; Dickhout, J.G. TDAG51 induces renal interstitial fibrosis through modulation of TGF-beta receptor 1 in chronic kidney disease. *Cell Death Dis.* **2021**, *12*, 921. [CrossRef] [PubMed]
56. Bignon, Y.; Rinaldi, A.; Nadour, Z.; Poindessous, V.; Nemazanyy, I.; Lenoir, O.; Fohlen, B.; Weill-Raynal, P.; Hertig, A.; Karras, A.; et al. Cell stress response impairs de novo NAD+ biosynthesis in the kidney. *JCI Insight* **2022**, *7*, e153019. [CrossRef]
57. Gorisse, L.; Jaisson, S.; Pietrement, C.; Gillery, P. Carbamylated Proteins in Renal Disease: Aggravating Factors or Just Biomarkers? *Int. J. Mol. Sci.* **2022**, *23*, 574. [CrossRef]
58. Zhang, X.; Li, X. Abnormal Iron and Lipid Metabolism Mediated Ferroptosis in Kidney Diseases and Its Therapeutic Potential. *Metabolites* **2022**, *12*, 58. [CrossRef]
59. Lombard, D.B.; Chua, K.F.; Mostoslavsky, R.; Franco, S.; Gostissa, M.; Alt, F.W. DNA repair, genome stability, and aging. *Cell* **2005**, *120*, 497–512. [CrossRef]

60. Park, M.R.; Li, K.; Lin, S.Y.; Hung, W.C. Connecting the Dots: From DNA Damage and Repair to Aging. *Int. J. Mol. Sci.* **2016**, *17*, 385. [CrossRef]
61. Kishi, S.; Brooks, C.R.; Taguchi, K.; Ichimura, T.; Mori, Y.; Akinfolarin, A.; Gupta, N.; Galichon, P.; Elias, B.C.; Suzuki, T.; et al. Proximal tubule ATR regulates DNA repair to prevent maladaptive renal injury responses. *J. Clin. Investig.* **2019**, *129*, 4797–4816. [CrossRef]
62. Campisi, J. Aging, cellular senescence, and cancer. *Annu. Rev. Physiol.* **2013**, *75*, 685–705. [CrossRef]
63. Castellano, G.; Franzin, R.; Sallustio, F.; Stasi, A.; Banelli, B.; Romani, M.; De Palma, G.; Lucarelli, G.; Divella, C.; Battaglia, M.; et al. Complement component C5a induces aberrant epigenetic modifications in renal tubular epithelial cells accelerating senescence by Wnt4/betacatenin signaling after ischemia/reperfusion injury. *Aging* **2019**, *11*, 4382–4406. [CrossRef] [PubMed]
64. Kuilman, T.; Michaloglou, C.; Vredeveld, L.C.; Douma, S.; van Doorn, R.; Desmet, C.J.; Aarden, L.A.; Mooi, W.J.; Peeper, D.S. Oncogene-induced senescence relayed by an interleukin-dependent inflammatory network. *Cell* **2008**, *133*, 1019–1031. [CrossRef] [PubMed]
65. Chu, A.Y.; Tin, A.; Schlosser, P.; Ko, Y.A.; Qiu, C.; Yao, C.; Joehanes, R.; Grams, M.E.; Liang, L.; Gluck, C.A.; et al. Epigenome-wide association studies identify DNA methylation associated with kidney function. *Nat. Commun.* **2017**, *8*, 1286. [CrossRef] [PubMed]
66. Morgado-Pascual, J.L.; Marchant, V.; Rodrigues-Diez, R.; Dolade, N.; Suarez-Alvarez, B.; Kerr, B.; Valdivielso, J.M.; Ruiz-Ortega, M.; Rayego-Mateos, S. Epigenetic Modification Mechanisms Involved in Inflammation and Fibrosis in Renal Pathology. *Mediat. Inflamm.* **2018**, *2018*, 2931049. [CrossRef]
67. Stenvinkel, P.; Karimi, M.; Johansson, S.; Axelsson, J.; Suliman, M.; Lindholm, B.; Heimburger, O.; Barany, P.; Alvestrand, A.; Nordfors, L.; et al. Impact of inflammation on epigenetic DNA methylation—A novel risk factor for cardiovascular disease? *J. Intern. Med.* **2007**, *261*, 488–499. [CrossRef]
68. Zhang, H.; Cai, X.; Yi, B.; Huang, J.; Wang, J.; Sun, J. Correlation of CTGF gene promoter methylation with CTGF expression in type 2 diabetes mellitus with or without nephropathy. *Mol. Med. Rep.* **2014**, *9*, 2138–2144. [CrossRef]
69. Franzin, R.; Stasi, A.; Ranieri, E.; Netti, G.S.; Cantaluppi, V.; Gesualdo, L.; Stallone, G.; Castellano, G. Targeting Premature Renal Aging: From Molecular Mechanisms of Cellular Senescence to Senolytic Trials. *Front. Pharmacol.* **2021**, *12*, 630419. [CrossRef]
70. Sanchez-Navarro, A.; Perez-Villalva, R.; Murillo-de-Ozores, A.R.; Martinez-Rojas, M.A.; Rodriguez-Aguilera, J.R.; Gonzalez, N.; Castaneda-Bueno, M.; Gamba, G.; Recillas-Targa, F.; Bobadilla, N.A. Vegfa promoter gene hypermethylation at HIF1alpha binding site is an early contributor to CKD progression after renal ischemia. *Sci. Rep.* **2021**, *11*, 8769. [CrossRef]
71. Quach, A.; Levine, M.E.; Tanaka, T.; Lu, A.T.; Chen, B.H.; Ferrucci, L.; Ritz, B.; Bandinelli, S.; Neuhouser, M.L.; Beasley, J.M.; et al. Epigenetic clock analysis of diet, exercise, education, and lifestyle factors. *Aging* **2017**, *9*, 419–446. [CrossRef]
72. Bechtel, W.; McGoohan, S.; Zeisberg, E.M.; Muller, G.A.; Kalbacher, H.; Salant, D.J.; Muller, C.A.; Kalluri, R.; Zeisberg, M. Methylation determines fibroblast activation and fibrogenesis in the kidney. *Nat. Med.* **2010**, *16*, 544–550. [CrossRef]
73. Wing, M.R.; Ramezani, A.; Gill, H.S.; Devaney, J.M.; Raj, D.S. Epigenetics of progression of chronic kidney disease: Fact or fantasy? *Semin. Nephrol.* **2013**, *33*, 363–374. [CrossRef] [PubMed]
74. Lee, C.G.; Kim, J.G.; Kim, H.J.; Kwon, H.K.; Cho, I.J.; Choi, D.W.; Lee, W.H.; Kim, W.D.; Hwang, S.J.; Choi, S.; et al. Discovery of an integrative network of microRNAs and transcriptomics changes for acute kidney injury. *Kidney Int.* **2014**, *86*, 943–953. [CrossRef] [PubMed]
75. Zhao, H.; Ma, S.X.; Shang, Y.Q.; Zhang, H.Q.; Su, W. microRNAs in chronic kidney disease. *Clin. Chim. Acta* **2019**, *491*, 59–65. [CrossRef]
76. Hernandez-Segura, A.; Nehme, J.; Demaria, M. Hallmarks of Cellular Senescence. *Trends Cell Biol.* **2018**, *28*, 436–453. [CrossRef] [PubMed]
77. Wang, W.J.; Cai, G.Y.; Chen, X.M. Cellular senescence, senescence-associated secretory phenotype, and chronic kidney disease. *Oncotarget* **2017**, *8*, 64520–64533. [CrossRef] [PubMed]
78. Schmitt, R.; Melk, A. New insights on molecular mechanisms of renal aging. *Am. J. Transplant.* **2012**, *12*, 2892–2900. [CrossRef]
79. Baker, D.J.; Childs, B.G.; Durik, M.; Wijers, M.E.; Sieben, C.J.; Zhong, J.; Saltness, R.A.; Jeganathan, K.B.; Verzosa, G.C.; Pezeshki, A.; et al. Naturally occurring p16(Ink4a)-positive cells shorten healthy lifespan. *Nature* **2016**, *530*, 184–189. [CrossRef]
80. Sturmlechner, I.; Durik, M.; Sieben, C.J.; Baker, D.J.; van Deursen, J.M. Cellular senescence in renal ageing and disease. *Nat. Rev. Nephrol.* **2017**, *13*, 77–89. [CrossRef]
81. Valentijn, F.A.; Falke, L.L.; Nguyen, T.Q.; Goldschmeding, R. Cellular senescence in the aging and diseased kidney. *J. Cell Commun. Signal* **2018**, *12*, 69–82. [CrossRef]
82. Harley, C.B.; Futcher, A.B.; Greider, C.W. Telomeres shorten during ageing of human fibroblasts. *Nature* **1990**, *345*, 458–460. [CrossRef]
83. Kooman, J.P.; Dekker, M.J.; Usvyat, L.A.; Kotanko, P.; van der Sande, F.M.; Schalkwijk, C.G.; Shiels, P.G.; Stenvinkel, P. Inflammation and premature aging in advanced chronic kidney disease. *Am. J. Physiol. Ren. Physiol.* **2017**, *313*, F938–F950. [CrossRef] [PubMed]
84. Li, S.; Jiang, S.; Zhang, Q.; Jin, B.; Lv, D.; Li, W.; Zhao, M.; Jiang, C.; Dai, C.; Liu, Z. Integrin beta3 Induction Promotes Tubular Cell Senescence and Kidney Fibrosis. *Front. Cell Dev. Biol.* **2021**, *9*, 733831. [CrossRef] [PubMed]
85. Wen, Y.; Crowley, S.D. The varying roles of macrophages in kidney injury and repair. *Curr. Opin. Nephrol. Hypertens.* **2020**, *29*, 286–292. [CrossRef] [PubMed]
86. Hostetter, T.H. Hyperfiltration and glomerulosclerosis. *Semin. Nephrol.* **2003**, *23*, 194–199. [CrossRef] [PubMed]

87. Taal, M.W.; Omer, S.A.; Nadim, M.K.; Mackenzie, H.S. Cellular and molecular mediators in common pathway mechanisms of chronic renal disease progression. *Curr. Opin. Nephrol. Hypertens.* **2000**, *9*, 323–331. [CrossRef] [PubMed]
88. Jones, S.E.; Kelly, D.J.; Cox, A.J.; Zhang, Y.; Gow, R.M.; Gilbert, R.E. Mast cell infiltration and chemokine expression in progressive renal disease. *Kidney Int.* **2003**, *64*, 906–913. [CrossRef]
89. Kuppe, C.; Ibrahim, M.M.; Kranz, J.; Zhang, X.; Ziegler, S.; Perales-Paton, J.; Jansen, J.; Reimer, K.C.; Smith, J.R.; Dobie, R.; et al. Decoding myofibroblast origins in human kidney fibrosis. *Nature* **2021**, *589*, 281–286. [CrossRef]
90. Meng, X.M.; Tang, P.M.; Li, J.; Lan, H.Y. Macrophage Phenotype in Kidney Injury and Repair. *Kidney Dis.* **2015**, *1*, 138–146. [CrossRef]
91. DeWolf, S.E.; Kasimsetty, S.G.; Hawkes, A.A.; Stocks, L.M.; Kurian, S.M.; McKay, D.B. DAMPs Released From Injured Renal Tubular Epithelial Cells Activate Innate Immune Signals in Healthy Renal Tubular Epithelial Cells. *Transplantation* **2022**, *106*, 1589–1599. [CrossRef]
92. Liu, Y.; Dai, X.; Yang, S.; Peng, Y.; Hou, F.; Zhou, Q. High salt aggravates renal inflammation via promoting pro-inflammatory macrophage in 5/6-nephrectomized rat. *Life Sci.* **2021**, *274*, 119109. [CrossRef]
93. Montford, J.R.; Bauer, C.; Rahkola, J.; Reisz, J.A.; Floyd, D.; Hopp, K.; Soranno, D.E.; Klawitter, J.; Weiser-Evans, M.C.M.; Nemenoff, R.; et al. 15-Lipoxygenase worsens renal fibrosis, inflammation, and metabolism in a murine model of ureteral obstruction. *Am. J. Physiol. Ren. Physiol.* **2022**, *322*, F105–F119. [CrossRef]
94. Huang, C.C.; Chou, C.A.; Chen, W.Y.; Yang, J.L.; Lee, W.C.; Chen, J.B.; Lee, C.T.; Li, L.C. Empagliflozin Ameliorates Free Fatty Acid Induced-Lipotoxicity in Renal Proximal Tubular Cells via the PPARgamma/CD36 Pathway in Obese Mice. *Int. J. Mol. Sci.* **2021**, *22*, 12408. [CrossRef]
95. Tan, X.Y.; Jing, H.Y.; Ma, Y.R. Interleukin-33/Suppression of Tumorigenicity 2 in Renal Fibrosis: Emerging Roles in Prognosis and Treatment. *Front. Physiol.* **2021**, *12*, 792897. [CrossRef] [PubMed]
96. Molina, P.; Gavela, E.; Vizcaino, B.; Huarte, E.; Carrero, J.J. Optimizing Diet to Slow CKD Progression. *Front. Med.* **2021**, *8*, 654250. [CrossRef] [PubMed]
97. Grgic, I.; Duffield, J.S.; Humphreys, B.D. The origin of interstitial myofibroblasts in chronic kidney disease. *Pediatr. Nephrol.* **2012**, *27*, 183–193. [CrossRef]
98. Strutz, F.; Zeisberg, M. Renal fibroblasts and myofibroblasts in chronic kidney disease. *J. Am. Soc. Nephrol.* **2006**, *17*, 2992–2998. [CrossRef]
99. Liu, Y. Epithelial to mesenchymal transition in renal fibrogenesis: Pathologic significance, molecular mechanism, and therapeutic intervention. *J. Am. Soc. Nephrol.* **2004**, *15*, 1–12. [CrossRef]
100. Lovisa, S.; Zeisberg, M.; Kalluri, R. Partial Epithelial-to-Mesenchymal Transition and Other New Mechanisms of Kidney Fibrosis. *Trends Endocrinol. Metab. TEM* **2016**, *27*, 681–695. [CrossRef]
101. Zhou, J.; Jiang, H.; Jiang, H.; Fan, Y.; Zhang, J.; Ma, X.; Yang, X.; Sun, Y.; Zhao, X. The ILEI/LIFR complex induces EMT via the Akt and ERK pathways in renal interstitial fibrosis. *J. Transl. Med.* **2022**, *20*, 54. [CrossRef]
102. Ostendorf, T.; Boor, P.; van Roeyen, C.R.; Floege, J. Platelet-derived growth factors (PDGFs) in glomerular and tubulointerstitial fibrosis. *Kidney Int. Suppl. (2011)* **2014**, *4*, 65–69. [CrossRef]
103. Buhl, E.M.; Djudjaj, S.; Klinkhammer, B.M.; Ermert, K.; Puelles, V.G.; Lindenmeyer, M.T.; Cohen, C.D.; He, C.; Borkham-Kamphorst, E.; Weiskirchen, R.; et al. Dysregulated mesenchymal PDGFR-beta drives kidney fibrosis. *EMBO Mol. Med.* **2020**, *12*, e11021. [CrossRef] [PubMed]
104. WHO Ten Chemicals of Major Public Health Concern. Available online: http://www.who.int/ipcs/assessment/public_health/chemicals_phc/en/ (accessed on 23 July 2018).
105. ATSDR. *Public Health Statement: Arsenic*; Center for Disease Control and Prevention: Atlanta, GA, USA, 2007.
106. Nriagu, J.O.; Bhattacharya, P.; Mukherjee, A.B.; Bundschuh, J.; Zevenhoven, R.; Loeppert, R.H. Arsenic in soil and graoundwater: An overview. In *Trace Metals and Other Contaminants in the Environment*; Bhattacharya, P., Mukherjee, A.B., Bundschuh, J., Zevenhoven, R., Loeppert, R.H., Eds.; Elsevier: Amsterdam, The Netherlands, 2007; Volume 9, pp. 3–30.
107. Shankar, S.; Shanker, U.; Shikha. Arsenic contamination of groundwater: A review of sources, prevalence, health risks, and strategies for mitigation. *Sci. World J.* **2014**, *2014*, 304524. [CrossRef] [PubMed]
108. van Halem, D.; Bakker, S.A.; Amy, G.L.; van Dijk, J.C. Arsenic in drinking water: A worldwide quality concern for water supply companies. *Drink. Water Eng. Sci.* **2009**, *2*, 29–34. [CrossRef]
109. Hong, Y.S.; Song, K.H.; Chung, J.Y. Health effects of chronic arsenic exposure. *J. Prev. Med. Public Health* **2014**, *47*, 245–252. [CrossRef] [PubMed]
110. Howard, G. *Arsenic, Drinking-Water and Health Risks Substitution in Arsenic Mitigation: A Discussion Paper*; World Health Organization: Geneva, Switzerland, 2003.
111. Ratnaike, R.N. Acute and chronic arsenic toxicity. *Postgrad. Med. J.* **2003**, *79*, 391–396. [CrossRef]
112. Martinez, V.D.; Vucic, E.A.; Becker-Santos, D.D.; Gil, L.; Lam, W.L. Arsenic exposure and the induction of human cancers. *J. Toxicol.* **2011**, *2011*, 431287. [CrossRef]
113. Hafey, M.J.; Aleksunes, L.M.; Bridges, C.C.; Brouwer, K.R.; Chien, H.C.; Leslie, E.M.; Hu, S.; Li, Y.; Shen, J.; Sparreboom, A.; et al. Transporters and Toxicity: Insights from the International Transporter Consortium Workshop 4. *Clin. Pharmacol. Ther.* **2022**, *112*, 527–539. [CrossRef]

114. Jalili, C.; Kazemi, M.; Cheng, H.; Mohammadi, H.; Babaei, A.; Taheri, E.; Moradi, S. Associations between exposure to heavy metals and the risk of chronic kidney disease: A systematic review and meta-analysis. *Crit. Rev. Toxicol.* **2021**, *51*, 165–182. [CrossRef]
115. Robles-Osorio, M.L.; Sabath-Silva, E.; Sabath, E. Arsenic-mediated nephrotoxicity. *Ren. Fail.* **2015**, *37*, 542–547. [CrossRef]
116. Roggenbeck, B.A.; Banerjee, M.; Leslie, E.M. Cellular arsenic transport pathways in mammals. *J. Environ. Sci. (China)* **2016**, *49*, 38–58. [CrossRef]
117. Jin, W.; Xue, Y.; Xue, Y.; Han, X.; Song, Q.; Zhang, J.; Li, Z.; Cheng, J.; Guan, S.; Sun, S.; et al. Tannic acid ameliorates arsenic trioxide-induced nephrotoxicity, contribution of NF-kappaB and Nrf2 pathways. *Biomed. Pharmacother.* **2020**, *126*, 110047. [CrossRef] [PubMed]
118. Duan, X.; Xu, G.; Li, J.; Yan, N.; Li, X.; Liu, X.; Li, B. Arsenic Induces Continuous Inflammation and Regulates Th1/Th2/Th17/Treg Balance in Liver and Kidney In Vivo. *Mediat. Inflamm.* **2022**, *2022*, 8414047. [CrossRef] [PubMed]
119. Xu, G.; Gu, Y.; Yan, N.; Li, Y.; Sun, L.; Li, B. Curcumin functions as an anti-inflammatory and antioxidant agent on arsenic-induced hepatic and kidney injury by inhibiting MAPKs, NF-kappaB and activating Nrf2 pathways. *Environ. Toxicol.* **2021**, *36*, 2161–2173. [CrossRef]
120. Wang, Y.; Zhao, H.; Shao, Y.; Liu, J.; Li, J.; Xing, M. Copper or/and arsenic induce oxidative stress-cascaded, nuclear factor kappa B-dependent inflammation and immune imbalance, trigging heat shock response in the kidney of chicken. *Oncotarget* **2017**, *8*, 98103–98116. [CrossRef]
121. Bermejo, S.; Bolufer, M.; Riveiro-Barciela, M.; Soler, M.J. Immunotherapy and the Spectrum of Kidney Disease: Should We Individualize the Treatment? *Front. Med. (Lausanne)* **2022**, *9*, 906565. [CrossRef] [PubMed]
122. Yen, Y.P.; Tsai, K.S.; Chen, Y.W.; Huang, C.F.; Yang, R.S.; Liu, S.H. Arsenic induces apoptosis in myoblasts through a reactive oxygen species-induced endoplasmic reticulum stress and mitochondrial dysfunction pathway. *Arch. Toxicol.* **2012**, *86*, 923–933. [CrossRef] [PubMed]
123. Jomova, K.; Jenisova, Z.; Feszterova, M.; Baros, S.; Liska, J.; Hudecova, D.; Rhodes, C.J.; Valko, M. Arsenic: Toxicity, oxidative stress and human disease. *J. Appl. Toxicol.* **2011**, *31*, 95–107. [CrossRef]
124. ATSDR. *Toxicological Profile for Cadmium*; U.S. Department of Health and Human Services, Public Health Service, Centers for Disease Control: Atlanta, GA, USA, 2008.
125. WHO. *Cadmium—Environmental Health Criteria 134*; WHO: Geneva, Switzerland, 1992.
126. MartzEmerson, M. *FAQs about Cadmium in Fertilizer: Fertilizer Laws and Limits*; Pacific Northwest Pollution Prevention Resource Center: Seattle, WA, USA, 2017; pp. 1–10.
127. Ashraf, M.W. Levels of heavy metals in popular cigarette brands and exposure to these metals via smoking. *Sci. World J.* **2012**, *2012*, 729430. [CrossRef]
128. Adams, S.V.; Newcomb, P.A. Cadmium blood and urine concentrations as measures of exposure: NHANES 1999-2010. *J. Expo. Sci. Environ. Epidemiol.* **2014**, *24*, 163–170. [CrossRef]
129. Souza, V.; Bucio, L.; Gutierrez-Ruiz, M.C. Cadmium uptake by a human hepatic cell line (WRL-68 cells). *Toxicology* **1997**, *120*, 215–220. [CrossRef]
130. Drobna, Z.; Styblo, M.; Thomas, D.J. An Overview of Arsenic Metabolism and Toxicity. *Curr. Protoc. Toxicol.* **2009**, *42*, 4–31.
131. Khairul, I.; Wang, Q.Q.; Jiang, Y.H.; Wang, C.; Naranmandura, H. Metabolism, toxicity and anticancer activities of arsenic compounds. *Oncotarget* **2017**, *8*, 23905–23926. [CrossRef]
132. Fujishiro, H.; Yano, Y.; Takada, Y.; Tanihara, M.; Himeno, S. Roles of ZIP8, ZIP14, and DMT1 in transport of cadmium and manganese in mouse kidney proximal tubule cells. *Met. Integr. Biomet. Sci.* **2012**, *4*, 700–708. [CrossRef]
133. Jarup, L.; Hellstrom, L.; Alfven, T.; Carlsson, M.D.; Grubb, A.; Persson, B.; Pettersson, C.; Spang, G.; Schutz, A.; Elinder, C.G. Low level exposure to cadmium and early kidney damage: The OSCAR study. *Occup. Environ. Med.* **2000**, *57*, 668–672. [CrossRef]
134. Ginsberg, G.L. Cadmium risk assessment in relation to background risk of chronic kidney disease. *J. Toxicol. Environ. Health A* **2012**, *75*, 374–390. [CrossRef]
135. Ferraro, P.M.; Costanzi, S.; Naticchia, A.; Sturniolo, A.; Gambaro, G. Low level exposure to cadmium increases the risk of chronic kidney disease: Analysis of the NHANES 1999-2006. *BMC Public Health* **2010**, *10*, 304. [CrossRef]
136. Edwards, J.R.; Prozialeck, W.C. Cadmium, diabetes and chronic kidney disease. *Toxicol. Appl. Pharm.* **2009**, *238*, 289–293. [CrossRef]
137. Nguyen, J.; Patel, A.; Gensburg, A.; Bokhari, R.; Lamar, P.; Edwards, J. Diabetogenic and Obesogenic Effects of Cadmium in Db/Db Mice and Rats at a Clinically Relevant Level of Exposure. *Toxics* **2022**, *10*, 107. [CrossRef]
138. Li, M.; Liu, X.; Zhang, Z. Hyperglycemia exacerbates cadmium-induced glomerular nephrosis. *Toxicol. Ind. Health* **2021**, *37*, 555–563. [CrossRef]
139. Aramjoo, H.; Arab-Zozani, M.; Feyzi, A.; Naghizadeh, A.; Aschner, M.; Naimabadi, A.; Farkhondeh, T.; Samarghandian, S. The association between environmental cadmium exposure, blood pressure, and hypertension: A systematic review and meta-analysis. *Environ. Sci. Pollut. Res. Int.* **2022**, *29*, 35682–35706. [CrossRef]
140. Giridhar, J.; Isom, G.E. Alteration of atrial natriuretic peptide levels by short term cadmium treatment. *Toxicology* **1991**, *70*, 185–194. [CrossRef]
141. Giridhar, J.; Rathinavelu, A.; Isom, G.E. Interaction of cadmium with atrial natriuretic peptide receptors: Implications for toxicity. *Toxicology* **1992**, *75*, 133–143. [CrossRef]

142. Nishida, K.; Watanabe, H.; Miyahisa, M.; Hiramoto, Y.; Nosaki, H.; Fujimura, R.; Maeda, H.; Otagiri, M.; Maruyama, T. Systemic and sustained thioredoxin analogue prevents acute kidney injury and its-associated distant organ damage in renal ischemia reperfusion injury mice. *Sci. Rep.* **2020**, *10*, 20635. [CrossRef]
143. Oner, G.; Senturk, U.K.; Izgut-Uysal, V.N. Role of cadmium-induced lipid peroxidation in the kidney response to atrial natriuretic hormone. *Nephron* **1996**, *72*, 257–262. [CrossRef]
144. Liu, Q.; Zhang, R.; Wang, X.; Shen, X.; Wang, P.; Sun, N.; Li, X.; Li, X.; Hai, C. Effects of sub-chronic, low-dose cadmium exposure on kidney damage and potential mechanisms. *Ann. Transl. Med.* **2019**, *7*, 177. [CrossRef]
145. Ikediobi, C.O.; Badisa, V.L.; Ayuk-Takem, L.T.; Latinwo, L.M.; West, J. Response of antioxidant enzymes and redox metabolites to cadmium-induced oxidative stress in CRL-1439 normal rat liver cells. *Int. J. Mol. Med.* **2004**, *14*, 87–92. [CrossRef]
146. Li, J.R.; Ou, Y.C.; Wu, C.C.; Wang, J.D.; Lin, S.Y.; Wang, Y.Y.; Chen, W.Y.; Liao, S.L.; Chen, C.J. Endoplasmic reticulum stress and autophagy contributed to cadmium nephrotoxicity in HK-2 cells and Sprague-Dawley rats. *Food Chem. Toxicol. Int. J. Publ. Br. Ind. Biol. Res. Assoc.* **2020**, *146*, 111828. [CrossRef]
147. Wang, Q.W.; Wang, Y.; Wang, T.; Zhang, K.B.; Yuan, Y.; Bian, J.C.; Liu, X.Z.; Gu, J.H.; Zhu, J.Q.; Liu, Z.P. Cadmium-induced autophagy is mediated by oxidative signaling in PC-12 cells and is associated with cytoprotection. *Mol. Med. Rep.* **2015**, *12*, 4448–4454. [CrossRef]
148. So, K.Y.; Park, B.H.; Oh, S.H. Cytoplasmic sirtuin 6 translocation mediated by p62 polyubiquitination plays a critical role in cadmium-induced kidney toxicity. *Cell Biol. Toxicol.* **2021**, *37*, 193–207. [CrossRef]
149. Dong, W.; Liu, G.; Zhang, K.; Tan, Y.; Zou, H.; Yuan, Y.; Gu, J.; Song, R.; Zhu, J.; Liu, Z. Cadmium exposure induces rat proximal tubular cells injury via p62-dependent Nrf2 nucleus translocation mediated activation of AMPK/AKT/mTOR pathway. *Ecotoxicol. Environ. Saf.* **2021**, *214*, 112058. [CrossRef]
150. Fan, R.F.; Tang, K.K.; Wang, Z.Y.; Wang, L. Persistent activation of Nrf2 promotes a vicious cycle of oxidative stress and autophagy inhibition in cadmium-induced kidney injury. *Toxicology* **2021**, *464*, 152999. [CrossRef]
151. Lee, H.Y.; Oh, S.H. Autophagy-mediated cytoplasmic accumulation of p53 leads to apoptosis through DRAM-BAX in cadmium-exposed human proximal tubular cells. *Biochem. Biophys. Res. Commun.* **2021**, *534*, 128–133. [CrossRef]
152. Go, Y.-M.; Orr, M.; Jones, D.P. Increased Nuclear Thioredoxin-1 Potentiates Cadmium-Induced Cytotoxicity. *Toxicol. Sci.* **2012**, *131*, 84–94. [CrossRef]
153. Yang, Z.; Wang, S.; Liu, H.; Xu, S. MAPK/iNOS pathway is involved in swine kidney necrosis caused by cadmium exposure. *Environ. Pollut.* **2021**, *274*, 116497. [CrossRef] [PubMed]
154. Prozialeck, W.C.; Edwards, J.R. Mechanisms of cadmium-induced proximal tubule injury: New insights with implications for biomonitoring and therapeutic interventions. *J. Pharmacol. Exp. Ther.* **2012**, *343*, 2–12. [CrossRef]
155. Kothinti, R.K.; Blodgett, A.B.; Petering, D.H.; Tabatabai, N.M. Cadmium down-regulation of kidney Sp1 binding to mouse SGLT1 and SGLT2 gene promoters: Possible reaction of cadmium with the zinc finger domain of Sp1. *Toxicol. Appl. Pharmacol.* **2010**, *244*, 254–262. [CrossRef]
156. Gage, J.C. Distribution and Excretion of Methyl and Phenyl Mercury Salts. *Br. J. Ind. Med.* **1964**, *21*, 197–202. [CrossRef]
157. Norseth, T.; Clarkson, T.W. Studies on the biotransformation of 203Hg-labeled methyl mercury chloride in rats. *Arch. Environ. Health* **1970**, *21*, 717–727. [CrossRef]
158. Norseth, T.; Clarkson, T.W. Biotransformation of methylmercury salts in the rat studied by specific determination of inorganic mercury. *Biochem. Pharmacol.* **1970**, *19*, 2775–2783. [CrossRef]
159. Omata, S.; Sato, M.; Sakimura, K.; Sugano, H. Time-dependent accumulation of inorganic mercury in subcellular fractions of kidney, liver, and brain of rats exposed to methylmercury. *Arch. Toxicol.* **1980**, *44*, 231–241. [CrossRef]
160. Houser, M.T.; Berndt, W.O. The effect of unilateral nephrectomy on the nephrotoxicity of mercuric chloride in the rat. *Toxicol. Appl. Pharmacol.* **1986**, *83*, 506–515. [CrossRef]
161. Ramos-Frendo, B.; Perez-Garcia, R.; Lopez-Novoa, J.M.; Hernando-Avendano, L. Increased severity of the acute renal failure induced by HgCl2 on rats with reduced renal mass. *Biomedicine* **1979**, *31*, 167–170. [PubMed]
162. Zalups, R.K.; Diamond, G.L. Mercuric chloride-induced nephrotoxicity in the rat following unilateral nephrectomy and compensatory renal growth. *Virchows Arch. B Cell Pathol. Incl. Mol. Pathol.* **1987**, *53*, 336–346. [CrossRef] [PubMed]
163. Zalups, R.K. Reductions in renal mass and the nephropathy induced by mercury. *Toxicol. Appl. Pharmacol.* **1997**, *143*, 366–379. [CrossRef] [PubMed]
164. Zalups, R.K.; Bridges, C.C. Seventy-five percent nephrectomy and the disposition of inorganic mercury in 2,3-dimercaptopropane-sulfonic acid-treated rats lacking functional multidrug-resistance protein 2. *J. Pharmacol. Exp. Ther.* **2010**, *332*, 866–875. [CrossRef] [PubMed]
165. Miller, S.; Pallan, S.; Gangji, A.S.; Lukic, D.; Clase, C.M. Mercury-associated nephrotic syndrome: A case report and systematic review of the literature. *Am. J. Kidney Dis.* **2013**, *62*, 135–138. [CrossRef]
166. Gao, Z.; Wu, N.; Du, X.; Li, H.; Mei, X.; Song, Y. Toxic Nephropathy Secondary to Chronic Mercury Poisoning: Clinical Characteristics and Outcomes. *Kidney Int. Rep.* **2022**, *7*, 1189–1197. [CrossRef]
167. Alok, A.; Yadav, A. *Membranous Nephropathy*; StatPearls Publishing: Treasure Island, FL, USA, 2022.
168. Qin, A.B.; Lin, Z.S.; Wang, S.X.; Wang, H.; Cui, Z.; Zhou, F.D.; Zhao, M.H. Comparison of Ultrastructural Features between Patients with Mercury-associated Membranous Nephropathy and Idiopathic Membranous Nephropathy. *Am. J. Med. Sci.* **2021**, *361*, 327–335. [CrossRef]

169. Molina, A.; Sanchez-Madrid, F.; Bricio, T.; Martin, A.; Barat, A.; Alvarez, V.; Mampaso, F. Prevention of mercuric chloride-induced nephritis in the brown Norway rat by treatment with antibodies against the alpha 4 integrin. *J. Immunol.* **1994**, *153*, 2313–2320.
170. Bowman, C.; Peters, D.K.; Lockwood, C.M. Anti-glomerular basement membrane autoantibodies in the Brown Norway rat: Detection by a solid-phase radioimmunoassay. *J. Immunol. Methods* **1983**, *61*, 325–333. [CrossRef]
171. Molina, A.; Sanchez-Madrid, F.; Bricio, T.; Martin, A.; Escudero, E.; Alvarez, V.; Mampaso, F. Abrogation of mercuric chloride-induced nephritis in the Brown Norway rat by treatment with antibodies against TNFalpha. *Mediat. Inflamm.* **1995**, *4*, 444–451. [CrossRef]
172. Guery, J.C.; Druet, E.; Glotz, D.; Hirsch, F.; Mandet, C.; De Heer, E.; Druet, P. Specificity and cross-reactive idiotypes of anti-glomerular basement membrane autoantibodies in HgCl$_2$-induced autoimmune glomerulonephritis. *Eur. J. Immunol.* **1990**, *20*, 93–100. [CrossRef]
173. Mathieson, P.W.; Thiru, S.; Oliveira, D.B. Mercuric chloride-treated brown Norway rats develop widespread tissue injury including necrotizing vasculitis. *Lab. Investig.* **1992**, *67*, 121–129. [PubMed]
174. Pelletier, L.; Rossert, J.; Pasquier, R.; Vial, M.C.; Druet, P. Role of CD8+ T cells in mercury-induced autoimmunity or immunosuppression in the rat. *Scand. J. Immunol.* **1990**, *31*, 65–74. [CrossRef] [PubMed]
175. Kosuda, L.L.; Wayne, A.; Nahounou, M.; Greiner, D.L.; Bigazzi, P.E. Reduction of the RT6.2+ subset of T lymphocytes in brown Norway rats with mercury-induced renal autoimmunity. *Cell. Immunol.* **1991**, *135*, 154–167. [CrossRef]
176. Escudero, E.; Martin, A.; Nieto, M.; Nieto, E.; Navarro, E.; Luque, A.; Cabanas, C.; Sanchez-Madrid, F.; Mampaso, F. Functional relevance of activated beta1 integrins in mercury-induced nephritis. *J. Am. Soc. Nephrol.* **2000**, *11*, 1075–1084. [CrossRef] [PubMed]
177. Tang, J.; Zhu, Q.; Xu, Y.; Zhou, Y.; Zhu, L.; Jin, L.; Wang, W.; Gao, L.; Chen, G.; Zhao, H. Total arsenic, dimethylarsinic acid, lead, cadmium, total mercury, methylmercury and hypertension among Asian populations in the United States: NHANES 2011–2018. *Ecotoxicol. Environ. Saf.* **2022**, *241*, 113776. [CrossRef]
178. Simoes, R.P.; Fardin, P.B.A.; Simoes, M.R.; Vassallo, D.V.; Padilha, A.S. Long-term Mercury Exposure Accelerates the Development of Hypertension in Prehypertensive Spontaneously Hypertensive Rats Inducing Endothelial Dysfunction: The Role of Oxidative Stress and Cyclooxygenase-2. *Biol. Trace Elem. Res.* **2020**, *196*, 565–578. [CrossRef]
179. Fardin, P.B.A.; Simoes, R.P.; Schereider, I.R.G.; Almenara, C.C.P.; Simoes, M.R.; Vassallo, D.V. Chronic Mercury Exposure in Prehypertensive SHRs Accelerates Hypertension Development and Activates Vasoprotective Mechanisms by Increasing NO and H$_2$O$_2$ Production. *Cardiovasc. Toxicol.* **2020**, *20*, 197–210. [CrossRef]
180. Vassallo, D.V.; Simoes, M.R.; Giuberti, K.; Azevedo, B.F.; Ribeiro Junior, R.F.; Salaices, M.; Stefanon, I. Effects of Chronic Exposure to Mercury on Angiotensin-Converting Enzyme Activity and Oxidative Stress in Normotensive and Hypertensive Rats. *Arq. Bras. Cardiol.* **2019**, *112*, 374–380. [CrossRef]
181. Habeeb, E.; Aldosari, S.; Saghir, S.A.; Cheema, M.; Momenah, T.; Husain, K.; Omidi, Y.; Rizvi, S.A.A.; Akram, M.; Ansari, R.A. Role of environmental toxicants in the development of hypertensive and cardiovascular diseases. *Toxicol. Rep.* **2022**, *9*, 521–533. [CrossRef] [PubMed]
182. Orr, S.E.; Barnes, M.C.; Joshee, L.; Uchakina, O.; McKallip, R.J.; Bridges, C.C. Potential mechanisms of cellular injury following exposure to a physiologically relevant species of inorganic mercury. *Toxicol. Lett.* **2019**, *304*, 13–20. [CrossRef] [PubMed]
183. Lund, B.O.; Miller, D.M.; Woods, J.S. Studies on Hg(II)-induced H$_2$O$_2$ formation and oxidative stress in vivo and in vitro in rat kidney mitochondria. *Biochem. Pharmacol.* **1993**, *45*, 2017–2024. [CrossRef]
184. Ma, L.; Bi, K.D.; Fan, Y.M.; Jiang, Z.Y.; Zhang, X.Y.; Zhang, J.W.; Zhao, J.; Jiang, F.L.; Dong, J.X. In vitro modulation of mercury-induced rat liver mitochondria dysfunction. *Toxicol. Res.* **2018**, *7*, 1135–1143. [CrossRef] [PubMed]
185. Han, B.; Lv, Z.; Han, X.; Li, S.; Han, B.; Yang, Q.; Wang, X.; Wu, P.; Li, J.; Deng, N. et al. Harmful Effects of Inorganic Mercury Exposure on Kidney Cells: Mitochondrial Dynamics Disorder and Excessive Oxidative Stress. *Biol. Trace Elem. Res.* **2022**, *200*, 1591–1597. [CrossRef] [PubMed]
186. Khan, H.; Singh, R.D.; Tiwari, R.; Gangopadhyay, S.; Roy, S.K.; Singh, D.; Srivastava, V. Mercury exposure induces cytoskeleton disruption and loss of renal function through epigenetic modulation of MMP9 expression. *Toxicology* **2017**, *386*, 28–39. [CrossRef]
187. Zhong, Y.; Wang, B.; Hu, S.; Wang, T.; Zhang, Y.; Wang, J.; Liu, Y.; Zhang, H. The role of endoplasmic reticulum stress in renal damage caused by acute mercury chloride poisoning. *J. Toxicol. Sci.* **2020**, *45*, 589–598. [CrossRef]
188. Rojas-Franco, P.; Franco-Colin, M.; Torres-Manzo, A.P.; Blas-Valdivia, V.; Thompson-Bonilla, M.D.R.; Kandir, S.; Cano-Europa, E. Endoplasmic reticulum stress participates in the pathophysiology of mercury-caused acute kidney injury. *Ren. Fail.* **2019**, *41*, 1001–1010. [CrossRef]
189. Vieira, J.; Marques, V.B.; Vieira, L.V.; Crajoinas, R.O.; Shimizu, M.H.M.; Seguro, A.C.; Carneiro, M.; Girardi, A.C.C.; Vassallo, D.V.; Dos Santos, L. Changes in the renal function after acute mercuric chloride exposure in the rat are associated with renal vascular endothelial dysfunction and proximal tubule NHE3 inhibition. *Toxicol. Lett.* **2021**, *341*, 23–32. [CrossRef]
190. Kramer, H.J.; Gonick, H.C.; Lu, E. In vitro inhibition of Na-K-ATPase by trace metals: Relation to renal and cardiovascular damage. *Nephron* **1986**, *44*, 329–336. [CrossRef]
191. Savage, D.F.; Stroud, R.M. Structural basis of aquaporin inhibition by mercury. *J. Mol. Biol.* **2007**, *368*, 607–617. [CrossRef] [PubMed]

192. Devuyst, O.; Burrow, C.R.; Smith, B.L.; Agre, P.; Knepper, M.A.; Wilson, P.D. Expression of aquaporins-1 and -2 during nephrogenesis and in autosomal dominant polycystic kidney disease. *Am. J. Physiol.* **1996**, *271 Pt 2*, F169–F183. [CrossRef] [PubMed]
193. Su, W.; Cao, R.; Zhang, X.Y.; Guan, Y. Aquaporins in the kidney: Physiology and pathophysiology. *Am. J. Physiol. Ren. Physiol.* **2020**, *318*, F193–F203. [CrossRef] [PubMed]

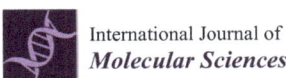

Review

The Signaling Pathway of TNF Receptors: Linking Animal Models of Renal Disease to Human CKD

Irina Lousa [1,2], Flávio Reis [3,4,5], Alice Santos-Silva [1,2] and Luís Belo [1,2,*]

1 Associate Laboratory i4HB-Institute for Health and Bioeconomy, Faculty of Pharmacy, University of Porto, 4050-313 Porto, Portugal; irina.filipa@hotmail.com (I.L.); assilva@ff.up.pt (A.S.-S.)
2 UCIBIO—Applied Molecular Biosciences Unit, Laboratory of Biochemistry, Department of Biological Sciences, Faculty of Pharmacy, University of Porto, 4050-313 Porto, Portugal
3 Institute of Pharmacology & Experimental Therapeutics & Coimbra Institute for Clinical and Biomedical Research (iCBR), Faculty of Medicine, University of Coimbra, 3000-548 Coimbra, Portugal; freis@fmed.uc.pt
4 Center for Innovative Biomedicine and Biotechnology (CIBB), University of Coimbra, 3004-504 Coimbra, Portugal
5 Clinical Academic Center of Coimbra (CACC), 3000-075 Coimbra, Portugal
* Correspondence: luisbelo@ff.up.pt

Abstract: Chronic kidney disease (CKD) has been recognized as a global public health problem. Despite the current advances in medicine, CKD-associated morbidity and mortality remain unacceptably high. Several studies have highlighted the contribution of inflammation and inflammatory mediators to the development and/or progression of CKD, such as tumor necrosis factor (TNF)-related biomarkers. The inflammation pathway driven by TNF-α, through TNF receptors 1 (TNFR1) and 2 (TNFR2), involves important mediators in the pathogenesis of CKD. Circulating levels of TNFRs were associated with changes in other biomarkers of kidney function and injury, and were described as predictors of disease progression, cardiovascular morbidity, and mortality in several cohorts of patients. Experimental studies describe the possible downstream signaling pathways induced upon TNFR activation and the resulting biological responses. This review will focus on the available data on TNFR1 and TNFR2, and illustrates their contributions to the pathophysiology of kidney diseases, their cellular and molecular roles, as well as their potential as CKD biomarkers. The emerging evidence shows that TNF receptors could act as biomarkers of renal damage and as mediators of the disease. Furthermore, it has been suggested that these biomarkers could significantly improve the discrimination of clinical CKD prognostic models.

Keywords: CKD; inflammation; TNF-alpha; TNFR; biomarkers

1. Chronic Kidney Disease—A Public Health Issue

In the last decade, chronic kidney disease (CKD) has been recognized as a global public health problem, due to its increasing incidence and prevalence rates [1,2]. Additionally, CKD is a significant contributor to early morbidity and mortality worldwide, as well as an important risk factor for cardiovascular diseases (CVD). In 2017, CKD was the 12th leading cause of death, globally, rising from 17th in 1990 [3].

CKD is a pathological condition that results from a gradual and permanent loss of renal function over time, characterized by the presence of kidney dysfunction and injury markers, over a period of at least three months. According to the '2012 Kidney Disease: Improving Global Outcomes' (KDIGO) guidelines, the severity of CKD is classified into five stages, according to glomerular filtration rate (GFR) and urinary albumin excretion [4].
Increased CKD severity is indicated by lower GFR and/or increased albuminuria levels.

The etiology of CKD depends on the setting, with diabetes and hypertension being the two major causes of kidney injury in developed countries [3]. However, irrespective of the

Citation: Lousa, I.; Reis, F.; Santos-Silva, A.; Belo, L. The Signaling Pathway of TNF Receptors: Linking Animal Models of Renal Disease to Human CKD. *Int. J. Mol. Sci.* **2022**, *23*, 3284. https://doi.org/10.3390/ijms23063284

Academic Editor: Andrea Huwiler

Received: 28 February 2022
Accepted: 16 March 2022
Published: 18 March 2022

Publisher's Note: MDPI stays neutral with regard to jurisdictional claims in published maps and institutional affiliations.

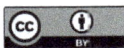

Copyright: © 2022 by the authors. Licensee MDPI, Basel, Switzerland. This article is an open access article distributed under the terms and conditions of the Creative Commons Attribution (CC BY) license (https://creativecommons.org/licenses/by/4.0/).

primary disease cause, CKD initiation and progression involves different pathophysiological pathways leading to kidney function decline [5], which involves a complex interaction between hemodynamic, metabolic, immunologic, and inflammatory mechanisms.

CKD is associated with a decreased quality of life, increased risk of hospitalization, cardiovascular complications and mortality, independently of other risk factors [1,3,6,7]. Importantly, CKD and its related comorbidities are largely preventable and manageable, if detected at an initial stage. Thus, early identification of CKD is essential, not only to predict and prevent CKD progression, but also to further improve patients' survival and reduce associated morbidities. Hence, more sensitive and earlier biomarkers of detection are necessary to achieve that goal, since the traditional biomarkers only increase when a significant filtration capacity has already been lost and kidney damage is advanced [8].

Several studies in the literature suggest that activation of inflammatory processes in the early stages of CKD drives kidney function impairment [5], meaning that the assessment of inflammatory markers might help in earlier diagnosis of CKD. Associations between biomarkers of inflammation and changes in GFR have been widely reported. Moreover, inflammation is a risk factor for CKD-associated morbidity and appears to contribute to cardiovascular mortality in CKD patients [9–12].

2. Inflammation as an Essential Component of CKD

The persistent low-grade inflammatory status that characterizes CKD plays a key role in the pathophysiology of the disease. Inflammation starts early in the onset of renal diseases [13,14] and worsens with disease progression [15], being particularly marked in hemodialysis patients [16]. Interestingly, inflammation can be identified either as a trigger or a consequence of CKD. The etiology of inflammation is multifactorial and can result from a primary cause of disease (diabetes, obesity) [17], from renal dysfunction comorbidities (uremia, metabolic acidosis, intestinal dysbiosis, vitamin D deficiency, oxidative stress) [17–19], and/or from dialysis procedures (intercurrent infections and thrombotic events) [20].

Inflammation is a well-established risk factor of both morbidity and mortality in CKD patients [21–23], leading to renal function deterioration and fibrosis. CKD patients present low to moderate levels of circulating inflammatory mediators [24,25] as a result of a deregulation of their synthesis, increased release, and/or impaired renal clearance [15,26]. It is broadly accepted that inflammation plays a role in CKD progression, but the association between disease initiation and the establishment of inflammation is debatable. Glomerular hypertrophy, endothelial dysfunction, podocytes damage, proteinuria, and tubular cells injury are some of the identified kidney insults that can trigger the development of inflammation [27].

The initial inflammatory response occurs to overcome renal injury, promote tissue remodeling and wound healing. However, when this process outreaches the physiological limit, a chronic inflammatory state may arise, with undesirable systemic consequences [14]. The dysregulated immune response results in a continuous activation of inflammatory mediators, contributing to renal scarring and fibrosis [24], the final common pathological manifestation of renal diseases.

The inflammatory state is characterized by activation of inflammatory cells, releasing an array of acute phase proteins, cytokines, and chemokines [19,25], which are able to interact with renal parenchymal cells and resident immune cells, and trigger the recruitment and activation of circulating monocytes, lymphocytes, and neutrophils, into renal tissue [13,14]. The activation of inflammatory response and the infiltration of inflammatory cells induce cellular transdifferentiation into myofibroblasts, which are responsible for the production and deposition of extracellular matrix components and cytoskeletal components, which leads to renal remodeling. In renal fibrosis, myofibroblasts seem to be derived from different cell types, such as tubular epithelial cells, interstitial fibroblasts, macrophages, as well as pericytes and endothelial cells [28]. The imbalance in matrix formation/degradation leads to accumulation of an extracellular matrix, which might lead to glomerulosclerosis and/or tubulointerstitial fibrosis and a consequent GFR decline [25,29]. Under chronic inflammatory activation, resident kidney cells exhibiting a proinflammatory phenotype, coupled with the activated immune cells, are responsible for perpetuating the ongoing inflammatory process, leading to renal fibrosis. Once renal fibrosis sets in, CKD progression is irreversible, irrespective of the initial cause [29]. Kidney hypoxia/ischemia, inflammation, and oxidative stress are simultaneously a cause and an effect of renal damage and fibrosis. Those events form a vicious cycle in CKD progression.

Cytokines and acute phase proteins are simultaneously key mediators and biomarkers of inflammation. Even though their circulating concentrations show a tendency to increase with the worsening of disease, the rate and magnitude of the increase depends on the molecule itself. It has been shown in several CKD models, that the classical proinflammatory signaling pathway, the NF-kB system [18,30], is activated by multiple inflammatory mediators, mainly by tumor necrosis factor alpha (TNF-α).

3. The TNF Signaling Pathway

Tumor necrosis factor alpha (TNF-α), also known as TNF superfamily member 2 (TNFSF2) or simply TNF, is a pleiotropic cytokine that can mediate the inflammatory response, regulate immune function by promoting immune cells activation and recruitment, and may trigger cell proliferation, differentiation, apoptosis, and necroptosis [31]. TNF-α is primarily produced by activated immune cells, and its increase in the circulation can be detected within minutes after the pro-inflammatory stimuli [32]; TNF-α can also be expressed by activated endothelial cells [33], fibroblasts [34], adipose tissue [35], cardiac myocytes [36], and neurons [37]. Abnormally elevated production, and/or sustained higher values of TNF-α, have been associated with autoimmune diseases, such as rheumatoid arthritis, multiple sclerosis, inflammatory bowel diseases [38,39], and chronic inflammatory disease states, such as sepsis, CKD, obesity, and diabetes [35,40,41].

TNF-α can be found in two bioactive homotrimeric forms: as a 26 kDa transmembrane peptide, or as a 17 kDa soluble form that is released into circulation upon cleavage by the metalloproteinase TNF-α converting enzyme (TACE) [31,42]. The pleotropic actions of TNF-α are mediated by either one of its two TNF receptors, TNFR1 and TNFR2 [32], which engage shared and distinct downstream signaling pathways; therefore, both exhibit common and divergent biological functions. While TNFR1 is basally expressed across all human cells [43] and is more efficiently triggered by soluble TNF-α, TNFR2 is mostly expressed in immune cells, endothelial cells, and neurons and has more affinity for the TNF-α membrane-bound form [44]. Besides its independent functions, TNFR2 acts as a ligand presenting TNF-α to TNFR1, potentiating its response [45]. Through the activity of TACE enzymes, TNFR1 and TNFR2 membrane receptors can also be converted into soluble forms, which act as antagonists of TNF-α [46].

TNF-α exerts both homeostatic and pro-inflammatory roles. However, TNF-α binding to TNFR1 mostly promotes inflammation and tissue injury [47], while binding to TNFR2 has been mainly implicated in immune modulation and tissue regeneration. TNFR2 is also essential for epithelial-to-mesenchymal transition and cell proliferation [47,48]. Thus, the immunoregulatory functions of TNF-α involve multiple mechanisms and depend on the regulation and relative expression of the two receptors, as well as their shedding [49].

TNFR1 and TNFR2 present different intracellular domains [50] that can interact with common and diverse downstream signaling molecules [47]. Figure 1 illustrates the TNFR1 and TNFR1 signaling pathways. The role of each receptor is context-dependent and can also be cell or tissue specific.

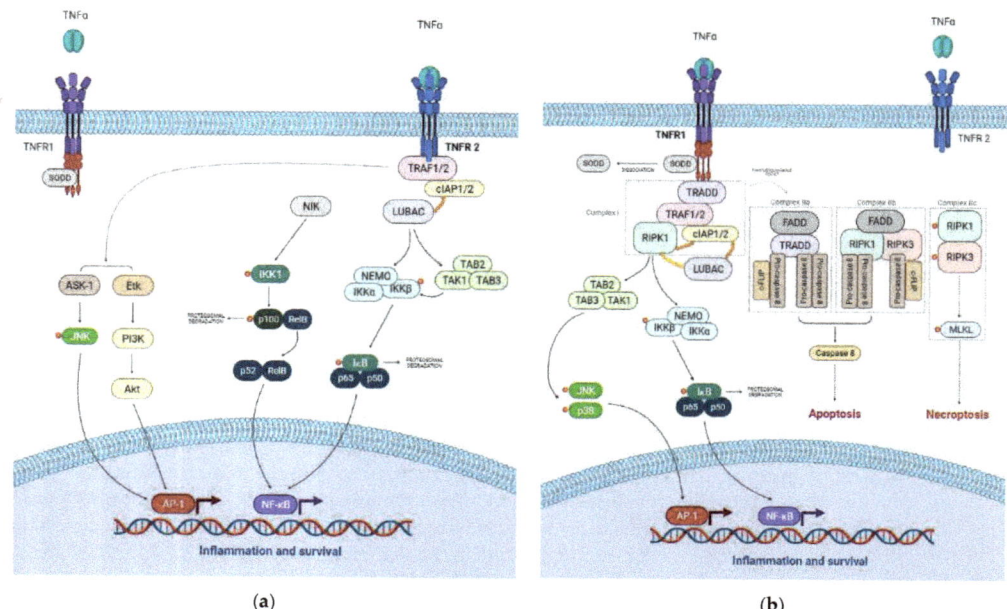

Figure 1. TNFR1 (**a**) and TNFR2 (**b**) mediated signaling pathways. Akt, protein kinase B; AP-1, activator protein-1; ASK-1, apoptosis signal-regulating kinase-1; c-FLIP, cellular FLICE-inhibitory protein; cIAP1/2, cellular inhibitor of apoptosis protein 1 or 2; Etk, endothelial/epithelial protein tyrosine kinase; FADD, Fas-associated death domain; IKK, inhibitor of kappa B kinase; IκB, NF-κB inhibitor; JNK, c-jun kinase; LUBAC, linear ubiquitin chain assembly complex; MAPK, mitogen activated protein kinase; MLKL, mixed lineage kinase domain-like protein; NEMO, NF-κB essential modulator; NF-kB, nuclear factor kappa B; NIK, NF-κB inducing kinase; PI3K, phosphatidylinositol 3-kinase; RIPK1/3, receptor interacting serine/threonine-protein kinase 1 or 3; SODD, silencer of death domains; TAB, TAK-binding proteins; TAK1, transforming growth factor-beta-activated kinase 1; TNFR1, tumor necrosis factor receptor 1; TNFR2, tumor necrosis factor receptor 2; TNF-α, tumor necrosis factor alpha; TRADD, TNF receptor-associated death domain; TRAF1/2, TNF receptor-associated factor 1 or 2.

3.1. TNFR1 Signaling Pathways

The pathways triggered upon TNFR1 activation are better known. TNFR1 contains an intracellular death domain (DD) that, in the absence of ligand, interacts with a cytosolic silencer of death domains (SODD) [50]. Upon binding to TNF-α, the inhibitory protein SODD is released and the DD of TNFR1 is recognized by the TNF receptor-associated death domain, TRADD, which recruits two additional adaptor proteins, TNF receptor-associated factor 1 or 2 (TRAF1/2) and receptor interacting serine/threonine-protein kinase 1 (RIPK1) [51–53]. The assembling of different signaling pathways that activate distinct downstream responses will depend on the ubiquitination state of RIPK1 [54]. Thus, RIPK1 is the major regulator of the cellular decision between TNF-mediated pro-survival signaling or death.

Ubiquitinated RIPK1 allows the activation of complex I, comprising TRADD, RIPK1, TRAF2, cellular inhibitor of apoptosis protein 1 or 2 (cIAP1/2), and linear ubiquitin chain assembly complex (LUBAC) [55,56]. Both cIAPs and LUBAC promote poly-ubiquitination of RIPK1 [55,56], which leads to the recruitment of two complexes: transforming growth factor-beta-activated kinase 1 (TAK1) complex, comprising TAK-binding proteins (TAB) 2 and 3; and inhibitor of kappa B kinase (IKK) complex, involving two kinases IKKα and IKKβ, and the regulatory subunit NF-κB essential modulator (NEMO, also known as

IKKγ) [57]. The recruitment of these two complexes (TAK1 and IKK) leads to the activation of mitogen activated protein kinases (MAPKs) and the canonical NF-κB pathway.

The activation of the IKK complex requires NEMO ubiquitination, by LUBAC [55,58], and IKKβ phosphorylation, by TAK1 [55,59]. In turn, the phosphorylated IKKβ initiates phosphorylation and proteosomal degradation of NF-kB inhibitor (IκB), unmasking the p65 subunit of NF-κB and enabling the translocation of the NF-κB heterodimer, composed of a p65 and a p50 subunit, into the nucleus, where it activates the transcription of various proinflammatory, anti-apoptotic, and pro-survival genes [60]. Another TAK1-dependent mechanism that upregulates proinflammatory gene expression involves the phosphorylation of mitogen activated protein kinases (MAPKs), such as c-jun kinase (JNK) and p38 [59,61], which further induces activator protein-1 (AP-1) transcription factor [62]

Alternatively, TNF-α binding to TNFR1 can induce two types of programmed cell death, apoptosis or necroptosis, when death-inducing signaling complexes (IIa, IIb, or IIc) are assembled in the cytosol [43]. TNF-TNFR1 mediated NF-κB signaling induces cell survival and requires polyubiquitination of RIPK1 bound to TRADD [63,64]. Therefore, when RIPK1 is not ubiquitinated, it dissociates from complex I, which favors the formation of death complexes. In these NF-κB inhibited conditions, TRADD recruits Fas-associated death domain (FADD) [53], a pro-caspase 8 dimer, and a heterodimer of pro-caspase 8 and the long form of cellular FLICE-inhibitory protein (c-FLIP) [57], forming complex IIa.

The depletion of the cIAP1 and 2 also reduces, or prevents, RIPK1 ubiquitination [65], resulting in apoptosis, through complex IIb. This cytoplasmic complex, formed by nonubiquitinated RIPK1 and FADD, recruits RIPK3, pro-caspase 8 dimer, and c-FLIP-pro-caspase 8 heterodimer, and induces apoptotic cell death, similarly to complex IIa [57].

Furthermore, the aggregation of RIPK1 and RIPK3 leads to the activation of mixed lineage kinase domain-like protein (MLKL) [66,67], through complex IIc. Several mechanisms by which phosphorylated MLKL induces necrotic cell death have been proposed [68], such as mitochondrial fragmentation and/or plasma membrane rupture with a subsequent influx of positively charged ions.

Ubiquitination of the proteins involved in TNFR1-signaling cascades has a major role in determining TNF-induced downstream outcomes. Ubiquitination status of RIPK1 determines whether TNF-TNFR1 signaling mediates cell survival or apoptosis, since RIPK1 ubiquitination prevents complex IIa and IIb from assembling. Several ubiquitin-modifying proteins that act on RIPK1 have been identified. The ubiquitin-modifying enzyme A20 is able to bind and remove polyubiquitin chains from RIPK1 and LUBAC, blocking NF-kB activation. Cylindromatosis (CYLD) is another deubiquitylating enzyme that acts on several proteins, such as TRAF2, RIPK1, and IKKγ, to regulate the NF-kB and JNK pathways [43,69]. In addition, cellular degradation or depletion of cIAPs prevents RIPK1 ubiquitination.

3.2. TNFR2 Signaling Pathways

Unlike TNFR1, TNFR2 does not have a DD, being unable to recruit TRADD [53]. Upon TNF-α binding, TNFR2 interacts directly with TRAF 1 or TRAF2, which recruits cIAP1 and 2, along with LUBAC [70,71]. Accordingly with the events triggered by TNFR1 signaling, the ubiquitin chains formed by LUBAC allow the recruitment of TAK1 and IKK complexes; therefore, activating the canonical NF-κB signaling pathway.

However, TNFR2 may also trigger non-canonical NF-κB signaling [72], by promoting activation of the NF-κB inducing kinase (NIK) [73]. In the absence of stimuli, NIK is ubiquitinated by intracellular TRAF/cIAPs complexes, and undergoes proteasomal degradation. However, upon TNF-α binding, the subsequent recruitment of these complexes by TNFRs, leads to NIK stabilization and activation. Activated NIK phosphorylates and induces the processing of p100, a protein that acts as an IκB-like molecule, which allows the nuclear translocation of p52/RelB [73]. This evidence confirms earlier studies that showed that the TNFR2 signaling involved in NF-kB activation occurs independently of TNFR1 signaling, which highlights distinct molecular pathways not shared with TNFR1 [74].

Furthermore, TNFR2 is able to activate JNK and protein kinase B (Akt) pathways [75,76]. TNFR2-mediated JNK activation seems to be TRAF2-dependent [76]. TNFR2 associates with apoptosis signal-regulating kinase-1 (ASK-1), an upstream MAPK critical for JNK activation [77]. TNFR2 mediated endothelial/epithelial protein tyrosine kinase (Etk) activation, subsequently stimulates phosphatidylinositol 3-kinase (PI3K) and its effector Akt, promoting pro-survival and reparative cascades [78]. These pathways are likely to be involved in the TNF-dependent activation of mesenchymal stem cells and T cells [44].

In endothelial cells, TNFR2 also signals through interferon regulatory factor-1 (IRF1), inducing interferon-β (IFN-β), promoting the transcription of inflammatory cytokines and monocytes recruitment during a TNF-induced inflammatory response [79].

TNFR2 can induce cell death indirectly by crosstalk with TNFR1. Depletion of TRAF2 by TNFR2 inhibits the NF-kB and MAPK signaling pathways mediated by TNFR1, favoring the formation of death complexes [80].

When TNFR1 and TNFR2 are co-expressed in the same cells, intracellular crosstalk between both signaling pathways seems to be mainly shaped by intracellular constraints, such as the availability of downstream effectors of each pathway, such as TRAF2 and ASK-1 [81,82]. However, there are other factors that contribute to the complexity of this cross-talk, such as the differential expression of both receptors in different cell types and the fact that the two signaling pathways are linked by positive and negative feedback mechanisms [44].

4. Involvement of TNF Receptors on Renal Deterioration

The inflammation pathway driven by TNF-α is important in the pathogenesis of CKD [83,84]. However, the role of TNF-α and its receptors in renal diseases is not completely clarified. Upon an inflammatory stimulus, TNF-α was shown to be overproduced in podocytes, mesangial cells, proximal tubules, glomerular cells, and also in infiltrating macrophages [84], amplifying the overall injury response. While TNFR1 is generally found in glomerular and peritubular endothelial cells, TNFR2 expression in renal cells has been shown to be transcriptionally induced after renal injury [84,85].

In this review, we summarize the more important results from published studies on the contribution of TNF-α and its receptors to the development and/or progression of CKD (Tables 1 and 2). A search in Pubmed was conducted, including animal and human studies, using the keywords "renal disease", "chronic kidney disease", or "CKD", and the biomarkers name "TNF-α", "TNFR1", and "TNFR2", to search the title and/or abstract. From the retrieved articles, and after title and abstract screening, we selected studies that evaluated the validity of these biomarkers in CKD diagnosis and prognosis, in different renal disease models and patients with different backgrounds. Furthermore, we searched for additional publications in the references of the selected articles.

4.1. Studies Addressing TNF-α and TNFRs in Animal Models

Animal studies are the primary source of evidence for the role of TNF-α in the development of kidney diseases (Table 1). In the classical 5/6 nephrectomy CKD model, NF-kB is activated and other proinflammatory genes are upregulated [86]. The systemic administration of TNF-α in rat models of anti-glomerular basement membrane antibody-mediated nephritis worsened the severity of glomerular injury by increasing neutrophil influx, albuminuria, and the prevalence of glomerular capillary thrombi [83]. TNF-α blockade reduced proteinuria, inflammation status, and renal scaring in mice [87] and rat [88] models of glomerulonephritis. It was also shown that TNF-α blockade prevented the development of crescents in a rat model of crescentic glomerulonephritis [88] and reduced renal tubular cell apoptosis, caspase activity, and several markers of renal fibrosis, in a model of unilateral ureteral obstruction [89,90].

Studies addressing the deletion of TNFR1 and/or TNFR2 genes, in animal models, also illustrated the contributions of the TNFRs in the pathophysiology of kidney diseases. The deletion of TNFR1 was associated with an increase in GFR, in an angiotensin II-induced model of hypertension [91]. Data from the same study showed that renal TNFR2 mRNA expression is increased in hypertensive TNFR1 knockout mice, along with increased urinary albumin excretion, compared to wild type mice and to TNFR1 knockout mice without induced hypertension. The authors suggested that TNFR2 has a leading role in the development of albuminuria [91]. Accordingly, TNFR2 knockout mice subjected to immune complex-mediated glomerulonephritis did not exhibit increased albuminuria and were protected from renal injury, despite preserving intact the immune system response [92]. In a model of unilateral ureteral obstruction, both TNFR1 and TNFR2 knockout mice showed a significantly reduced relative volume of the cortical interstitium, in the obstructed kidney, compared with the wild-type mice, as a result of the decreased deposition of pro-fibrotic proteins [93]. Additionally, the individual knockout of TNFR1 or TNFR2 resulted in decreased inflammation, demonstrated by the reduced activation of the NF-κB pathway. TNFR deletion was found to have comparable favorable effects in kidney disease development in several other animal studies [94–97].

TNFR participation in diabetic kidney disease has been the subject of specific research. Previous studies reported that the TNF-α inhibition protects against tubular injuries [97] and prevents renal hypertrophy [98] in diabetic rats. A diabetic mice model treated with a TNF-α inhibitor, Etanercept, showed improvements in albuminuria, decreased expression of inflammatory molecules, and decreased macrophage infiltration into the kidney [99]; renal levels of TNFR2, but not TNF-α or TNFR1, were decreased compared to non-treated mice [99]. The authors suggested that diabetic nephropathy is predominantly associated with the inflammatory action of TNF-α via the TNFR2 pathway. Other works also demonstrated that the administration of TNF antagonists inhibits salt retention, renal hypertrophy [98], and albuminuria [100], suggesting that TNF inhibition may slow the progression of diabetic nephropathy.

Transcriptomics further showed that both oxidative stress and inflammation play a role in the pathogenesis of CKD, and are correlated with cellular alterations that lead to systemic complications [101]. In ischemia–reperfusion mice models, proximal tubule cells at a late injury stage that mimic chronic progression confirmed a marked activation of the TNF, NF-κB, and AP-1 signaling pathways [102].

Table 1. Association of TNF-α and TNF receptors with renal dysfunction and disease in animal models.

Year	Study Model	Methods	Study Outcomes	Reference
1989	Anti GBM nephritis rat model	Pretreatment with human TNF-α	Pretreatment of rats with TNF-α increased the glomerular neutrophil influx and exacerbated glomerular injury, judged by the increased albuminuria and the prevalence of glomerular capillary thrombi.	[83]
1998	Anti-GBM nephritis mice model	Tnf-α knockout mice	In TNF-deficient mice, the influx of lymphocytes was reduced, the development of proteinuria was delayed and the formation of crescents was almost completely prevented.	[87]
1999	UUO mice model	Tnfr1 and Tnfr2 knockout	Individual knockout of the TNFRs genes resulted in significantly less NF-kB activation compared with the WT. Tnfr1 knockout showed a significant reduction in Tnf-α mRNA levels compared with WT or Tnfr2 knockout mice.	[93]
2001	Rat model of crescentic glomerulonephritis	TNF-α blockade with sTNFR1	Treatment with sTNFR1 caused a marked reduction in albuminuria, reduced glomerular cell infiltration, activation, and proliferation, and prevented the development of crescents.	[88]

Table 1. Cont.

Year	Study Model	Methods	Study Outcomes	Reference
2003	Mice model of cisplatin-induced acute renal failure	$Tnfr1$ and $Tnfr2$ knockout	$Tnfr2$-deficient mice developed less-severe renal dysfunction and showed reduced necrosis, apoptosis, and leukocyte infiltration into the kidney, and lower renal and serum TNF levels compared with either $Tnfr1$-deficient or WT mice.	[94]
2003	Streptozotocin (STZ)-induced diabetic rats	Administration of a TNF antagonist (TNFR:Fc)	Administration of a TNF antagonist reduces urinary TNF-α excretion and prevents sodium retention and renal hypertrophy. TNF-α contributes to early diabetic nephropathy, and its inhibition may attenuate early pathological changes.	[98]
2005	Rat model of nephrotoxic nephritis	Administration of anti-TNF-α antibody	Neutralization of endogenous TNF-α reduces glomerular inflammation, crescent formation, and tubulointerstitial scarring, with preservation of renal function.	[103]
2005	Anti-GBM nephritis mice model	$Tnfr1$ or $Tnfr2$ knockout	Lack of Tnfr1 resulted in excessive renal T cell accumulation and an associated reduction in apoptosis of these cells. $Tnfr2$-deficient mice were completely protected from glomerulonephritis, despite an intact systemic immune response.	[92]
2005	UUO rat model	TNF-α blockade with PEG-sTNFR1	Treatment with PEG-sTNFR1 reduced tissue Tnf-α and protein production, renal tubular cell apoptosis, and caspase activity.	[89]
2007	UUO rat model	TNF-α blockade with PEG-sTNFR1	Renal obstruction induced increased tissue TNF-α and several markers of renal fibrosis, whereas treatment with PEG-sTNFR1 significantly reduced each of these markers of renal fibrosis.	[90]
2007	Rat model of kidney transplantation	Treatment with cyclsporine	In rats with acute allograft rejection, significantly elevated expression of TNFR2 was observed in tubular epithelial cells, podocytes, B cells, and monocytes/macrophages. TNFR2 expression levels were associated with renal function.	[104]
2007	STZ-induced diabetic rats	Administration TNF-α inhibitors, Infliximab and FR167653	TNF-α inhibition with infliximab and FR167653 decreased urinary albumin excretion, suggesting the role of TNF-α in the pathogenesis of diabetic nephropathy, with TNF-α inhibition is a potential therapeutic strategy.	[100]
2008	UUO mice model	Tnf-α knockout	Tnf-deficient mice showed an increase of extracellular matrix in the kidneys and infiltrating macrophages, explained by the increased TNFR2 expression level.	[105]
2009	SLE prone mice models	$Tnfr1$, $Tnfr2$ and double $Tnfr1/2$ knockout	Doubly-deficient mice developed accelerated pathological and clinical nephritis, while mice deficient in either TNFR, alone, did not differ from each other or from WT controls.	[106]

Table 1. Cont.

Year	Study Model	Methods	Study Outcomes	Reference
2010	ANG II-dependent mice model of hypertension	Tnfr1 knockout	Angiotensin II inhibited renal Tnfr1 mRNA accumulation, while increasing that of Tnfr2. Deletion of Tnfr1 was associated with increased albuminuria and creatinine clearance, in response to ANG II infusion.	[91]
2013	Anti-GBM nephritis mice model	Tnf-α, Tnfr1 and Tnfr2 knockout	Tnfr2 deficiency resulted in a reduction in renal macrophage but not neutrophil accumulation, while Tnfr1 deletion prevented the influx of both leukocyte subsets.	[79]
2013	TNF-induced inflammation mice model	Tnfr1, Tnfr2 and double Tnfr1/2 knockout	TNF-induced glomerular leukocyte infiltration was abrogated in Tnfr1-deficient mice, whereas Tnfr2-deficiency decreased mononuclear phagocytes infiltrates, but not neutrophils.	[107]
2014	Mice models of LPS- or TNF-induced acute endotoxemia	Tnfr1 knockout	LPS and TNF-treated WT models showed alterations of glomerular endothelium, increased albuminuria, and decreased GFR. The effects of LPS on the glomerular endothelial surface layer, GFR, and albuminuria were diminished in Tnfr1 knockout mice.	[108]
2014	Type 2 diabetic model of the KK-Ay mouse	TNF-α inhibition with Etanercept (ETN)	Renal mRNA and/or protein levels of Tnfr2, but not Tnf-α and Tnfr1, in ETN-treated mice were significantly decreased. ETN may exert a renal protective effect via inhibition of the inflammatory pathway activated by TNFR2 rather than TNFR1.	[99]
2017	Mice with CaOx nephrocalcinosis-related CKD	Tnfr1, Tnfr2 and double Tnfr1/2 knockout	WT mice developed progressive CKD, while Tnfr1-, Tnfr2-, and Tnfr1/2-deficient mice lacked intrarenal CaOx deposition and tubular damage, despite exhibiting similar levels of hyperoxaluria.	[95]
2019	STZ-induced diabetic rats	Treatment with adalimumabe, a TNF-α inhibitor	TNF-α inhibition reduced albuminuria, glomerular injury, and tubular injury in STZ-induced diabetic rats. TNF-α inhibition reduced the NLRP3 inflammasome in tubules and decreased expression of tubular IL-6 and IL-17A mRNA.	[97]
2020	Rodent models of 2,8-DHA crystal nephropathy	Tnfr1 and Tnfr2 knockout	Deletion of Tnfr1 significantly reduced tubular inflammation, thereby ameliorating the disease course. In contrast, genetic deletion of Tnfr2 had no effect on the manifestations of 2,8-DHA nephropathy.	[96]
2021	Ischemia-reperfusion mice model	Clamping of the renal pedicles	Proximal tubular cells exhibited a profibrotic and proinflammatory profile, and a marked transcriptional activation of NF-κB and AP-1 signaling pathways.	[102]

Abbreviations: ANG II, angiotensin II; AP-1, activator protein 1; CaOx, calcium oxalate; DHA, 2,8-dihydroxyadenine; ETN, Etanercept; GBM, glomerular basement membrane; LPS, lipopolysaccharide; NF-κB: factor nuclear kappa B; SLE, systemic lupus erythematosus; sTNFR1, soluble tumor necrosis factor receptor 1; STZ, Streptozotocin; TNFR1, tumor necrosis factor receptor 1; TNFR2, tumor necrosis factor receptor 2; TNF-α, tumor necrosis factor alpha; UUO, unilateral ureteral obstruction; WT, wild type.

4.2. Studies Addressing TNF-α and TNFRs in Human Kidney Disease and Related Clinical Outcomes

In clinical studies, circulating TNFR1 and TNFR2 were shown to be increased in several cohorts of patients, with different CKD etiologies and diverse age-groups and races (Table 2). Despite being responsible for engaging different downstream signaling pathways, the strength of associations with renal function is similar for both receptors.

The first study assessing the serum levels of a TNFR (unidentified either as TNFR1 or TNFR2) in CKD patients was published in 1994, and showed a strong correlation between the receptor levels and serum creatinine, in a group of 26 non-dialyzed CKD patients [109]. TNFR1 and TNFR2 were further associated with eGFR and with albuminuria in several subsequent studies [110–113]. In a prospective cohort that included 984 CKD patients, eGFR was negatively correlated with the serum levels of TNFR1 and TNFR2 [113]. To a lesser extent, both biomarkers were also positively correlated with urinary protein-to-creatinine ratio. Furthermore, in a cohort of patients, with a diverse set of kidney diseases and undergoing native kidney biopsy, TNFR1 and TNFR2 plasma levels were associated with underlying histopathologic lesions and adverse clinical outcomes, such as disease progression and death [114].

In a group of 106 biopsy-proven IgA nephropathy patients, higher serum levels of TNFR1 and TNFR2 were present in patients with more severe renal interstitial fibrosis [112]. Increased circulating levels of TNF receptors were similarly described as prognostic markers of idiopathic membranous nephropathy [115] and contrast-induced nephropathy [116]. Patients with systemic lupus erythematosus (SLE) have also been studied, with urinary TNFR1 [117] and serum TNFR2 [118] levels being elevated in cases of lupus nephritis.

The predictive value of TNFRs was mostly described in diabetic nephropathy, as reviewed by Murakoshi et al. (2020) [119]. Several results from the Joslin Kidney Center studies showed that the TNFRs seem to be candidate biomarkers of renal function decline in both type 1 [120] and type 2 [121] diabetic patients. Moreover, in type 1 diabetic patients, the increased circulating levels of TNFR1 and TNFR2 were the strongest determinants of CKD progression, preceding the onset of microalbuminuria and/or its progression to macroalbuminuria [122]. Higher baseline circulating levels of TNFR1 and TNFR2 were associated with a higher risk of eGFR worsening in patients with both early and established diabetic nephropathy [123]. A systematic review and meta-analysis highlighted the reliability of TNFRs in predicting diabetic kidney disease progression. The results seem to be consistent across different cohorts of diabetic patients [124–127]. A recently published study, evaluated a composite risk score termed KidneyIntelX for predicting the progression of diabetic kidney disease, in a large multinational cohort. KidneyIntelX comprises clinical variables and the circulating levels of three biomarkers, TNFR1, TNFR2, and kidney injury molecule 1 (KIM-1). KidneyIntelX successfully stratified patients for disease progression, showing that, after 1 year, a greater reduction in eGFR was observed in patients with higher changes in KidneyIntelX risk scores, independently of the baseline risk score value and the treatment option [128].

CKD patients have an increased risk of mortality due to CVD, which is independent of the traditional risk factors, possibly due to the chronic inflammatory state. Both circulating TNFRs were described as predictors of CVD risk [113,129] and all-cause mortality [129,130] in CKD populations, independently of eGFR and albuminuria, and irrespective of the cause of kidney disease. Some studies [131–133] have also addressed the prognostic value of circulating TNFRs in HD patients. Despite TFNRs being substantially linked with other inflammatory markers, Carlsson et al. observed no significant connection between either TNFRs and death, in a longitudinal cohort analysis of 207 prevalent HD patients [131]; two more recent studies, including one from our team, reported that circulating levels of TNFR1 and TNFR2 are independent predictors of all-cause mortality in ESKD patients under chronic HD [132,133] (REF 2017 and 2021), although for cardiovascular mortality, the significance was only observed for TNFR1 [132].

In the last 15 years, proteomic and transcriptomic studies have proven useful in discovering new insights into the TNF-α signaling pathway in CKD, as well as the associated-comorbidities. In a proteomic analysis of human serum from patients with CKD, TNF-α was associated with disease severity [134,135], as well as with vascular changes [134]. The circulating extracellular vesicles of CKD patients showed a pro-inflammatory profile, that included markers of the TNF signaling pathways. Niewczas et al. measured 194 circulating inflammatory proteins using aptamer-based proteomics analysis of different cohorts of diabetic patients [136]. The results showed that, out of the 194 measured proteins, 17 were TNFR superfamily-related, and also that TNFR1 and TNFR2 were strong predictors of renal function decline [136]. Accordingly, Ihara et al. showed that a profile of multiple circulating TNF receptors, including TNFR1 and TNFR2, was associated with early progressive renal decline in type 1 diabetes [137]. Tubular cells of IgA nephropathy patients also overexpressed genes of the inflammatory TNF signaling pathway [138].

4.3. Anti-TNF-α Therapy in Patients with Impaired Kidney Function

The huge amount of scientific evidence linking TNF signaling with the pathophysiology of CKD raises questions regarding the utility and safety of therapeutic strategies targeting TNF-α in humans with impaired kidney function.

Nephrotoxicity is a rare side effect of anti-TNF-α medications, and a few reports of this occurrence have been described in the literature. Premužić et al. reported an association of TNF-α inhibitors (adalimumab and golimumab) and the development of IgA nephropathy in three patients with both rheumatoid arthritis and diabetes, but without history of renal disease [139]. Moreover, Stokes et al. showed that a subset of patients on anti-TNF-α therapy who had no prior evidence of renal diseases, developed glomerulonephritis. This was supported by serologic abnormalities and by the presence and formation of autoantibodies [140].

However, other studies demonstrated the therapeutic benefit of TNF-α blocking in improving renal inflammation and function. In patients with rheumatoid arthritis and CKD, the administration of anti-TNF-α was associated with less renal function decline [141]. In addition, the use of anti-TNF-α agents showed promising results in renal vasculitis [142] and kidney transplant recipients with rheumatic disease [143].

There is a limitation to the beneficial effects of anti-TNF-α agents, which seems to be related to their ability to induce autoimmunity by disrupting TNF-α normal immune regulation. Their use in clinical practice would require surveillance for complications. Indeed, the biological functions of cytokines are complex, and, thereby, blocking of cytokines might induce other unexpected and unclear effects in vivo. Furthermore, the effects of anti-TNF-α agents might be modulated by other factors, such as their distribution into diseased tissues, and degradation by proteases. Given the potential benefits of these therapies, a deeper understanding of the TNF signaling pathway and the mechanisms of action of the anti-TNF-α agents and their correlation with the clinical settings is needed for a more appropriate and personalized selection of therapeutic agents, and even for the development of new biological preparations, to be applied in the treatment of inflammatory diseases.

Table 2. Association of TNF-α and TNF receptors with renal dysfunction and disease, as well as with adverse clinical outcomes in human studies.

Year	Study Type	Study Population	Biomarkers	Study Outcomes	Reference
1994	Cross-sectional	26 non-HD CKD patients, 61 HD patients, 43 renal transplant recipients and 34 healthy controls	Serum levels of TNFR?	All patient groups showed significantly higher TNFR levels compared to the control group. A correlation of TNFR and creatinine levels was only found in the group of non-dialyzed CKD patients.	[109]
2005	Retrospective cohort	687 individuals from the CARE trial study, with CKD and previous myocardial, infarction,	Serum levels of TNFR2	Higher TNFR2 is independently associated with faster rates of kidney function loss in CKD. Inflammation may mediate the loss of kidney function among subjects with CKD and concomitant coronary disease.	[110]
2007	Cross-sectional	38 patients with SLE and 15 healthy controls	Urinary levels of TNFR1	Urinary TNFR1 levels were elevated in patients with lupus nephritis and correlated with proteinuria and SLE disease activity index scores.	[117]
2007	Prospective cohort	3075 adults aged 70 to 79	Serum levels of TNF-α, TNFR1 and TNFR2	In an elderly cohort of patients with eGFR $\geq$ 60 mL/min/1.73 m^2, cystatin C was strongly associated with TNF-α and the TNFRs.	[144]
2008	Cross-sectional	6814 participants free of cardiovascular disease, from the MESA study	Circulating levels of TNFR1	Creatinine-based eGFR had significant correlations with TNFR1, in both participants with and without CKD.	[145]
2009	Cross-sectional	96 human renal allograft biopsies	Renal TNFR2 expression	In human renal transplant biopsies, there was an increase in the number of TNFR2-positive podocytes, in tubular epithelial cells, B cells, and monocytes/macrophages.	[104]
2009	Cross-sectional	667 participants with diabetes	Serum levels of TNF-α, TNFR1 and TNFR2	Elevated concentrations of serum markers of the TNF-α pathway were strongly associated with decreased renal function in T1D patients without proteinuria.	[146]
2010	Prospective cohort	55 patients with biopsy-proven primary glomerulonephritis and 20 healthy controls	Urinary levels of TNFR1	Elevated TNFR1 urinary levels predicted renal function decline and advanced renal interstitial fibrosis in patients with primary nephropathy.	[147]
2010	Cross-sectional	3294 participants from the Framingham Offspring Study, 291 of them with CKD	Serum levels of TNF-α and TNFR2	A significant proportion of variability in TNFR2 concentration was explained by CKD status and higher cystatin C quartiles. Higher concentrations of TNF and TNFR2 were associated with CKD status, higher cystatin C, and higher UACR.	[148]
2011	Prospective cohort	4926 patients followed for 15 years	Serum levels of TNFR2	For the risk of developing incident CKD among those who were CKD-free at baseline, only TNFR2 and IL-6 levels, but not CRP, were positively associated with incident CKD.	[149]
2012	Prospective cohort	3939 participants with established CKD	Plasma levels of TNF-α	Biomarkers of inflammation (cytokines and acute phase proteins) were higher in participants with lower levels of kidney function and higher levels of albuminuria.	[9]

Table 2. Cont.

Year	Study Type	Study Population	Biomarkers	Study Outcomes	Reference
2012	Prospective cohort	628 patients with T1D normal renal function, and no proteinuria	Serum levels of TNFR1 and TNFR2	Elevated serum concentrations of TNFR1 and TNFR2 were strongly associated with early renal function loss, progression to CKD stage 3 or higher, in patients with T1D who had normal renal function.	[120]
2012	Prospective cohort	410 patients with T2D	Serum levels of TNFR1 and TNFR2	Elevated concentrations of circulating TNFRs in patients with T2D at baseline were very strong predictors of the subsequent progression to ESRD in subjects with and without proteinuria.	[121]
2012	Prospective cohort	12 patients with active lupus nephritis, 14 with inactive SLE, and 14 healthy subjects	Serum levels of TNF-α and TNFR2	TNFR2 serum levels were elevated in all patients with active lupus nephritis and declined after clinical remission.	[113]
2013	Prospective cohort	84 glomerulonephritis patients under immunosuppressive therapy and 18 healthy controls	Serum and urine levels of TNFR1 and TNFR2	Urinary levels, but not serum levels, of TNFR1 and TNFR2 were effective in predicting a favorable response to immunosuppressive treatment in patients with primary glomerulonephritis.	[150]
2014	Prospective cohort	Patients with T1D and normoalbuminuria (286) or microalbuminuria (248)	Serum levels of TNF-α, TNFR1 and TNFR2	In both groups, the strongest determinants of renal decline were baseline serum concentrations of uric acid and TNFRs. Renal decline was not associated with sex or baseline serum concentration of the other measured markers.	[122]
2014	Prospective cohort	113 patients with biopsy-proven iMN and 43 healthy volunteers	Serum levels of TNFR1 and TNFR2	Estimated glomerular filtration rate and proteinuria tended to worsen as the TNFRs levels increased. Renal tubular TNFRs expression was associated with circulating TNFRs levels.	[115]
2014	Prospective cohort	522 T2D patients with DKD	Serum levels of TNFR1	TNFR1 is a strong prognostic factor for all-cause mortality in T2D with renal dysfunction, and its clinical utility is suggested in addition to established risk factors for all-cause mortality.	[130]
2014	Prospective cohort	429 patients with T1D and overt nephropathy	Plasma levels of TNFR1	Circulating levels of TNFR1 were highly correlated with eGFR, especially in patients with an eGFR < 60 mL/min/1.73 m^2. Circulating levels of the TNFR1 also remained associated with ESRD after adjusting for the competing risk of death.	[151]
2014	Prospective cohort	349 T1D patients with proteinuria and CKD staged 1–3	Serum levels of TNFR2	Serum TNFR2 was the strongest determinant of renal decline and ESRD risk. The rate of eGFR loss became steeper with rising concentration of TNFR2, and elevated HbA1c augmented the strength of this association.	[152]

Table 2. Cont.

Year	Study Type	Study Population	Biomarkers	Study Outcomes	Reference
2015	Prospective cohort	223 biopsy-proven primary IgA nephropathy patients	Serum levels of TNFR1 and TNFR2	Both TNFRs levels were significantly higher in patients with eGFR < 60 mL/min/1.73 m^2 than in patients with higher eGFR. Both TNFRs were associated with renal function decline, independent of age and uric acid levels.	[153]
2015	Prospective cohort	262 patients admitted for a CAG and/or a PCI	Serum levels of TNFR1 and TNFR2	Markedly elevated concentrations of circulating TNFRs were correlated with the occurrence of contrast-induced nephropathy (CIN) and significantly associated with prolonged renal dysfunction, regardless of the development of CIN.	[116]
2015	Prospective cohort	131 patients with CKD at stages 4 and 5	Serum levels of TNFR1 and TNFR2	Both TNFRs were independently associated with all-cause mortality or an increased risk for cardiovascular events in advanced CKD, irrespective of the cause of kidney disease.	[129]
2015	Prospective cohort	347 patients with newly diagnosed biopsy-proven primary IgA nephropt2athy	Plasma levels of TNFR1 and TNFR2	eGFR decreased and proteinuria worsened proportionally as TNFR1 and TNFR2 levels increased. Tubulointerstitial lesions, such as interstitial fibrosis and tubular atrophy, were significantly more severe as concentrations of circulating TNFRs increased, regardless of eGFR levels.	[154]
2015	Prospective cohort	193 Pima Indians with T2D	Serum levels of TNFR1 and TNFR2	Elevated serum concentrations of TNFR1 or TNFR2 were associated with increased risk of ESRD in American Indians with type 2 diabetes, after accounting for traditional risk factors including UACR and mGFR.	[155]
2015	Cross- sectional	106 biopsy-proven IgA nephropathy patients and 34 healthy subjects	Serum and urinary levels of TNFR1 and TNFR2	Elevated serum TNFR1 or TNFR2 levels were significantly associated with the severity of renal interstitial fibrosis after adjusting for eGFR, UPCR, and other markers of tubular damage.	[112]
2015	Prospective cohort	207 patients undergoing HD	Serum levels of TNFR1 and TNFR2	Prevalent hemodialysis patients had several-fold higher levels of sTNFRs compared to previous studies in CKD stage-4 patients. However, no consistent association between TNFR and mortality was observed.	[131]
2016	Prospective cohort	2220 Chinese patients aged 50–70 years old with eGFR > 60 mL/min/1.73 m^2	Plasma levels of TNFR2	Elevated levels of TNFR2 were independently associated with a greater risk of kidney function decline in middle-aged and elderly Chinese.	[156]
2016	Prospective cohort	83 Pima Indians with T2D	Serum levels of TNF-α, TNFR1 and TNFR2	TNFR1 and TNFR2 significantly correlated inversely with the percentage of endothelial cell fenestration and the total filtration surface per glomerulus. Thus, TNFRs may be involved in the pathogenesis of early glomerular lesions in DN.	[124]

Table 2. Cont.

Year	Study Type	Study Population	Biomarkers	Study Outcomes	Reference
2016	Prospective cohort	86 patients with CKD stages 2–4	A panel of biomarkers, including TNF-α	The panel of proteomic inflammatory and mineral and bone disorder biomarkers showed a better performance in detecting early CKD stages, disease progression, and vascular changes, than each single biomarker.	[134]
2016	Prospective cohort	3430 participants with eGFR of 20–70 mL/min/1.73 m^2	Plasma levels of TNF-α	Elevated plasma levels of TNF-α and decreased serum albumin were associated with rapid loss of kidney function in patients with CKD.	[10]
2016	Prospective cohort	543 patients with stage 5 CKD	Serum levels TNF-α	TNF-α could, independently of other biomarkers, predict all-cause mortality, but not clinical CVD.	[157]
2016	Prospective cohort	607 Swedish patients with T2D	Circulating levels of TNFR1 and TNFR2	Higher levels of both TNFR1 and TNFR2 were associated with prevalent diabetic kidney disease, as well as with worsened kidney function and higher urinary albumin/creatinine ratio.	[127]
2017	Nested case-control	380 participants with early DKD (190 matched case-control pairs) from the ACCORD study	Plasma levels of TNFR1 and TNFR2	At baseline, median levels of TNFR1 and TNFR2 were roughly two-fold higher in the advanced than in the early cohort. TNFR1 and TNFR2 levels were associated with higher risk of eGFR decline in T2DM persons with both early (ACCORD) and established (VA-NEPHRON-D) DKD. In both cohorts, patients who reached the renal outcome had higher baseline TNFRs levels.	[123]
	Prospective cohort	1256 participants with advanced DKD from the VA-NEPHRON-D Cohort			
2017	Prospective cohort	984 patients with CKD	Serum levels of TNFR1 and TNFR2	TNFR1 and TNFR2 predicted CVD risk, even after adjustment for clinical covariates, such as urinary protein/creatinine ratio, eGFR, and high-sensitivity CRP.	[113]
2017	Prospective cohort	1.135 French patients with T2D	Serum levels of TNFR1	In addition to established risk factors, TNFR1 improves risk prediction of loss of renal function in patients with T2D.	[125]
2017	Prospective cohort	319 patients receiving maintenance hemodialysis	Serum levels of TNF-α, TNFR1 and TNFR2	Elevated TNFRs levels were associated with an increased risk of cardiovascular and/or all-cause mortality, independently of other studied covariates, in patients undergoing HD.	[102]
2017	Prospective cohort	122 patients with confirmed DN	Renal tissue expression of TNFR1 and TNFR2	No correlations were found between glomerular or tubular expressions of TNFRs, and clinical parameters, including GFR decline slopes.	[158]

Table 2. Cont.

Year	Study Type	Study Population	Biomarkers	Study Outcomes	Reference
2018	Prospective cohort	453 Indigenous Australians with and without diabetes and/or CKD	Serum levels of TNFR1	Circulating levels of TNFR1 were associated with greater kidney disease progression, independently of albuminuria and eGFR, in Indigenous Australians with diabetes.	[126]
2018	Prospective cohort	594 Japanese patients with T2D and eGFR > 30 mL/min/1.73 m2 (stages 1 to 3)	Serum levels of TNF-α, TNFR1 and TNFR2	Circulating TNF-related inflammatory biomarkers were associated with urinary albumin/creatinine ratio and eGFR. Among the biomarkers, the association of TNFRs with eGFR was the strongest after adjustment for relevant covariates.	[111]
2018	Prospective cohort	2399 patients with CKD and no history of cardiovascular disease	Plasma levels of TNF-α	A composite inflammation score with 4 biomarkers (IL-6, TNF-a, fibrinogen, and albumin) was associated with a graded increase in risk for incident atherosclerotic vascular disease events and death in patients with CKD.	[23]
2018	Prospective cohort	2871 participants multiethnic cohort	Serum levels of TNFR1	Elevated serum TNFR1 concentrations were associated with faster declines in eGFR over the course of a decade in a multiethnic population, independently of previously known risk factors for kidney disease progression.	[159]
2019	Prospective cohort	525 diabetic participants of 3 independent cohorts	194 proteins, including TNFR1 and TNFR2	Kidney risk inflammatory signature (KRIS) comprising 17 circulating inflammatory proteins, including TNFR1 and TNFR2, were associated with incident ESRD in diabetic patients.	[136]
2019	Systematic review and Meta-analysis	6526 participants from 11 cohorts for TNFR1 measurements and 5385 participants from 10 prospective for TNFR2 measurements	Circulating levels of TNFR1 and TNFR2	Circulating TNFR-1 and TNFR-2 are reliable predictors of DKD progression.	[160]
2019	Prospective cohort	47 patients with diabetes and eGFR > 60 mL/min/1.73	Serum levels of TNFR1	In patients with an early decline in renal function, TNFR1 values increased as eGFR decreased, over an 8-year period. In contrast, there were no significant changes in soluble TNFR1 levels in patients with stable renal function.	[161]
2020	Prospective cohort	165 case participants from the ADVANCE trial and 330 matched control	Plasma levels of TNFR1 and TNFR2	Elevated circulating TNFR1 and TNFR2 levels were associated with poor kidney outcome.	[162]
2020	Cross-sectional	26 adults with terminal stage CKD and 10 healthy controls	Serum levels of 27 cytokines, including TNF-α	Serum levels of TNF-α were increased 6 to 12 times in patients with CKD, as compared to controls. TNF-α levels positively correlated with complement systems components.	[135]
2020	Prospective cohort	894 CRIC Study participants with diabetes and an eGFR of < 60 mL/min/1.73 m^2	Plasma levels of TNFR1 and TNFR2	Higher plasma levels of TNFR1 and TNFR2 were associated with increased risk of progression of DN. TNFR2 had the highest risk after accounting for the other biomarkers.	[163]

Table 2. Cont.

Year	Study Type	Study Population	Biomarkers	Study Outcomes	Reference
2020	Prospective cohort	651 children with 1–16 years old with an eGFR of 30–90 mL/min/1.73 m^2	Plasma levels of TNFR1 and TNFR2	Children with a plasma TNFR1 or TNFR2 concentration in the highest quartile were at significantly higher risk of CKD progression, compared with children with a concentration for the respective biomarker in the lowest quartile.	[164]
2021	Prospective cohort	139 adults with CKD stages 1 to 5	Serum levels of 11 markers, including TNFR1 and TNFR2	Patients with high TNFR1, coupled with low complement 3a desarginine, almost universally (96%) developed the composite renal and mortality endpoint.	[165]
2021	Prospective cohort	346 T1D patients, 198 with macroalbuminuria and 148 with microalbuminuria	25 TNF family proteins, including TNFR1 and TNFR2	Levels of TNR1 and TNFR2 were associated with increased risk of early progressive renal decline in T1D diabetic patients with macro and microalbuminuria.	[137]
2021	Prospective cohort	523 CKD patients undergoing kidney biopsy with a diverse set of kidney diseases	Plasma levels of TNFR1 and TNFR2	Both TNFR1 and TNFR2 were associated with tubulointerstitial and glomerular lesions; each doubling of TNFR1 and TNFR2 was associated with an increased risk of CKD progression, but only TNFR2 was associated with risk of death.	[114]
2021	Prospective cohort	2553 patients with T2D and normoalbuminuria	Plasma levels of TNFR1 and TNFR2	Each doubling of baseline TNFR1 and TNFR2 was associated with a higher risk of kidney outcome (40% reduction in eGFR or kidney failure), in normoalbuminuric patients.	[166]
2021	Prospective cohort	3523 participants from the CANVAS placebo-controlled trial	Plasma levels of TNFR1 and TNFR2	Each doubling in baseline TNFR1 and TNFR2 was associated with a higher risk of kidney outcomes. Early decreases in TNFR1 and TNFR2 during treatment were associated with a lower risk of disease progression.	[167]
2021	Cross-sectional	499 patients with T2D and eGFR $\geq$ 60 mL/min/1.73 m^2	Serum and urinary TNFR1 and TNFR2 levels	Kidney measures appear to be strongly associated with serum TNFRs, rather than urinary TNFRs in patients with type 2 diabetes and normal renal function.	[168]
2021	Prospective cohort	594 participants with T2D and eGFR < 60 mL/min/1.73 m^2	Plasma levels of TNFR1 and TNFR2	TNFR1 and TNFR2 were associated with risk of incident kidney failure needing RRT, in adults with diabetes and an eGFR < 60 mL/min/1.73 m^2, after adjustment for established risk factors.	[169]
2021	Cross-sectional	5 human renal biopsy specimens from IgA nephropathy patients and 1 healthy control	Transcriptomic analysis of single-cell RNA	Tubular cells of IgA nephropathy patients were enriched in inflammatory pathways, including TNF-α signaling.	[138]
2021	Prospective cohort	289 ESRD patients under chronic HD therapy	Several biomarkers circulating levels, including TNFR2	TNFR2 levels were an independent predictor of all-cause mortality (1-year follow-up study). Circulating levels of cfDNA emerged as the best predictor of mortality.	[133]

Table 2. Cont.

Year	Study Type	Study Population	Biomarkers	Study Outcomes	Reference
2022	Prospective cohort	1325 participants from the CANVAS trial with prevalent DKD	KidneyIntelX score, including plasma levels of TNFR1 and TNFR2	Changes in the KidneyIntelX score from baseline to 1 year were associated with future risk of CKD progression, independently of the baseline risk score and treatment arm.	[128]

Abbreviations: ACCORD, Action to Control Cardiovascular Risk in Diabetes trial; ADVANCE, Action in Diabetes and Vascular Disease; CAG, coronary angiography; CARE, The Cholesterol and Recurrent Events trial; cfDNA, cell-free DNA; CIN, contrast-induced nephropathy; CKD, chronic kidney disease; CRIC, chronic Renal Insufficiency Cohort; CRP, C-reactive protein; CVD, cardiovascular disease; DN, diabetic nephropathy; eGFR, estimated glomerular filtration rate; ESRD, end-stage renal disease; Hba1c, hemoglobina glicada; HD, hemodialysis; IgAN, IgA nephropathy; IL-6, Interleukin-6; iMN, idiopathic membranous nephropathy; KRIS, kidney risk inflammatory signature; MESA, Multi-ethnic study of atherosclerosis; mGFR, measured glomerular filtration rate; PCI, percutaneous coronary intervention; SLE, systemic lupus erythematosus; T1D, type 1 diabetes; T2D, type 2 diabetes; TNFR1, tumor necrosis factor receptor 1; TNFR2, tumor necrosis factor receptor 2; TNF-α, tumor necrosis factor alpha; UACR, urinary albumin-to-creatinine ratio; UPCR, urinary protein-to-creatinine ratio; VA-NEPHRON, Veterans Administration NEPHROpathy iN Diabetes study.

5. Considerations for Future Research

Despite recent breakthroughs in CKD care, the rates of morbidity and mortality are still unacceptable. Chronic inflammation is a common feature in kidney diseases, regardless of its etiology, and which plays a key role in disease pathophysiology, progression, and development of associated complications. Unresolved inflammatory processes generally lead to renal fibrosis and ESRD.

The role of TNF-α in the pathogenesis of kidney diseases depends on the engagement of receptor-specific and/or common signaling cascades. The differential expression of both receptors in different cell types, and the fact that soluble and transmembrane TNF-α present different affinities to each receptor, are other factors that contribute to the complexity of TNF-α signaling.

Circulating TNFRs have been associated with renal damage in several animal and human studies. Based on the available data, increased levels of TNFRs associate with decreased eGFR and increased albuminuria. Overall, TNFRs have proven to be useful and effective in predicting renal function decline and CKD progression, as well as CKD-associated morbidity and mortality, among different cohorts of patients in both cross-sectional and longitudinal studies. The consistency of the published literature evidences their potential role as prognostic and risk-predictive biomarkers in CKD, along with the traditional markers already used in clinical practice.

The mechanisms by which the TNFRs initiate and perpetuate renal damage are not completely understood. In fact, there is evidence that TNF-α is not the only molecule involved in the regulation of its receptors during renal function decline [84], suggesting that other molecules and chemokines act as potential downstream effectors on TNFRs. Moreover, the interplay between TNFR1 and TNFR2, the role of each receptor in specific kidney diseases (particularly in more rare diseases), and their prognostic value in patient outcomes deserve further investigation.

To date, there are no anti-inflammatory treatments for CKD patients. Treating inflammation and preventing the progression of renal fibrosis is complex, due to the crosstalk between the inflammatory signaling pathways. The approved therapeutic use of anti-TNF monoclonal antibodies is currently limited to autoimmune diseases, such as rheumatoid arthritis, Chron's disease, or psoriatic arthritis [170]. Considering the relevance of the TNF signaling pathways in CKD pathophysiology, studies on the efficacy of the existing TNF biologics in renal diseases would be useful. Furthermore, individual inhibition of TNFR1 or TNFR2 may further clarify the balance of proinflammatory/immunomodulatory roles for each of these receptors.

Future research should focus on validating the promising findings in large, multi-centered studies, with standardized methodologies, to allow their translation into clinical practice. TNFRs could be important tools to improve CKD patient's characterization and management, with direct implications for strategies to prevent or postpone the progression of CKD. This may possibly result in a better prognosis for patients, as well as in financial benefits, lowering healthcare costs in CKD management.

Author Contributions: Conceptualization, I.L., A.S.-S., L.B. and F.R.; writing—original draft preparation, I.L.; writing—review and editing, I.L., A.S.-S., L.B., F.R. and L.B.; supervision, A.S.-S., L.B. and F.R. All authors have read and agreed to the published version of the manuscript.

Funding: This work was financially supported by national funds from FCT—Fundação para a Ciência e a Tecnologia, I.P., in the scope of the project UIDP/04378/2020 and UIDB/04378/2020 of the Research Unit on Applied Molecular Biosciences—UCIBIO and the project LA/P/0140/2020 of the Associate Laboratory Institute for Health and Bioeconomy—i4HB.

Acknowledgments: This work was financially supported by national funds from FCT—Fundação para a Ciência e a Tecnologia, I.P., in the scope of the project UIDP/04378/2020 and UIDB/04378/2020 of the Research Unit on Applied Molecular Biosciences—UCIBIO and the project LA/P/0140/2020 of the Associate Laboratory Institute for Health and Bioeconomy—i4HB; by FEDER COMPETE2020 funds UIDP/04539/2020 (CIBB); by PTDC/SAU-NUT/31712/2017, POCI-01-0145-FEDER-007440 and POCI-01-0145-FEDER-031712, and by FCT doctoral grant SFRH/BD/145939/2019; by funds from Portugal Regional Coordination and Development Commissions (Norte-01-0145-FEDER-000024; Centro-01-0145-FEDER-000012) and FEDER/COMPETE 2020 (POCI-01-0145-FEDER-031322)]. Figure 1 was created with BioRender.

Conflicts of Interest: The authors declare no conflict of interest.

References

1. Crews, D.C.; Bello, A.K.; Saadi, G.; World Kidney Day Steering Committee. Burden, access, and disparities in kidney disease. *Braz. J. Med. Biol. Res.* **2019**, *52*, e8338. [CrossRef] [PubMed]
2. Jager, K.J.; Kovesdy, C.; Langham, R.; Rosenberg, M.; Jha, V.; Zoccali, C. A single number for advocacy and communication—Worldwide more than 850 million individuals have kidney diseases. *Nephrol. Dial. Transplant.* **2019**, *34*, 1803–1805. [CrossRef] [PubMed]
3. GBD Chronic Kidney Disease Collaboration. Global, regional, and national burden of chronic kidney disease, 1990-2017: A systematic analysis for the Global Burden of Disease Study 2017. *Lancet* **2020**, *395*, 709–733. [CrossRef]
4. Levin, A.; Stevens, P.E.; Bilous, R.W.; Coresh, J.; De Francisco, A.L.M.; De Jong, P.E.; Griffith, K.E.; Hemmelgarn, B.R.; Iseki, K.; Lamb, E.J.; et al. Kidney disease: Improving global outcomes (KDIGO) CKD work group. KDIGO 2012 clinical practice guideline for the evaluation and management of chronic kidney disease. *Kidney Int. Suppl.* **2013**, *3*, 1–150.
5. Schlondorff, D.O. Overview of factors contributing to the pathophysiology of progressive renal disease. *Kidney Int.* **2008**, *74*, 860–866. [CrossRef] [PubMed]
6. Jankowski, J.; Floege, J.; Fliser, D.; Böhm, M.; Marx, N. Cardiovascular Disease in Chronic Kidney Disease: Pathophysiological Insights and Therapeutic Options. *Circulation* **2021**, *143*, 1157–1172. [CrossRef]
7. Go, A.S.; Chertow, G.M.; Fan, D.; McCulloch, C.E.; Hsu, C.Y. Chronic kidney disease and the risks of death, cardiovascular events, and hospitalization. *N. Engl. J. Med.* **2004**, *351*, 1296–1305. [CrossRef]
8. Zhang, W.R.; Parikh, C.R. Biomarkers of Acute and Chronic Kidney Disease. *Annu. Rev. Physiol.* **2019**, *81*, 309–333. [CrossRef]
9. Gupta, J.; Mitra, N.; Kanetsky, P.A.; Devaney, J.; Wing, M.R.; Reilly, M.; Shah, V.O.; Balakrishnan, V.S.; Guzman, N.J.; Girndt, M.; et al. Association between albuminuria, kidney function, and inflammatory biomarker profile in CKD in CRIC. *Clin. J. Am. Soc. Nephrol.* **2012**, *7*, 1938–1946. [CrossRef]
10. Amdur, R.L.; Feldman, H.I.; Gupta, J.; Yang, W.; Kanetsky, P.; Shlipak, M.; Rahman, M.; Lash, J.P.; Townsend, R.R.; Ojo, A.; et al. Inflammation and Progression of CKD: The CRIC Study. *Clin. J. Am. Soc. Nephrol.* **2016**, *11*, 1546–1556. [CrossRef]
11. Schei, J.; Stefansson, V.T.; Eriksen, B.O.; Jenssen, T.G.; Solbu, M.D.; Wilsgaard, T.; Melsom, T. Association of TNF Receptor 2 and CRP with GFR Decline in the General Nondiabetic Population. *Clin. J. Am. Soc. Nephrol.* **2017**, *12*, 624–634. [CrossRef] [PubMed]
12. Mihai, S.; Codrici, E.; Popescu, I.D.; Enciu, A.M.; Albulescu, L.; Necula, L.G.; Mambet, C.; Anton, G.; Tanase, C. Inflammation-Related Mechanisms in Chronic Kidney Disease Prediction, Progression, and Outcome. *J. Immunol. Res.* **2018**, *2018*, 2180373. [CrossRef] [PubMed]
13. Fanelli, C.; Noreddin, A.; Nunes, A. Inflammation in Nonimmune-Mediated Chronic Kidney Disease. In *Chronic Kidney Disease—From Pathophysiology to Clinical Improvements*; Rath, T., Ed.; IntechOpen: London, UK, 2017. [CrossRef]
14. Kurts, C.; Panzer, U.; Anders, H.J.; Rees, A.J. The immune system and kidney disease: Basic concepts and clinical implications. *Nat. Rev. Immunol.* **2013**, *13*, 738–753. [CrossRef] [PubMed]

15. Mihai, S.; Codrici, E.; Popescu, I.D.; Enciu, A.-M.; Rusu, E.; Zilisteanu, D.; Necula, L.G.; Anton, G.; Tanase, C. Inflammation-Related Patterns in the Clinical Staging and Severity Assessment of Chronic Kidney Disease. *Dis. Markers* **2019**, *2019*, 1814304. [CrossRef]
16. Valente, M.J.; Rocha, S.; Coimbra, S.; Catarino, C.; Rocha-Pereira, P.; Bronze-da-Rocha, E.; Oliveira, J.G.; Madureira, J.; Fernandes, J.C.; do Sameiro-Faria, M.; et al. Long Pentraxin 3 as a Broader Biomarker for Multiple Risk Factors in End-Stage Renal Disease: Association with All-Cause Mortality. *Mediat. Inflamm.* **2019**, *2019*, 3295725. [CrossRef]
17. Imig, J.D.; Ryan, M.J. Immune and inflammatory role in renal disease. *Compr. Physiol.* **2013**, *3*, 957–976. [CrossRef]
18. Andrade-Oliveira, V.; Foresto-Neto, O.; Watanabe, I.K.M.; Zatz, R.; Câmara, N.O.S. Inflammation in Renal Diseases: New and Old Players. *Front. Pharmacol.* **2019**, *10*, 1192. [CrossRef]
19. Raj, D.S.; Pecoits-Filho, R.; Kimmel, P.L. Chapter 17—Inflammation in Chronic Kidney Disease. In *Chronic Renal Disease*; Kimmel, P.L., Rosenberg, M.E., Eds.; Academic Press: San Diego, CA, USA, 2015; pp. 199–212. [CrossRef]
20. Yao, Q.; Axelsson, J.; Stenvinkel, P.; Lindholm, B. Chronic Systemic Inflammation in Dialysis Patients: An Update on Causes and Consequences. *ASAIO J.* **2004**, *50*, Iii–Ivii. [CrossRef]
21. Avesani, C.M.; Carrero, J.J.; Axelsson, J.; Qureshi, A.R.; Lindholm, B.; Stenvinkel, P. Inflammation and wasting in chronic kidney disease: Partners in crime. *Kidney Int.* **2006**, *70*, S8–S13. [CrossRef]
22. Mazzaferro, S.; De Martini, N.; Rotondi, S.; Tartaglione, L.; Ureña-Torres, P.; Bover, J.; Pasquali, M. Bone, inflammation and chronic kidney disease. *Clin. Chim. Acta* **2020**, *506*, 236–240. [CrossRef]
23. Amdur, R.L.; Feldman, H.I.; Dominic, E.A.; Anderson, A.H.; Beddhu, S.; Rahman, M.; Wolf, M.; Reilly, M.; Ojo, A.; Townsend, R.R.; et al. Use of Measures of Inflammation and Kidney Function for Prediction of Atherosclerotic Vascular Disease Events and Death in Patients With CKD: Findings From the CRIC Study. *Am. J. Kidney Dis.* **2019**, *73*, 344–353. [CrossRef] [PubMed]
24. Lv, W.; Booz, G.W.; Wang, Y.; Fan, F.; Roman, R.J. Inflammation and renal fibrosis: Recent developments on key signaling molecules as potential therapeutic targets. *Eur. J. Pharmacol.* **2018**, *820*, 65–76. [CrossRef] [PubMed]
25. Meng, X.M. Inflammatory Mediators and Renal Fibrosis. *Adv. Exp. Med. Biol.* **2019**, *1165*, 381–406. [CrossRef] [PubMed]
26. Castillo-Rodríguez, E.; Pizarro-Sánchez, S.; Sanz, A.B.; Ramos, A.M.; Sanchez-Niño, M.D.; Martin-Cleary, C.; Fernandez-Fernandez, B.; Ortiz, A. Inflammatory Cytokines as Uremic Toxins: "Ni Son Todos Los Que Estan, Ni Estan Todos Los Que Son". *Toxins* **2017**, *9*, 114. [CrossRef]
27. Hodgkins, K.S.; Schnaper, H.W. Tubulointerstitial injury and the progression of chronic kidney disease. *Pediatr. Nephrol.* **2012**, *27*, 901–909. [CrossRef]
28. Falke, L.L.; Gholizadeh, S.; Goldschmeding, R.; Kok, R.J.; Nguyen, T.Q. Diverse origins of the myofibroblast—Implications for kidney fibrosis. *Nat. Rev. Nephrol.* **2015**, *11*, 233–244. [CrossRef]
29. Humphreys, B.D. Mechanisms of Renal Fibrosis. *Annu. Rev. Physiol.* **2018**, *80*, 309–326. [CrossRef]
30. Nogueira, A.; Pires, M.J.; Oliveira, P.A. Pathophysiological Mechanisms of Renal Fibrosis: A Review of Animal Models and Therapeutic Strategies. *In Vivo* **2017**, *31*, 1–22. [CrossRef]
31. Sellati, T.J.; Sahay, B. Cells of Innate Immunity: Mechanisms of Activation. In *Pathobiology of Human Disease*; McManus, L.M., Mitchell, R.N., Eds.; Academic Press: San Diego, CA, USA, 2014; pp. 258–274. [CrossRef]
32. Idriss, H.T.; Naismith, J.H. TNF alpha and the TNF receptor superfamily: Structure-function relationship(s). *Microsc. Res. Tech.* **2000**, *50*, 184–195. [CrossRef]
33. Imaizumi, T.; Itaya, H.; Fujita, K.; Kudoh, D.; Kudoh, S.; Mori, K.; Fujimoto, K.; Matsumiya, T.; Yoshida, H.; Satoh, K. Expression of tumor necrosis factor-alpha in cultured human endothelial cells stimulated with lipopolysaccharide or interleukin-1alpha. *Arterioscler. Thromb. Vasc. Biol.* **2000**, *20*, 410–415. [CrossRef]
34. Fahey, T.J., 3rd; Turbeville, T.; McIntyre, K. Differential TNF secretion by wound fibroblasts compared to normal fibroblasts in response to LPS. *J. Surg. Res.* **1995**, *58*, 759–764. [CrossRef] [PubMed]
35. Hotamisligil, G.S.; Shargill, N.S.; Spiegelman, B.M. Adipose expression of tumor necrosis factor-alpha: Direct role in obesity-linked insulin resistance. *Science* **1993**, *259*, 87–91. [CrossRef] [PubMed]
36. Kubota, T.; McTiernan, C.F.; Frye, C.S.; Demetris, A.J.; Feldman, A.M. Cardiac-specific overexpression of tumor necrosis factor-alpha causes lethal myocarditis in transgenic mice. *J. Card. Fail.* **1997**, *3*, 117–124. [CrossRef]
37. Gahring, L.C.; Carlson, N.G.; Kulmar, R.A.; Rogers, S.W. Neuronal expression of tumor necrosis factor alpha in the murine brain. *Neuroimmunomodulation* **1996**, *3*, 289–303. [CrossRef]
38. Jang, D.I.; Lee, A.H.; Shin, H.Y.; Song, H.R.; Park, J.H.; Kang, T.B.; Lee, S.R.; Yang, S.H. The Role of Tumor Necrosis Factor Alpha (TNF-α) in Autoimmune Disease and Current TNF-α Inhibitors in Therapeutics. *Int. J. Mol. Sci.* **2021**, *22*, 2719. [CrossRef]
39. Göbel, K.; Ruck, T.; Meuth, S.G. Cytokine signaling in multiple sclerosis: Lost in translation. *Mult. Scler.* **2018**, *24*, 432–439. [CrossRef]
40. Schulte, W.; Bernhagen, J.; Bucala, R. Cytokines in sepsis: Potent immunoregulators and potential therapeutic targets—An updated view. *Mediat. Inflamm.* **2013**, *2013*, 165974. [CrossRef]
41. Tinti, F.; Lai, S.; Noce, A.; Rotondi, S.; Marrone, G.; Mazzaferro, S.; Di Daniele, N.; Mitterhofer, A.P. Chronic Kidney Disease as a Systemic Inflammatory Syndrome: Update on Mechanisms Involved and Potential Treatment. *Life* **2021**, *11*, 419. [CrossRef]

42. Black, R.A.; Rauch, C.T.; Kozlosky, C.J.; Peschon, J.J.; Slack, J.L.; Wolfson, M.F.; Castner, B.J.; Stocking, K.L.; Reddy, P.; Srinivasan, S.; et al. A metalloproteinase disintegrin that releases tumour-necrosis factor-alpha from cells. *Nature* **1997**, *385*, 729–733. [CrossRef]
43. Holbrook, J.; Lara-Reyna, S.; Jarosz-Griffiths, H.; McDermott, M. Tumour necrosis factor signalling in health and disease. *F1000Research* **2019**, *8*, 23. [CrossRef]
44. Medler, J.; Wajant, H. Tumor necrosis factor receptor-2 (TNFR2): An overview of an emerging drug target. *Expert Opin. Ther. Targets* **2019**, *23*, 295–307. [CrossRef] [PubMed]
45. Tartaglia, L.A.; Pennica, D.; Goeddel, D.V. Ligand passing: The 75-kDa tumor necrosis factor (TNF) receptor recruits TNF for signaling by the 55-kDa TNF receptor. *J. Biol. Chem.* **1993**, *268*, 18542–18548. [CrossRef]
46. Aderka, D.; Engelmann, H.; Maor, Y.; Brakebusch, C.; Wallach, D. Stabilization of the bioactivity of tumor necrosis factor by its soluble receptors. *J. Exp. Med.* **1992**, *175*, 323–329 [CrossRef] [PubMed]
47. Gough, P.; Myles, I.A. Tumor Necrosis Factor Receptors: Pleiotropic Signaling Complexes and Their Differential Effects. *Front. Immunol.* **2020**, *11*, 585880. [CrossRef] [PubMed]
48. Yang, S.; Wang, J.; Brand, D.D.; Zheng, S.G. Role of TNF-TNF Receptor 2 Signal in Regulatory T Cells and Its Therapeutic Implications. *Front. Immunol.* **2018**, *9*, 784. [CrossRef] [PubMed]
49. Xanthoulea, S.; Pasparakis, M.; Kousteni, S.; Brakebusch, C.; Wallach, D.; Bauer, J.; Lassmann, H.; Kollias, G. Tumor necrosis factor (TNF) receptor shedding controls thresholds of innate immune activation that balance opposing TNF functions in infectious and inflammatory diseases. *J. Exp. Med.* **2004**, *200*, 367–376. [CrossRef]
50. Dembic, Z.; Loetscher, H.; Gubler, U.; Pan, Y.C.; Lahm, H.W.; Gentz, R.; Brockhaus, M.; Lesslauer, W. Two human TNF receptors have similar extracellular, but distinct intracellular, domain sequences. *Cytokine* **1990**, *2*, 231–237. [CrossRef]
51. Hsu, H.; Xiong, J.; Goeddel, D.V. The TNF receptor 1-associated protein TRADD signals cell death and NF-kappa B activation. *Cell* **1995**, *81*, 495–504. [CrossRef]
52. Hsu, H.; Huang, J.; Shu, H.B.; Baichwal, V.; Goeddel, D.V. TNF-dependent recruitment of the protein kinase RIP to the TNF receptor-1 signaling complex. *Immunity* **1996**, *4*, 387–396. [CrossRef]
53. Hsu, H.; Shu, H.B.; Pan, M.G.; Goeddel, D.V. TRADD-TRAF2 and TRADD-FADD interactions define two distinct TNF receptor 1 signal transduction pathways. *Cell* **1996**, *84*, 299–308. [CrossRef]
54. Humphries, F.; Yang, S.; Wang, B.; Moynagh, P.N. RIP kinases: Key decision makers in cell death and innate immunity. *Cell Death Differ.* **2015**, *22*, 225–236. [CrossRef]
55. Mahoney, D.J.; Cheung, H.H.; Mrad, R.L.; Plenchette, S.; Simard, C.; Enwere, E.; Arora, V.; Mak, T.W.; Lacasse, E.C.; Waring, J.; et al. Both cIAP1 and cIAP2 regulate TNFalpha-mediated NF-kappaB activation. *Proc. Natl. Acad. Sci. USA* **2008**, *105*, 11778–11783. [CrossRef] [PubMed]
56. Haas, T.L.; Emmerich, C.H.; Gerlach, B.; Schmukle, A.C.; Cordier, S.M.; Rieser, E.; Feltham, R.; Vince, J.; Warnken, U.; Wenger, T.; et al. Recruitment of the linear ubiquitin chain assembly complex stabilizes the TNF-R1 signaling complex and is required for TNF-mediated gene induction. *Mol. Cell* **2009**, *36*, 831–844. [CrossRef] [PubMed]
57. Brenner, D.; Blaser, H.; Mak, T.W. Regulation of tumour necrosis factor signalling: Live or let die. *Nat. Rev. Immunol.* **2015**, *15*, 362–374. [CrossRef] [PubMed]
58. Ea, C.K.; Deng, L.; Xia, Z.P.; Pineda, G.; Chen, Z.J. Activation of IKK by TNFalpha requires site-specific ubiquitination of RIP1 and polyubiquitin binding by NEMO. *Mol. Cell* **2006**, *22*, 245–257. [CrossRef] [PubMed]
59. Wang, C.; Deng, L.; Hong, M.; Akkaraju, G.R.; Inoue, J.; Chen, Z.J. TAK1 is a ubiquitin-dependent kinase of MKK and IKK. *Nature* **2001**, *412*, 346–351. [CrossRef] [PubMed]
60. Wajant, H.; Scheurich, P. TNFR1-induced activation of the classical NF-κB pathway. *FEBS J.* **2011**, *278*, 862–876. [CrossRef] [PubMed]
61. Chen, I.T.; Hsu, P.-H.; Hsu, W.-C.; Chen, N.-J.; Tseng, P.-H. Polyubiquitination of Transforming Growth Factor β-activated Kinase 1 (TAK1) at Lysine 562 Residue Regulates TLR4-mediated JNK and p38 MAPK Activation. *Sci. Rep.* **2015**, *5*, 12300. [CrossRef]
62. Karin, M. The regulation of AP-1 activity by mitogen-activated protein kinases. *J. Biol. Chem.* **1995**, *270*, 16483–16486. [CrossRef]
63. Fujita, K.; Srinivasula, S.M. Ubiquitination and TNFR1 signaling. *Results Probl. Cell Differ.* **2009**, *49*, 87–114. [CrossRef]
64. Li, X.; Zhang, M.; Huang, X.; Liang, W.; Li, G.; Lu, X.; Li, Y.; Pan, H.; Shi, L.; Zhu, H.; et al. Ubiquitination of RIPK1 regulates its activation mediated by TNFR1 and TLRs signaling in distinct manners. *Nat. Commun.* **2020**, *11*, 6364. [CrossRef] [PubMed]
65. Zhang, J.; Webster, J.D.; Dugger, D.L.; Goncharov, T.; Roose-Girma, M.; Hung, J.; Kwon, Y.C.; Vucic, D.; Newton, K.; Dixit, V.M. Ubiquitin Ligases cIAP1 and cIAP2 Limit Cell Death to Prevent Inflammation. *Cell Rep.* **2019**, *27*, 2679–2689.e2673. [CrossRef] [PubMed]
66. Newton, K. RIPK1 and RIPK3: Critical regulators of inflammation and cell death. *Trends Cell Biol.* **2015**, *25*, 347–353. [CrossRef] [PubMed]
67. Sun, L.; Wang, H.; Wang, Z.; He, S.; Chen, S.; Liao, D.; Wang, L.; Yan, J.; Liu, W.; Lei, X.; et al. Mixed lineage kinase domain-like protein mediates necrosis signaling downstream of RIP3 kinase. *Cell* **2012**, *148*, 213–227. [CrossRef] [PubMed]
68. Li, L.; Tong, A.; Zhang, Q.; Wei, Y.; Wei, X. The molecular mechanisms of MLKL-dependent and MLKL-independent necrosis. *J. Mol. Cell Biol.* **2020**, *13*, 3–14. [CrossRef] [PubMed]
69. Kalliolias, G.D.; Ivashkiv, L.B. TNF biology, pathogenic mechanisms and emerging therapeutic strategies. *Nat. Rev. Rheumatol.* **2016**, *12*, 49–62. [CrossRef]

70. Rothe, M.; Pan, M.G.; Henzel, W.J.; Ayres, T.M.; Goeddel, D.V. The TNFR2-TRAF signaling complex contains two novel proteins related to baculoviral inhibitor of apoptosis proteins. *Cell* **1995**, *83*, 1243–1252. [CrossRef]
71. Borghi, A.; Haegman, M.; Fischer, R.; Carpentier, I.; Bertrand, M.J.M.; Libert, C.; Afonina, I.S.; Beyaert, R. The E3 ubiquitin ligases HOIP and cIAP1 are recruited to the TNFR2 signaling complex and mediate TNFR2-induced canonical NF-κB signaling. *Biochem. Pharmacol.* **2018**, *153*, 292–298. [CrossRef]
72. Rauert, H.; Wicovsky, A.; Müller, N.; Siegmund, D.; Spindler, V.; Waschke, J.; Kneitz, C.; Wajant, H. Membrane tumor necrosis factor (TNF) induces p100 processing via TNF receptor-2 (TNFR2). *J. Biol. Chem.* **2010**, *285*, 7394–7404. [CrossRef]
73. Sun, S.-C. Non-canonical NF-κB signaling pathway. *Cell Res.* **2011**, *21*, 71–85. [CrossRef]
74. Thommesen, L.; Laegreid, A. Distinct differences between TNF receptor 1- and TNF receptor 2-mediated activation of NFkappaB. *J. Biochem. Mol. Biol.* **2005**, *38*, 281–289. [CrossRef] [PubMed]
75. Al-Lamki, R.S.; Wang, J.; Vandenabeele, P.; Bradley, J.A.; Thiru, S.; Luo, D.; Min, W.; Pober, J.S.; Bradley, J.R. TNFR1- and TNFR2-mediated signaling pathways in human kidney are cell type-specific and differentially contribute to renal injury. *FASEB J.* **2005**, *19*, 1637–1645. [CrossRef] [PubMed]
76. Reinhard, C.; Shamoon, B.; Shyamala, V.; Williams, L.T. Tumor necrosis factor alpha-induced activation of c-jun N-terminal kinase is mediated by TRAF2. *EMBO J.* **1997**, *16*, 1080–1092. [CrossRef]
77. Ji, W.; Li, Y.; Wan, T.; Wang, J.; Zhang, H.; Chen, H.; Min, W. Both internalization and AIP1 association are required for tumor necrosis factor receptor 2-mediated JNK signaling. *Arterioscler. Thromb. Vasc. Biol.* **2012**, *32*, 2271–2279. [CrossRef] [PubMed]
78. So, T.; Croft, M. Regulation of PI-3-Kinase and Akt Signaling in T Lymphocytes and Other Cells by TNFR Family Molecules. *Front. Immunol.* **2013**, *4*, 139. [CrossRef] [PubMed]
79. Venkatesh, D.; Ernandez, T.; Rosetti, F.; Batal, I.; Cullere, X.; Luscinskas, F.W.; Zhang, Y.; Stavrakis, G.; García-Cardeña, G.; Horwitz, B.H.; et al. Endothelial TNF receptor 2 induces IRF1 transcription factor-dependent interferon-β autocrine signaling to promote monocyte recruitment. *Immunity* **2013**, *38*, 1025–1037. [CrossRef] [PubMed]
80. Fotin-Mleczek, M.; Henkler, F.; Samel, D.; Reichwein, M.; Hausser, A.; Parmryd, I.; Scheurich, P.; Schmid, J.A.; Wajant, H. Apoptotic crosstalk of TNF receptors: TNF-R2-induces depletion of TRAF2 and IAP proteins and accelerates TNF-R1-dependent activation of caspase-8. *J. Cell Sci.* **2002**, *115*, 2757–2770. [CrossRef]
81. Pimentel-Muiños, F.X.; Seed, B. Regulated commitment of TNF receptor signaling: A molecular switch for death or activation. *Immunity* **1999**, *11*, 783–793. [CrossRef]
82. Naudé, P.J.; den Boer, J.A.; Luiten, P.G.; Eisel, U.L. Tumor necrosis factor receptor cross-talk. *FEBS J.* **2011**, *278*, 888–898. [CrossRef]
83. Tomosugi, N.I.; Cashman, S.J.; Hay, H.; Pusey, C.D.; Evans, D.J.; Shaw, A.; Rees, A.J. Modulation of antibody-mediated glomerular injury in vivo by bacterial lipopolysaccharide, tumor necrosis factor, and IL-1. *J. Immunol.* **1989**, *142*, 3083–3090.
84. Al-Lamki, R.S.; Mayadas, T.N. TNF receptors: Signaling pathways and contribution to renal dysfunction. *Kidney Int.* **2015**, *87*, 281–296. [CrossRef] [PubMed]
85. Al-Lamki, R.S.; Wang, J.; Skepper, J.N.; Thiru, S.; Pober, J.S.; Bradley, J.R. Expression of tumor necrosis factor receptors in normal kidney and rejecting renal transplants. *Lab. Investig.* **2001**, *81*, 1503–1515. [CrossRef] [PubMed]
86. Ribeiro, S.; Garrido, P.; Fernandes, J.; Vala, H.; Rocha-Pereira, P.; Costa, E.; Belo, L.; Reis, F.; Santos-Silva, A. Renal risk-benefit determinants of recombinant human erythropoietin therapy in the remnant kidney rat model—Hypertension, anaemia, inflammation and drug dose. *Clin. Exp. Pharmacol. Physiol.* **2016**, *43*, 343–354. [CrossRef] [PubMed]
87. Le Hir, M.; Haas, C.; Marino, M.; Ryffel, B. Prevention of crescentic glomerulonephritis induced by anti-glomerular membrane antibody in tumor necrosis factor-deficient mice. *Lab. Investig.* **1998**, *78*, 1625–1631.
88. Karkar, A.M.; Smith, J.; Pusey, C.D. Prevention and treatment of experimental crescentic glomerulonephritis by blocking tumour necrosis factor-alpha. *Nephrol. Dial. Transplant.* **2001**, *16*, 518–524. [CrossRef] [PubMed]
89. Misseri, R.; Meldrum, D.R.; Dinarello, C.A.; Dagher, P.; Hile, K.L.; Rink, R.C.; Meldrum, K.K. TNF-alpha mediates obstruction-induced renal tubular cell apoptosis and proapoptotic signaling. *Am. J. Physiol.-Ren. Physiol.* **2005**, *288*, F406–F411. [CrossRef]
90. Meldrum, K.K.; Misseri, R.; Metcalfe, P.; Dinarello, C.A.; Hile, K.L.; Meldrum, D.R. TNF-alpha neutralization ameliorates obstruction-induced renal fibrosis and dysfunction. *Am. J. Physiol.-Regul. Integr. Comp. Physiol.* **2007**, *292*, R1456–R1464. [CrossRef]
91. Chen, C.C.; Pedraza, P.L.; Hao, S.; Stier, C.T.; Ferreri, N.R. TNFR1-deficient mice display altered blood pressure and renal responses to ANG II infusion. *Am. J. Physiol.-Ren. Physiol.* **2010**, *299*, F1141–F1150. [CrossRef]
92. Vielhauer, V.; Stavrakis, G.; Mayadas, T.N. Renal cell-expressed TNF receptor 2, not receptor 1, is essential for the development of glomerulonephritis. *J. Clin. Investig.* **2005**, *115*, 1199–1209. [CrossRef]
93. Guo, G.; Morrissey, J.; McCracken, R.; Tolley, T.; Klahr, S. Role of TNFR1 and TNFR2 receptors in tubulointerstitial fibrosis of obstructive nephropathy. *Am. J. Physiol.* **1999**, *277*, F766–F772. [CrossRef]
94. Ramesh, G.; Reeves, W.B. TNFR2-mediated apoptosis and necrosis in cisplatin-induced acute renal failure. *Am. J. Physiol.-Ren. Physiol.* **2003**, *285*, F610–F618. [CrossRef]
95. Mulay, S.R.; Eberhard, J.N.; Desai, J.; Marschner, J.A.; Kumar, S.V.; Weidenbusch, M.; Grigorescu, M.; Lech, M.; Eltrich, N.; Müller, L.; et al. Hyperoxaluria Requires TNF Receptors to Initiate Crystal Adhesion and Kidney Stone Disease. *J. Am. Soc. Nephrol.* **2017**, *28*, 761–768. [CrossRef] [PubMed]

96. Klinkhammer, B.M.; Djudjaj, S.; Kunter, U.; Falsson, R.; Edvardsson, V.O.; Wiech, T.; Thorsteinsdottir, M.; Hardarson, S.; Foresto-Neto, O.; Mulay, S.R.; et al. Cellular and Molecular Mechanisms of Kidney Injury in 2,8-Dihydroxyadenine Nephropathy. *J. Am. Soc. Nephrol.* **2020**, *31*, 799–816. [CrossRef] [PubMed]
97. Cheng, D.; Liang, R.; Huang, B.; Hou, J.; Yin, J.; Zhao, T.; Zhou, L.; Wu, R.; Qian, Y.; Wang, F. Tumor necrosis factor-α blockade ameliorates diabetic nephropathy in rats. *Clin. Kidney J.* **2019**, *14*, 301–308. [CrossRef] [PubMed]
98. DiPetrillo, K.; Coutermarsh, B.; Gesek, F.A. Urinary tumor necrosis factor contributes to sodium retention and renal hypertrophy during diabetes. *Am. J. Physiol.-Ren. Physiol.* **2003**, *284*, F113–F121. [CrossRef]
99. Omote, K.; Gohda, T.; Murakoshi, M.; Sasaki, Y.; Kazuno, S.; Fujimura, T.; Ishizaka, M.; Sonoda, Y.; Tomino, Y. Role of the TNF pathway in the progression of diabetic nephropathy in KK-A(y) mice. *Am. J. Physiol.-Ren. Physiol.* **2014**, *306*, F1335–F1347. [CrossRef]
100. Moriwaki, Y.; Inokuchi, T.; Yamamoto, A.; Ka, T.; Tsutsumi, Z.; Takahashi, S.; Yamamoto, T. Effect of TNF-alpha inhibition on urinary albumin excretion in experimental diabetic rats. *Acta Diabetol.* **2007**, *44*, 215–218. [CrossRef]
101. Granata, S.; Dalla Gassa, A.; Bellin, G.; Lupo, A.; Zaza, G. Transcriptomics: A Step behind the Comprehension of the Polygenic Influence on Oxidative Stress, Immune Deregulation, and Mitochondrial Dysfunction in Chronic Kidney Disease. *Bio. Res. Int.* **2016**, *2016*, 9290857. [CrossRef]
102. Gerhardt, L.M.S.; Liu, J.; Koppitch, K.; Cippà, P.E.; McMahon, A.P. Single-nuclear transcriptomics reveals diversity of proximal tubule cell states in a dynamic response to acute kidney injury. *Proc. Natl. Acad. Sc. USA* **2021**, *118*, e2026684118. [CrossRef]
103. Khan, S.B.; Cook, H.T.; Bhangal, G.; Smith, J.; Tam, F.W.; Pusey, C.D. Antibody blockade of TNF-alpha reduces inflammation and scarring in experimental crescentic glomerulonephritis. *Kidney Int.* **2005**, *67*, 1812–1820. [CrossRef]
104. Hoffmann, U.; Bergler, T.; Rihm, M.; Pace, C.; Krüger, B.; Rümmele, P.; Stoelcker, B.; Banas, B.; Männel, D.N.; Krämer, B.K. Upregulation of TNF receptor type 2 in human and experimental renal allograft rejection. *Am. J. Transplant.* **2009**, *9*, 675–686. [CrossRef] [PubMed]
105. Morimoto, Y.; Gai, Z.; Tanishima, H.; Kawakatsu, M.; Itoh, S.; Hatamura, I.; Muragaki, Y. TNF-alpha deficiency accelerates renal tubular interstitial fibrosis in the late stage of ureteral obstruction. *Exp. Mol. Pathol.* **2008**, *85*, 207–213. [CrossRef] [PubMed]
106. Jacob, N.; Yang, H.; Pricop, L.; Liu, Y.; Gao, X.; Zheng, S.G.; Wang, J.; Gao, H.X.; Futterman, C.; Koss, M.N.; et al. Accelerated pathological and clinical nephritis in systemic lupus erythematosus-prone New Zealand Mixed 2328 mice doubly deficient in TNF receptor 1 and TNF receptor 2 via a Th17-associated pathway. *J. Immunol.* **2009**, *182*, 2532–2541. [CrossRef]
107. Taubitz, A.; Schwarz, M.; Eltrich, N.; Lindenmeyer, M.T.; Vielhauer, V. Distinct contributions of TNF receptor 1 and 2 to TNF-induced glomerular inflammation in mice. *PLoS ONE* **2013**, *8*, e68167. [CrossRef]
108. Xu, C.; Chang, A.; Hack, B.K.; Eadon, M.T.; Alper, S.L.; Cunningham, P.N. TNF-mediated damage to glomerular endothelium is an important determinant of acute kidney injury in sepsis. *Kidney Int.* **2014**, *85*, 72–81. [CrossRef] [PubMed]
109. Halwachs, G.; Tiran, A.; Reisinger, E.C.; Zach, R.; Sabin, K.; Fölsch, B.; Lanzer, H.; Holzer, H.; Wilders-Truschnig, M. Serum levels of the soluble receptor for tumor necrosis factor in patients with renal disease. *Clin. Investig.* **1994**, *72*, 473–476. [CrossRef] [PubMed]
110. Tonelli, M.; Sacks, F.; Pfeffer, M.; Jhangri, G.S.; Curhan, G. Biomarkers of inflammation and progression of chronic kidney disease. *Kidney Int.* **2005**, *68*, 237–245. [CrossRef]
111. Kamei, N.; Yamashita, M.; Nishizaki, Y.; Yanagisawa, N.; Nojiri, S.; Tanaka, K.; Yamashita, Y.; Shibata, T.; Murakoshi, M.; Suzuki, Y.; et al. Association between circulating tumor necrosis factor-related biomarkers and estimated glomerular filtration rate in type 2 diabetes. *Sci. Rep.* **2018**, *8*, 15302. [CrossRef]
112. Sonoda, Y.; Gohda, T.; Suzuki, Y.; Omote, K.; Ishizaka, M.; Matsuoka, J.; Tomino, Y. Circulating TNF receptors 1 and 2 are associated with the severity of renal interstitial fibrosis in IgA nephropathy. *PLoS ONE* **2015**, *10*, e0122212. [CrossRef]
113. Bae, E.; Cha, R.H.; Kim, Y.C.; An, J.N.; Kim, D.K.; Yoo, K.D.; Lee, S.M.; Kim, M.H.; Park, J.T.; Kang, S.W.; et al. Circulating TNF receptors predict cardiovascular disease in patients with chronic kidney disease. *Medicine* **2017**, *96*, e6666. [CrossRef]
114. Srivastava, A.; Schmidt, I.M.; Palsson, R.; Weins, A.; Bonventre, J.V.; Sabbisetti, V.; Stillman, I.E.; Rennke, H.G.; Waikar, S.S The Associations of Plasma Biomarkers of Inflammation With Histopathologic Lesions, Kidney Disease Progression, and Mortality-The Boston Kidney Biopsy Cohort Study. *Kidney Int. Rep.* **2021**, *6*, 685–694. [CrossRef]
115. Lee, S.M.; Yang, S.; Cha, R.H.; Kim, M.; An, J.N.; Paik, J.H.; Kim, D.K.; Kang, S.W.; Lim, C.S.; Kim, Y.S.; et al. Circulating TNF receptors are significant prognostic biomarkers for idiopathic membranous nephropathy. *PLoS ONE* **2014**, *9*, e104354. [CrossRef]
116. An, J.N.; Yoo, K.D.; Hwang, J.H.; Kim, H.L.; Kim, S.H.; Yang, S.H.; Kim, J.H.; Kim, D.K.; Oh, Y.K.; Kim, Y.S.; et al. Circulating tumour necrosis factor receptors 1 and 2 predict contrast-induced nephropathy and progressive renal dysfunction: A prospective cohort study. *Nephrology* **2015**, *20*, 552–559. [CrossRef]
117. Wu, T.; Xie, C.; Wang, H.W.; Zhou, X.J.; Schwartz, N.; Calixto, S.; Mackay, M.; Aranow, C.; Putterman, C.; Mohan, C. Elevated urinary VCAM-1, P-selectin, soluble TNF receptor-1, and CXC chemokine ligand 16 in multiple murine lupus strains and human lupus nephritis. *J. Immunol.* **2007**, *179*, 7166–7175. [CrossRef]
118. Koenig, K.F.; Groeschl, I.; Pesickova, S.S.; Tesar, V.; Eisenberger, U.; Trendelenburg, M. Serum cytokine profile in patients with active lupus nephritis. *Cytokine* **2012**, *60*, 410–416. [CrossRef]
119. Murakoshi, M.; Gohda, T.; Suzuki, Y. Circulating Tumor Necrosis Factor Receptors: A Potential Biomarker for the Progression of Diabetic Kidney Disease. *Int. J. Mol. Sci.* **2020**, *21*, 1957. [CrossRef]

120. Gohda, T.; Niewczas, M.A.; Ficociello, L.H.; Walker, W.H.; Skupien, J.; Rosetti, F.; Cullere, X.; Johnson, A.C.; Crabtree, G.; Smiles, A.M.; et al. Circulating TNF receptors 1 and 2 predict stage 3 CKD in type 1 diabetes. *J. Am. Soc. Nephrol.* **2012**, *23*, 516–524. [CrossRef]
121. Niewczas, M.A.; Gohda, T.; Skupien, J.; Smiles, A.M.; Walker, W.H.; Rosetti, F.; Cullere, X.; Eckfeldt, J.H.; Doria, A.; Mayadas, T.N.; et al. Circulating TNF receptors 1 and 2 predict ESRD in type 2 diabetes. *J. Am. Soc. Nephrol.* **2012**, *23*, 507–515. [CrossRef]
122. Krolewski, A.S.; Niewczas, M.A.; Skupien, J.; Gohda, T.; Smiles, A.; Eckfeldt, J.H.; Doria, A.; Warram, J.H. Early progressive renal decline precedes the onset of microalbuminuria and its progression to macroalbuminuria. *Diabetes Care* **2014**, *37*, 226–234. [CrossRef]
123. Coca, S.G.; Nadkarni, G.N.; Huang, Y.; Moledina, D.G.; Rao, V.; Zhang, J.; Ferket, B.; Crowley, S.T.; Fried, L.F.; Parikh, C.R. Plasma Biomarkers and Kidney Function Decline in Early and Established Diabetic Kidney Disease. *J. Am. Soc. Nephrol.* **2017**, *28*, 2786–2793. [CrossRef]
124. Pavkov, M.E.; Weil, E.J.; Fufaa, G.D.; Nelson, R.G.; Lemley, K.V.; Knowler, W.C.; Niewczas, M.A.; Krolewski, A.S. Tumor necrosis factor receptors 1 and 2 are associated with early glomerular lesions in type 2 diabetes. *Kidney Int.* **2016**, *89*, 226–234. [CrossRef]
125. Saulnier, P.J.; Gand, E.; Velho, G.; Mohammedi, K.; Zaoui, P.; Fraty, M.; Halimi, J.M.; Roussel, R.; Ragot, S.; Hadjadj, S. Association of Circulating Biomarkers (Adrenomedullin, TNFR1, and NT-proBNP) With Renal Function Decline in Patients With Type 2 Diabetes: A French Prospective Cohort. *Diabetes Care* **2017**, *40*, 367–374. [CrossRef]
126. Barr, E.L.M.; Barzi, F.; Hughes, J.T.; Jerums, G.; Hoy, W.E.; O'Dea, K.; Jones, G.R.D.; Lawton, P.D.; Brown, A.D.H.; Thomas, M.; et al. High Baseline Levels of Tumor Necrosis Factor Receptor 1 Are Associated With Progression of Kidney Disease in Indigenous Australians With Diabetes: The eGFR Follow-up Study. *Diabetes Care* **2018**, *41*, 739–747. [CrossRef]
127. Carlsson, A.C.; Östgren, C.J.; Nystrom, F.H.; Länne, T.; Jennersjö, P.; Larsson, A.; Ärnlöv, J. Association of soluble tumor necrosis factor receptors 1 and 2 with nephropathy, cardiovascular events, and total mortality in type 2 diabetes. *Cardiovasc. Diabetol.* **2016**, *15*, 40. [CrossRef]
128. Lam, D.; Nadkarni, G.N.; Mosoyan, G.; Neal, B.; Mahaffey, K.W.; Rosenthal, N.; Hansen, M.K.; Heerspink, H.J.L.; Fleming, F.; Coca, S.G. Clinical Utility of KidneyIntelX in Early Stages of Diabetic Kidney Disease in the CANVAS Trial. *Am. J. Nephrol.* **2022**, *53*, 21–31. [CrossRef]
129. Neirynck, N.; Glorieux, G.; Schepers, E.; Verbeke, F.; Vanholder, R. Soluble tumor necrosis factor receptor 1 and 2 predict outcomes in advanced chronic kidney disease: A prospective cohort study. *PLoS ONE* **2015**, *10*, e0122073. [CrossRef]
130. Saulnier, P.J.; Gand, E.; Ragot, S.; Ducrocq, G.; Halimi, J.M.; Hulin-Delmotte, C.; Llaty, P.; Montaigne, D.; Rigalleau, V.; Roussel, R.; et al. Association of serum concentration of TNFR1 with all-cause mortality in patients with type 2 diabetes and chronic kidney disease: Follow-up of the SURDIAGENE Cohort. *Diabetes Care* **2014**, *37*, 1425–1431. [CrossRef]
131. Carlsson, A.C.; Carrero, J.J.; Stenvinkel, P.; Bottai, M.; Barany, P.; Larsson, A.; Ärnlöv, J. High levels of soluble tumor necrosis factor receptors 1 and 2 and their association with mortality in patients undergoing hemodialysis. *Cardiorenal Med.* **2015**, *5*, 89–95. [CrossRef]
132. Gohda, T.; Maruyama, S.; Kamei, N.; Yamaguchi, S.; Shibata, T.; Murakoshi, M.; Horikoshi, S.; Tomino, Y.; Ohsawa, I.; Gotoh, H.; et al. Circulating TNF Receptors 1 and 2 Predict Mortality in Patients with End-stage Renal Disease Undergoing Dialysis. *Sci. Rep.* **2017**, *7*, 43520. [CrossRef]
133. Coimbra, S.; Rocha, S.; Nascimento, H.; Valente, M.J.; Catarino, C.; Rocha-Pereira, P.; Sameiro-Faria, M.; Oliveira, J.G.; Madureira, J.; Fernandes, J.C.; et al. Cell-free DNA as a marker for the outcome of end-stage renal disease patients on haemodialysis. *Clin. Kidney J.* **2021**, *14*, 1371–1378. [CrossRef]
134. Mihai, S.; Codrici, E.; Popescu, I.D.; Enciu, A.-M.; Rusu, E.; Zilisteanu, D.; Albulescu, R.; Anton, G.; Tanase, C. Proteomic Biomarkers Panel: New Insights in Chronic Kidney Disease. *Dis. Markers* **2016**, *2016*, 3185232. [CrossRef]
135. Romanova, Y.; Laikov, A.; Markelova, M.; Khadiullina, R.; Makseev, A.; Hasanova, M.; Rizvanov, A.; Khaiboullina, S.; Salafutdinov, I. Proteomic Analysis of Human Serum from Patients with Chronic Kidney Disease. *Biomolecules* **2020**, *10*, 257. [CrossRef]
136. Niewczas, M.A.; Pavkov, M.E.; Skupien, J.; Smiles, A.; Md Dom, Z.I.; Wilson, J.M.; Park, J.; Nair, V.; Schlafly, A.; Saulnier, P.J.; et al. A signature of circulating inflammatory proteins and development of end-stage renal disease in diabetes. *Nat. Med.* **2019**, *25*, 805–813. [CrossRef]
137. Ihara, K.; Skupien, J.; Krolewski, B.; Md Dom, Z.I.; O'Neil, K.; Satake, E.; Kobayashi, H.; Rashidi, N.M.; Niewczas, M.A.; Krolewski, A.S. A profile of multiple circulating tumor necrosis factor receptors associated with early progressive kidney decline in Type 1 Diabetes is similar to profiles in autoimmune disorders. *Kidney Int.* **2021**, *99*, 725–736. [CrossRef]
138. Tang, R.; Meng, T.; Lin, W.; Shen, C.; Ooi, J.D.; Eggenhuizen, P.J.; Jin, P.; Ding, X.; Chen, J.; Tang, Y.; et al. A Partial Picture of the Single-Cell Transcriptomics of Human IgA Nephropathy. *Front. Immunol.* **2021**, *12*, 645988. [CrossRef]
139. Premužić, V.; Padjen, I.; Cerovec, M.; Ćorić, M.; Jelaković, B.; Anić, B. The Association of TNF-Alpha Inhibitors and Development of IgA Nephropathy in Patients with Rheumatoid Arthritis and Diabetes. *Case Rep. Nephrol.* **2020**, *2020*, 9480860. [CrossRef]
140. Stokes, M.B.; Foster, K.; Markowitz, G.S.; Ebrahimi, F.; Hines, W.; Kaufman, D.; Moore, B.; Wolde, D.; D'Agati, V.D. Development of glomerulonephritis during anti-TNF-alpha therapy for rheumatoid arthritis. *Nephrol. Dial. Transplant.* **2005**, *20*, 1400–1406. [CrossRef]
141. Kim, H.W.; Lee, C.K.; Cha, H.S.; Choe, J.Y.; Park, E.J.; Kim, J. Effect of anti-tumor necrosis factor alpha treatment of rheumatoid arthritis and chronic kidney disease. *Rheumatol. Int.* **2015**, *35*, 727–734. [CrossRef] [PubMed]

142. Bartolucci, P.; Ramanoelina, J.; Cohen, P.; Mahr, A.; Godmer, P.; Le Hello, C.; Guillevin, L. Efficacy of the anti-TNF-alpha antibody infliximab against refractory systemic vasculitides: An open pilot study on 10 patients. *Rheumatology* **2002**, *41*, 1126–1132. [CrossRef]
143. Garrouste, C.; Anglicheau, D.; Kamar, N.; Bachelier, C.; Rivalan, J.; Pereira, B.; Caillard, S.; Aniort, J.; Gatault, P.; Soubrier, M. et al. Anti-TNFα therapy for chronic inflammatory disease in kidney transplant recipients: Clinical outcomes. *Medicine* **2016**, *95*, e5108. [CrossRef]
144. Keller, C.R.; Odden, M.C.; Fried, L.F.; Newman, A.B.; Angleman, S.; Green, C.A.; Cummings, S.R.; Harris, T.B.; Shlipak, M.G. Kidney function and markers of inflammation in elderly persons without chronic kidney disease: The health, aging, and body composition study. *Kidney Int.* **2007**, *71*, 239–244. [CrossRef]
145. Keller, C.; Katz, R.; Cushman, M.; Fried, L.F.; Shlipak, M. Association of kidney function with inflammatory and procoagulant markers in a diverse cohort: A cross-sectional analysis from the Multi-Ethnic Study of Atherosclerosis (MESA). *BMC Nephrol.* **2008**, *9*, 9. [CrossRef]
146. Niewczas, M.A.; Ficociello, L.H.; Johnson, A.C.; Walker, W.; Rosolowsky, E.T.; Rosnan, B.; Warram, J.H.; Krolewski, A.S. Serum concentrations of markers of TNFalpha and Fas-mediated pathways and renal function in nonproteinuric patients with type 1 diabetes. *Clin. J. Am. Soc. Nephrol.* **2009**, *4*, 62–70. [CrossRef]
147. Idasiak-Piechocka, I.; Oko, A.; Pawliczak, E.; Kaczmarek, E.; Czekalski, S. Urinary excretion of soluble tumour necrosis factor receptor 1 as a marker of increased risk of progressive kidney function deterioration in patients with primary chronic glomerulonephritis. *Nephrol. Dial. Transplant.* **2010**, *25*, 3948–3956. [CrossRef]
148. Upadhyay, A.; Larson, M.G.; Guo, C.Y.; Vasan, R.S.; Lipinska, I.; O'Donnell, C.J.; Kathiresan, S.; Meigs, J.B.; Keaney, J.F., Jr.; Rong, J.; et al. Inflammation, kidney function and albuminuria in the Framingham Offspring cohort. *Nephrol. Dial. Transplant.* **2011**, *26*, 920–926. [CrossRef]
149. Shankar, A.; Sun, L.; Klein, B.E.; Lee, K.E.; Muntner, P.; Nieto, F.J.; Tsai, M.Y.; Cruickshanks, K.J.; Schubert, C.R.; Brazy, P.C.; et al. Markers of inflammation predict the long-term risk of developing chronic kidney disease: A population-based cohort study. *Kidney Int.* **2011**, *80*, 1231–1238. [CrossRef]
150. Zwiech, R. Predictive value of conjointly examined IL-1ra, TNF-R I, TNF-R II, and RANTES in patients with primary glomerulonephritis. *J. Korean Med. Sci.* **2013**, *28*, 261–267. [CrossRef]
151. Forsblom, C.; Moran, J.; Harjutsalo, V.; Loughman, T.; Wadén, J.; Tolonen, N.; Thorn, L.; Saraheimo, M.; Gordin, D.; Groop, P.H.; et al. Added value of soluble tumor necrosis factor-α receptor 1 as a biomarker of ESRD risk in patients with type 1 diabetes. *Diabetes Care* **2014**, *37*, 2334–2342. [CrossRef]
152. Skupien, J.; Warram, J.H.; Niewczas, M.A.; Gohda, T.; Malecki, M.; Mychaleckyj, J.C.; Galecki, A.T.; Krolewski, A.S. Synergism between circulating tumor necrosis factor receptor 2 and HbA(1c) in determining renal decline during 5-18 years of follow-up in patients with type 1 diabetes and proteinuria. *Diabetes Care* **2014**, *37*, 2601–2608. [CrossRef]
153. Murakoshi, M.; Gohda, T.; Sonoda, Y.; Suzuki, H.; Tomino, Y.; Horikoshi, S.; Suzuki, Y. Effect of tonsillectomy with steroid pulse therapy on circulating tumor necrosis factor receptors 1 and 2 in IgA nephropathy. *Clin. Exp. Nephrol.* **2017**, *21*, 1068–1074. [CrossRef]
154. Oh, Y.J.; An, J.N.; Kim, C.T.; Yang, S.H.; Lee, H.; Kim, D.K.; Joo, K.W.; Paik, J.H.; Kang, S.W.; Park, J.T.; et al. Circulating Tumor Necrosis Factor α Receptors Predict the Outcomes of Human IgA Nephropathy: A Prospective Cohort Study. *PLoS ONE* **2015**, *10*, e0132826. [CrossRef] [PubMed]
155. Pavkov, M.E.; Nelson, R.G.; Knowler, W.C.; Cheng, Y.; Krolewski, A.S.; Niewczas, M.A. Elevation of circulating TNF receptors 1 and 2 increases the risk of end-stage renal disease in American Indians with type 2 diabetes. *Kidney Int.* **2015**, *87*, 812–819. [CrossRef] [PubMed]
156. Liu, G.; Deng, Y.; Sun, L.; Ye, X.; Yao, P.; Hu, Y.; Wang, F.; Ma, Y.; Li, H.; Liu, Y.; et al. Elevated plasma tumor necrosis factor-α receptor 2 and resistin are associated with increased incidence of kidney function decline in Chinese adults. *Endocrine* **2016**, *52*, 541–549. [CrossRef] [PubMed]
157. Sun, J.; Axelsson, J.; Machowska, A.; Heimbürger, O.; Bárány, P.; Lindholm, B.; Lindström, K.; Stenvinkel, P.; Qureshi, A.R. Biomarkers of Cardiovascular Disease and Mortality Risk in Patients with Advanced CKD. *Clin. J. Am. Soc. Nephrol.* **2016**, *11*, 1163–1172. [CrossRef] [PubMed]
158. Hwang, S.; Park, J.; Kim, J.; Jang, H.R.; Kwon, G.Y.; Huh, W.; Kim, Y.G.; Kim, D.J.; Oh, H.Y.; Lee, J.E. Tissue expression of tubular injury markers is associated with renal function decline in diabetic nephropathy. *J. Diabetes Complicat.* **2017**, *31*, 1704–1709. [CrossRef] [PubMed]
159. Bhatraju, P.K.; Zelnick, L.R.; Shlipak, M.; Katz, R.; Kestenbaum, B. Association of Soluble TNFR-1 Concentrations with Long-Term Decline in Kidney Function: The Multi-Ethnic Study of Atherosclerosis. *J. Am. Soc. Nephrol.* **2018**, *29*, 2713–2721. [CrossRef] [PubMed]
160. Ye, X.; Luo, T.; Wang, K.; Wang, Y.; Yang, S.; Li, Q.; Hu, J. Circulating TNF receptors 1 and 2 predict progression of diabetic kidney disease: A meta-analysis. *Diabetes Metab. Res. Rev.* **2019**, *35*, e3195. [CrossRef]
161. MacIsaac, R.J.; Farag, M.; Obeyesekere, V.; Clarke, M.; Boston, R.; Ward, G.M.; Jerums, G.; Ekinci, E.I. Changes in soluble tumor necrosis factor receptor type 1 levels and early renal function decline in patients with diabetes. *J. Diabetes Investig.* **2019**, *10*, 1537–1542. [CrossRef]

162. Oshima, M.; Hara, A.; Toyama, T.; Jun, M.; Pollock, C.; Jardine, M.; Harrap, S.; Poulter, N.; Cooper, M.E.; Woodward, M.; et al. Comparison of Circulating Biomarkers in Predicting Diabetic Kidney Disease Progression with Autoantibodies to Erythropoietin Receptor. *Kidney Int. Rep.* **2021**, *6*, 284–295. [CrossRef]
163. Schrauben, S.J.; Shou, H.; Zhang, X.; Anderson, A.H.; Bonventre, J.V.; Chen, J.; Coca, S.; Furth, S.L.; Greenberg, J.H.; Gutierrez, O.M.; et al. Association of Multiple Plasma Biomarker Concentrations with Progression of Prevalent Diabetic Kidney Disease: Findings from the Chronic Renal Insufficiency Cohort (CRIC) Study. *J. Am. Soc. Nephrol.* **2021**, *32*, 115–126. [CrossRef]
164. Greenberg, J.H.; Abraham, A.G.; Xu, Y.; Schelling, J.R.; Feldman, H.I.; Sabbisetti, V.S.; Gonzalez, M.C.; Coca, S.; Schrauben, S.J.; Waikar, S.S.; et al. Plasma Biomarkers of Tubular Injury and Inflammation Are Associated with CKD Progression in Children. *J. Am. Soc. Nephrol.* **2020**, *31*, 1067–1077. [CrossRef] [PubMed]
165. Martin, W.P.; Conroy, C.; Naicker, S.D.; Cormican, S.; Griffin, T.P.; Islam, M.N.; McCole, E.M.; McConnell, I.; Lamont, J.; FitzGerald, P.; et al. Multiplex Serum Biomarker Assays Improve Prediction of Renal and Mortality Outcomes in Chronic Kidney Disease. *Kidney360* **2021**, *2*, 1225–1239. [CrossRef] [PubMed]
166. Waijer, S.W.; Sen, T.; Arnott, C.; Neal, B.; Kosterink, J.G.W.; Mahaffey, K.W.; Parikh, C.R.; de Zeeuw, D.; Perkovic, V.; Neuen, B.L.; et al. Association between TNF Receptors and KIM-1 with Kidney Outcomes in Early-Stage Diabetic Kidney Disease. *Clin. J. Am. Soc. Nephrol.* **2021**, *17*, 251–259. [CrossRef] [PubMed]
167. Sen, T.; Li, J.; Neuen, B.L.; Neal, B.; Arnott, C.; Parikh, C.R.; Coca, S.G.; Perkovic, V.; Mahaffey, K.W.; Yavin, Y.; et al. Effects of the SGLT2 inhibitor canagliflozin on plasma biomarkers TNFR-1, TNFR-2 and KIM-1 in the CANVAS trial. *Diabetologia* **2021**, *64*, 2147–2158. [CrossRef] [PubMed]
168. Gohda, T.; Kamei, N.; Kubota, M.; Tanaka, K.; Yamashita, Y.; Sakuma, H.; Kishida, C.; Adachi, E.; Koshida, T.; Murakoshi, M.; et al. Fractional excretion of tumor necrosis factor receptor 1 and 2 in patients with type 2 diabetes and normal renal function. *J. Diabetes Investig.* **2021**, *12*, 382–389. [CrossRef] [PubMed]
169. Gutiérrez, O.M.; Shlipak, M.G.; Katz, R.; Waikar, S.S.; Greenberg, J.H.; Schrauben, S.J.; Coca, S.; Parikh, C.R.; Vasan, R.S.; Feldman, H.I.; et al. Associations of Plasma Biomarkers of Inflammation, Fibrosis, and Kidney Tubular Injury With Progression of Diabetic Kidney Disease: A Cohort Study. *Am. J. Kidney Dis.* **2021**, *9*, 18. [CrossRef] [PubMed]
170. Udalova, I.; Monaco, C.; Nanchahal, J.; Feldmann, M. Anti-TNF Therapy. *Microbiol. Spectr.* **2016**, *4*, 15. [CrossRef] [PubMed]

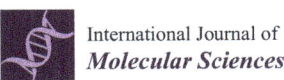

Article

Potential Urine Proteomic Biomarkers for Focal Segmental Glomerulosclerosis and Minimal Change Disease

Natalia V. Chebotareva [1,*], Anatoliy Vinogradov [2], Alexander G. Brzhozovskiy [3,4], Daria N. Kashirina [3,4], Maria I. Indeykina [4,5], Anna E. Bugrova [4,5], Marina Lebedeva [1], Sergey Moiseev [1], Evgeny N. Nikolaev [4] and Alexey S. Kononikhin [4,*]

1. Nephrology Department, Sechenov First Moscow State Medical University, Trubezkaya, 8, 119048 Moscow, Russia
2. Department of Internal Medicine, Lomonosov Moscow State University, GSP-1, Leninskie Gory, 119991 Moscow, Russia
3. Institute of Biomedical Problems—Russian Federation State Scientific Research Center, Russian Academy of Sciences, Khoroshevskoe Shosse, 76A, 123007 Moscow, Russia
4. Skolkovo Institute of Science and Technology, Bolshoy Boulevard 30, Bld. 1, 121205 Moscow, Russia
5. Emanuel Institute for Biochemical Physics, Russian Academy of Science, Kosygina Str., 4, 119334 Moscow, Russia
* Correspondence: natasha_tcheb@mail.ru (N.V.C.); a.kononikhin@skoltech.ru (A.S.K.)

Abstract: Primary focal segmental glomerulosclerosis (FSGS), along with minimal change disease (MCD), are diseases with primary podocyte damage that are clinically manifested by the nephrotic syndrome. The pathogenesis of these podocytopathies is still unknown, and therefore, the search for biomarkers of these diseases is ongoing. Our aim was to determine of the proteomic profile of urine from patients with FSGS and MCD. Patients with a confirmed diagnosis of FSGS (n = 30) and MCD (n = 9) were recruited for the study. For a comprehensive assessment of the severity of FSGS a special index was introduced, which was calculated as follows: the first score was assigned depending on the level of eGFR, the second score—depending on the proteinuria level, the third score—resistance to steroid therapy. Patients with the sum of these scores of less than 3 were included in group 1, with 3 or more—in group 2. The urinary proteome was analyzed using liquid chromatography/mass spectrometry. The proteome profiles of patients with severe progressive FSGS from group 2, mild FSGS from group 1 and MCD were compared. Results of the label free analysis were validated using targeted LC-MS based on multiple reaction monitoring (MRM) with stable isotope labelled peptide standards (SIS) available for 47 of the 76 proteins identified as differentiating between at least one pair of groups. Quantitative MRM SIS validation measurements for these 47 proteins revealed 22 proteins with significant differences between at least one of the two group pairs and 14 proteins were validated for both comparisons. In addition, all of the 22 proteins validated by MRM SIS analysis showed the same direction of change as at the discovery stage with label-free LC-MS analysis, i.e., up or down regulation in MCD and FSGS1 against FSGS2. Patients from the FSGS group 2 showed a significantly different profile from both FSGS group 1 and MCD. Among the 47 significantly differentiating proteins, the most significant were apolipoprotein A-IV, hemopexin, vitronectin, gelsolin, components of the complement system (C4b, factors B and I), retinol- and vitamin D-binding proteins. Patients with mild form of FSGS and MCD showed lower levels of Cystatin C, gelsolin and complement factor I.

Keywords: urine proteome; FSGS; MCD; podocyte dysfunction; mass spectrometry

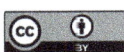

1. Introduction

Primary focal segmental glomerulosclerosis (FSGS) and minimal change disease (MCD) are diseases with primary damage to podocytes (primary podocytopathies), clinically manifested by high proteinuria and nephrotic syndrome [1,2]. FSGS is characterized by the presence of sclerosis in parts (segmental) of at least one glomerulus (focal) in a kidney biopsy specimen, when examined by light microscopy, immunofluorescence, or electron microscopy. Minimal change disease (MCD) is the leading cause of the nephrotic syndrome in children (approximately 90 percent) and in a minority of adults (approximately 10 percent) [3]. Light microscopy in case of MCD shows only a minor abnormality in the glomeruli, immunohistological methods display no deposits of immunoglobulins and complements, and electron microscopy reveals a diffuse loss of podocyte foot processes. Development of the nephrotic syndrome is due to the damage of the podocyte, foot process effacement and detachment of the podocyte from the glomerular basement membrane (GBM). As a result, proteins pass through the defects of the GBM and proteinuria develops. The onset of both diseases—FSGS and MCD, is usually acute with a severe nephrotic syndrome. A decrease in kidney function at the onset of the disease is diagnosed in 25–50% of patients, hematuria in 50%, and arterial hypertension in 20% of patients with FSGS [2,4].

Patients with MCD, as well as some patients with FSGS, respond well to steroid therapy [5]. However, 25–50% have steroid resistance—a severe form of FSGS. Severe FSGS is characterized by high proteinuria, renal impairment in the initial stages, and an unfavorable prognosis on the progression of renal dysfunction [2,4,6–8].

In primary FSGS, a putative circulating factor that is toxic to the podocyte causes generalized podocyte dysfunction. Secondary FSGS generally occurs as an adaptive phenomenon due to the reduction of the nephron mass or direct toxicity from drugs or viral infections. The circulating factor in FSGS and MCD is still unknown, and therefore the study of specific mechanisms that are involved in podocyte damage is ongoing. This knowledge could improve our understanding of the pathogenetic mechanisms of these diseases. Approaches based on mass spectrometry (MS) are the most objective and sensitive tools that have already provided most of the currently known information on the content of peptides and proteins in urine in various nephropathies [9–12]. The urinary proteome contains mainly (up to 70%) proteins and peptides of renal origin [13,14]. In general, this approach is the most appropriate for the search for potential biomarkers and mechanisms related to the development and progression of kidney diseases.

The aim of our study was to characterize changes in the urinary proteomic profiles of patients with different course of focal segmental glomerulosclerosis and minimal change disease to determine their specific biomarkers.

2. Results

2.1. Optimization of the Urine Preparation Protocol for Proteomic Analysis

All clinical urine samples were characterized by proteinuria of varying severity (Table 1). In order to select the optimal method of urine sample preparation for LC-MS/MS analysis 3 previously published methods for concentrating, purifying and hydrolyzing proteins were tested: (1) precipitation of proteins with ice-cold acetone [15]; (2) concentration and hydrolysis of proteins on filters (filter-aided sample preparation (FASP), Microcon (Millipore) filters were used) [16]; (3) ultrafiltration to purify proteins from low molecular weight components of urine [17]. The main criteria for the optimization of urine sample preparation were the robustness and ease of reproducibility of all steps; and the second the effectiveness of the protocol in the view of the number of detected proteins. It was decided not to use the third method due to its excessive laboriousness and poor reproducibility of the ultrafiltration stage for urine samples with proteinuria.

Table 1. Calculation of the FSGS severity index.

Parameters	Score
eGFR CKD-EPI, mL/min/1.73 m^2	
>60	0
45–59	1
35–45	2
<35	3
Proteinuria, g/24 h	
>2	0
2–3	0.5
3–4	1
4–5	1.5
5–6	2
6–7	2.5
>7	3
Steroid resistance	
Absent	0
Present	1

Comparison of the two remaining methods of sample preparation showed that more different proteins was detected using the acetone precipitation method (Table 2, Figure 1). The first protocol allowed to detect the highest number of proteins in the test samples with proteinuria (5, 7, 10 mg/mL of total protein) and was used for further studies with minor modifications.

Table 2. Efficiency of urine proteins extraction by two methods (Acetone precipitation by ice-cold acetone protein precipitation; FASP—protein concentration and hydrolysis on filters). The number of identified proteins is indicated in Table.

Method	Sample 1 (5 mg/mL)	Sample 1 (7 mg/mL)	Sample 1 (10 mg/mL)
Acetone precipitation	439	520	530
FASP	362	456	441

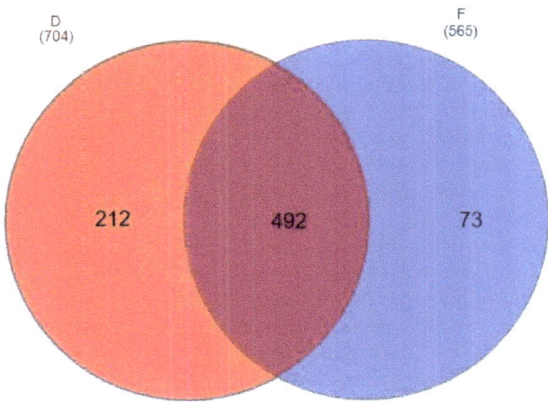

Figure 1. Venn diagram comparing different methods of urine sample preparation for proteomic analysis (D—ice-cold acetone protein precipitation method; F—protein concentration and hydrolysis on filters (FASP)).

2.2. Label Free Analysis of the Urine Proteome for Patients with FSGS and MCD

Comparison of proteomic profiles of patients with FSGS and and MCD showed no significant differences in the protein levels (Figure 2).

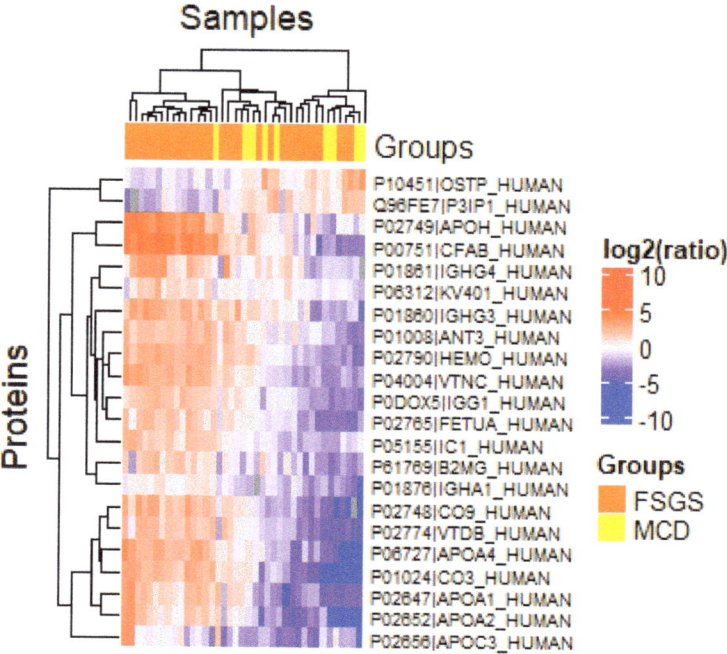

Figure 2. Hierarchical clustering of proteins identified in urine samples of patients with MCD and FSGS. The box denotes log2-transformed values of peak intensity.

However, the FSGS group in total showed a high variability between the patients inside the group. Thus for a comprehensive assessment of this cohort, a special index was introduced, which was calculated as follows: the first score was assigned depending on the level of eGFR, the second—depending on the severity of proteinuria, the third—steroid resistance of the nephrotic syndrome. Steroid-resistance was defined as the absence of a decrease in proteinuria levels after 16 weeks of prednisolone therapy or a decrease by less than 50% of the baseline level.

The renal function was considered "saved", if the estimated glomerular filtration rate, determined by the CKD-EPI formula (eGFR CKD-EPI), was above 60 mL/min/1.73 m^2; and "impaired"—if it was less.

Using this index the patients with FSGS were subdivided into two groups: with a sum of scores of less than 3—mild FSGS (1), and with 3 or higher—severe progressive FSGS (2) (Table 1).

These two subgroups did not differ significantly in the severity of the nephrotic syndrome and renal dysfunction at the onset of the disease. However, in the follow-ups, the patients of the second group were characterized by a more severe FSGS course, meaning impaired renal function and steroid resistance. A wide range of urine proteins was detected at elevated levels in group 2 (Figure 3). For example, an increase in urinary excretion of complement components C3, C4B, factor B, as well as components of the membrane attack complex C8a and C9 were found. The detection of retinol-binding protein 4 and vitamin D-binding proteins in the urine is a consequence of tubulo-interstitial inflammation and injury of the tubular epithelium secondary to glomerular proteinuria [18–21]. Simultaneously with the interstitial inflammation, the accumulation of extracellular matrix (ECM) components and tubulo-interstitial fibrosis are also activated. Alpha-2-HS-glycoprotein can be attributed to the group of proteins responsible for active processes of ECM accumulation, expression of receptors on cells, and ECM protein metabolism (Figure 3).

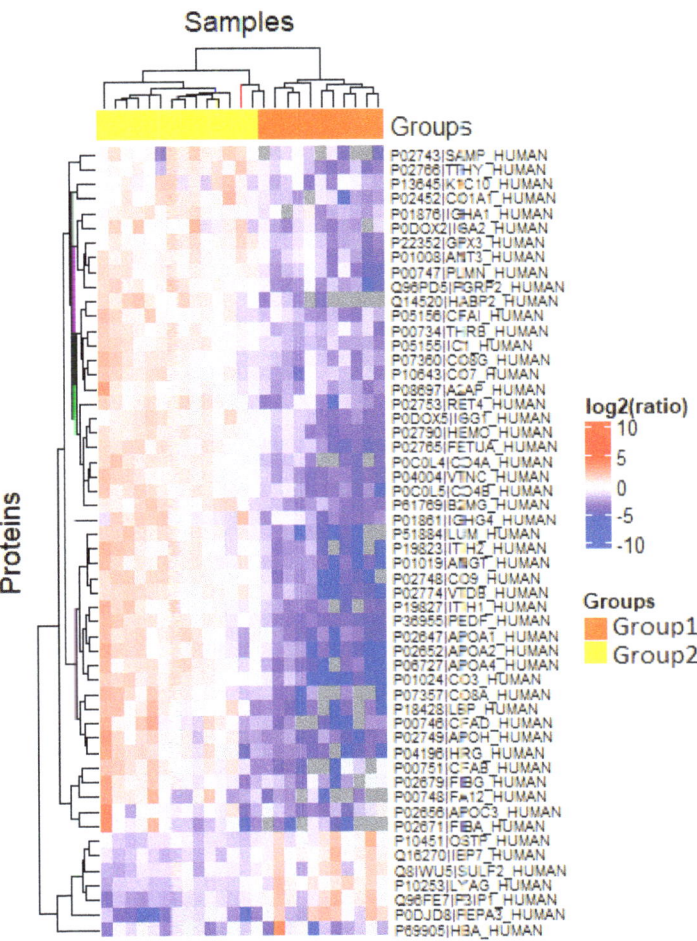

Figure 3. Hierarchical clustering of proteins identified in urine samples of patients with FSGS in group 1 and group 2. The box denotes log2-transformed values of peak intensity.

Considering patients with FSGS separately, we found some minor differences in the protein profiles of patients with saved and impaired renal function. In particular, patients with impaired renal function showed higher levels of thyroid hormone-binding protein, β2-microglobulin, vitamin D-binding protein, alpha-2-HS-glycoprotein (fetuin A) (Figure 4).

Proteins that differ between FSGS group 2 and MCD are by 83% identical to those differentiating the two FSGS groups (Figure 5). It can also be seen that like FSGS group 1 patients samples from MCD patients also have elevated levels of osteopontin and the inhibitor of phosphoinositide-3 kinase, while complement proteins, apolipoproteins, hemopexin, vitronectin, and other proteins in urine remain low (Figure 6).

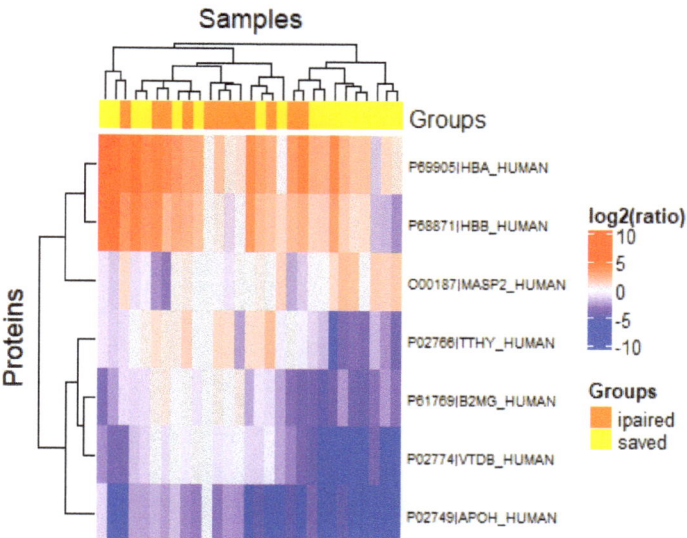

Figure 4. Hierarchical clustering of proteins identified in urine samples of FSGS patients with saved and impaired renal function. The color gradient denotes the log2-transformed ratio of the mean peak intensity values measured in the two groups.

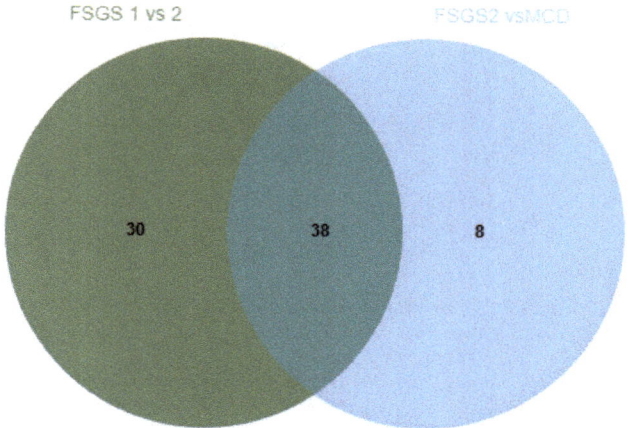

Figure 5. Proteins that differ between FSGS sub groups (1 and 2) and MCD.

Results of the label free analysis were validated using targeted LC-MS based on multiple reaction monitoring (MRM) with stable isotope labelled peptide standards (SIS) available for 47 of the 76 proteins identified as differentiating between at least one pair of groups (Supp. Table S1). Quantitative MRM SIS validation measurements for these 47 proteins revealed 22 proteins with significant differences between at least one of the two group pairs and 14 proteins were validated for both comparisons (Table 3). Also all of the 22 proteins validated by MRM SIS analysis showed the same direction of change as at the discovery stage with label-free LC-MS analysis, i.e., up or down regulation in MCD and FSGS1 against FSGS2. Moreover, it is worth to note that the absolute values of the measured proteins fold changes between groups for the two quantitation methods (label-free vs. MRM SIS) in their orders of magnitude are in good agreement (Supp. Table S1).

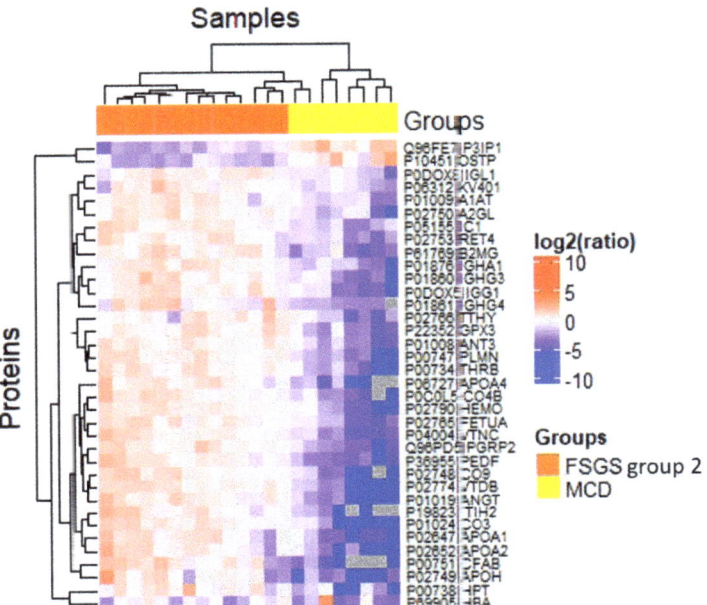

Figure 6. Hierarchical clustering of proteins identified in urine samples of patients with FSGS in group 2 and MCD. The color gradient denotes the log2-transformed ratio of the mean peak intensity values measured in the two groups.

The most important function and source of proteins are presented in Table 4. The levels of the most significant proteins in arbitrary units in FSGS group 1, FSGS group 2 and MCD are shown in Figures 7–9.

Table 3. Urinary proteins selected in this study for validation as perspective potential biomarkers for differentiating patients with MCD and FSGS (group 1—FSGS 1 and group 2—FSGS 2).

| | Protein ID | Description | FSGS 1 vs. FSGS 2 | | FSGS 2 vs. MCD | | Direction Change in FSGS 2 | Average Fold Change between Groups | Validated in at Least 1 Group | Validated in Both Groups |
			TIMS LFQ (Discovery Phase) Significant FSGS 1 vs. FSGS 2 (−10 × LOG(p) > 20)	QQQ SIS MRM (Validation Phase) Significant FSGS 1 vs. FSGS 2 (p < 0.05)	TIMS LFQ (Discovery Phase) Significant FSGS 2 vs. MCD (−10 × LOG(p) > 20)	QQQ SIS MRM (Validation Phase) Significant FSGS 2 vs. MCD (p < 0.05)				
1	P04004	Vitronectin	+	+	+	+	up	10	+	+
2	P06727	Apolipoprotein A-IV	+	+	+	+	up	10	+	+
3	P19823	Inter-alpha-trypsin inhibitor heavy chain H2	+	+	+	+	up	9	+	+
4	P02774	Vitamin D-binding protein	+	+	+	+	up	8	+	+
5	P61769	Beta-2-microglobulin	+	+	+	+	up	8	+	+
6	P0C0L5	Complement C4-B	+	+	+	+	up	7	+	+
7	P02765	Alpha-2-HS-glycoprotein	+	+	+	+	up	6	+	+
8	P02790	Hemopexin	+	+	+	+	up	6	+	+
9	P05155	Plasma protease C1 inhibitor	+	+	+	+	up	6	+	+
10	P02753	Retinol-binding protein 4	+	+	+	+	up	6	+	+
11	P00747	Plasminogen	+	+	+	+	up	6	+	+
12	P00734	Prothrombin	+	+	+	+	up	6	+	+
13	P02766	Transthyretin	+	+	+	+	up	5	+	+
14	P06312	Immunoglobulin kappa variable 4-1	+	+	+	+	up	3	+	+
15	P10909	Clusterin		+	+	+	up	3	+	
16	P02748	Complement component C9	+	+	+		up	11	+	
17	P00751	Complement factor B	+	+	+		up	11	+	
18	P51884	Lumican	+	+		+	up	9	+	

Table 3. Cont.

Protein ID		Description	FSGS 1 vs. FSGS 2			FSGS 2 vs. MCD		Direction Change in FSGS 2	Average Fold Change between Groups	Validated in at Least 1 Group	Validated in Both Groups
			TIMS LFQ (Discovery Phase) Significant FSGS 1 vs. FSGS 2 (−10 × LOG(p) > 20)	QQQ SIS MRM (Validation Phase) Significant FSGS 1 vs. FSGS 2 (p < 0.05)		TIMS LFQ (Discovery Phase) Significant FSGS 2 vs. MCD (−10 × LOG(p) > 20)	QQQ SIS MRM (Validation Phase) Significant FSGS 2 vs. MCD (p < 0.05)				
19	P05156	Complement factor I	+				+	up	6	+	
20	P01034	Cystatin-C	+	+			+	up	3	+	
21	P06396	Gelsolin	+	+				up	2	−	
22	Q08380	Galectin-3-binding protein	+	+				down	6	+	

Table 4. Description of urinary proteins selected in this study for differentiating patients with MCD and FSGS (group 1—FSGS 1 and group 2—FSGS 2).

Protein Group	Description	Clinical/Histological Form	Pathogenetic Role
1	Lumican	FSGS 2 group	Lumican, an extracellular matrix proteoglycan, related to ECM accumulation [22]
2	Vitamin D-binding protein	FSGS 2 group	Potential marker of renal interstitial inflammation and fibrosis, and steroid-resistant nephrotic syndrome [18–20]
3	Plasminogen	FSGS 2 group	Plasma abundant protein. Converts to plasmin, may activate epithelial sodium channels causing sodium retention and edema [23]
4	Hemopexin	FSGS 2 group	Hemopexin induces nephrin-dependent reorganization of the actin cytoskeleton in podocytes [24–26]
5	Prothrombin	FSGS 2 group	Plasma abundant protein
6	Complement factor I	FSGS 2 group	Plasma abundant protein
7	Inter-alpha-trypsin inhibitor heavy chain H2	FSGS 2 group	The inter-alpha-trypsin inhibitors (ITI) are a family of structurally related plasma serine protease inhibitors involved in extracellular matrix stabilization. ITIs are involved in the accumulation of tubulo-interstitial fibrosis in severe forms of FSGS and it activates CD44 + parietal profibrogenic cells in FSGS [27–29]
8	Transthyretin	FSGS 2 group	Plasma abundant protein

Table 4. Cont.

Protein Group	Description	Clinical/Histological Form	Pathogenetic Role
9	Complement factor B	FSGS 2 group	The complement components C4B showed a massive increase in protein abundance in FSGS [30,31]
10	Apolipoprotein A-I	FSGS 2 group	ApoA-1b is noted to be present in the urine of recurrent FSGS possibly correlating with disease activity [32–34]
	Apolipoprotein A-IV	FSGS 2	Plasma abundant protein
11	Complement component C9	FSGS 2	The complement components C1 and C4B, properdin (CFP) showed a massive increase in protein abundance in FSGS [30]
12	Plasma protease C1 inhibitor	FSGS 2	Activation of the C1 complex is under control of the C1-inhibitor. It forms a proteolytically inactive complex with the C1r or C1s proteases. May play a potentially crucial role in regulating important physiological pathways including complement activation, blood coagulation, fibrinolysis and the generation of kinins. Acute phase marker [35]
14	Alpha-2-HS-glycoprotein/Fetuin A	FSGS 2	In proteinuric patients, significant urinary losses of fetuin-A may cause low serum fetuin-A levels. However, its peptides are elevated in the urine of patients with a high percentage of TIF [36,37]
15	Retinol-binding protein 4	FSGS 2	It is filtered through the GBM and reabsorbed in the tubules, reflecting lysosomal proteolysis in the tubular epithelium. Its increase primarily indicates tubular damage. In addition, its level is associated with response to therapy. [21]
16	Vitronectin	FSGS 2	Vitronectin activates integrins, through which podocytes are attached to the GBM. Possibly vitronectin activation is involved in podocyte detachment from GBM [38]
17	Beta-2-microglobulin	FSGS 2	Plasma abundant protein
18	Immunoglobulin kappa variable 4-1	FSGS 2	Plasma abundant protein
19	Gelsolin	FSGS 2	Gelsolin, a Ca-dependent actin-binding protein, induces a change in the orientation of the actin filament, indicating a conformational change in actin [39,40]
20	Cystatin	FSGS 2	Urinary cystatin C as a specific marker of tubular dysfunction [41]
21	Clusterin	FSGS 2	Clusterin facilitates in vivo clearance of extracellular misfolded proteins and apoptosis. Clusterin has been postulated as a down modulator of the inflammatory response [42]
22	Complement C4-B	FSGS 2	The complement components C1 and C4B, properdin (CFP) showed a massive increase in protein abundance in FSGS [30,43]
23	Galectin-3-binding protein	FSGS 1 and MCD	Galectin-3-binding protein is a secreted, hyperglycosylated protein expressed by the majority of human cells. Urinary G3BP is a non-invasive biomarker for clinically and histologically reflecting lupus nephritis activity [44,45]

total 22 proteins

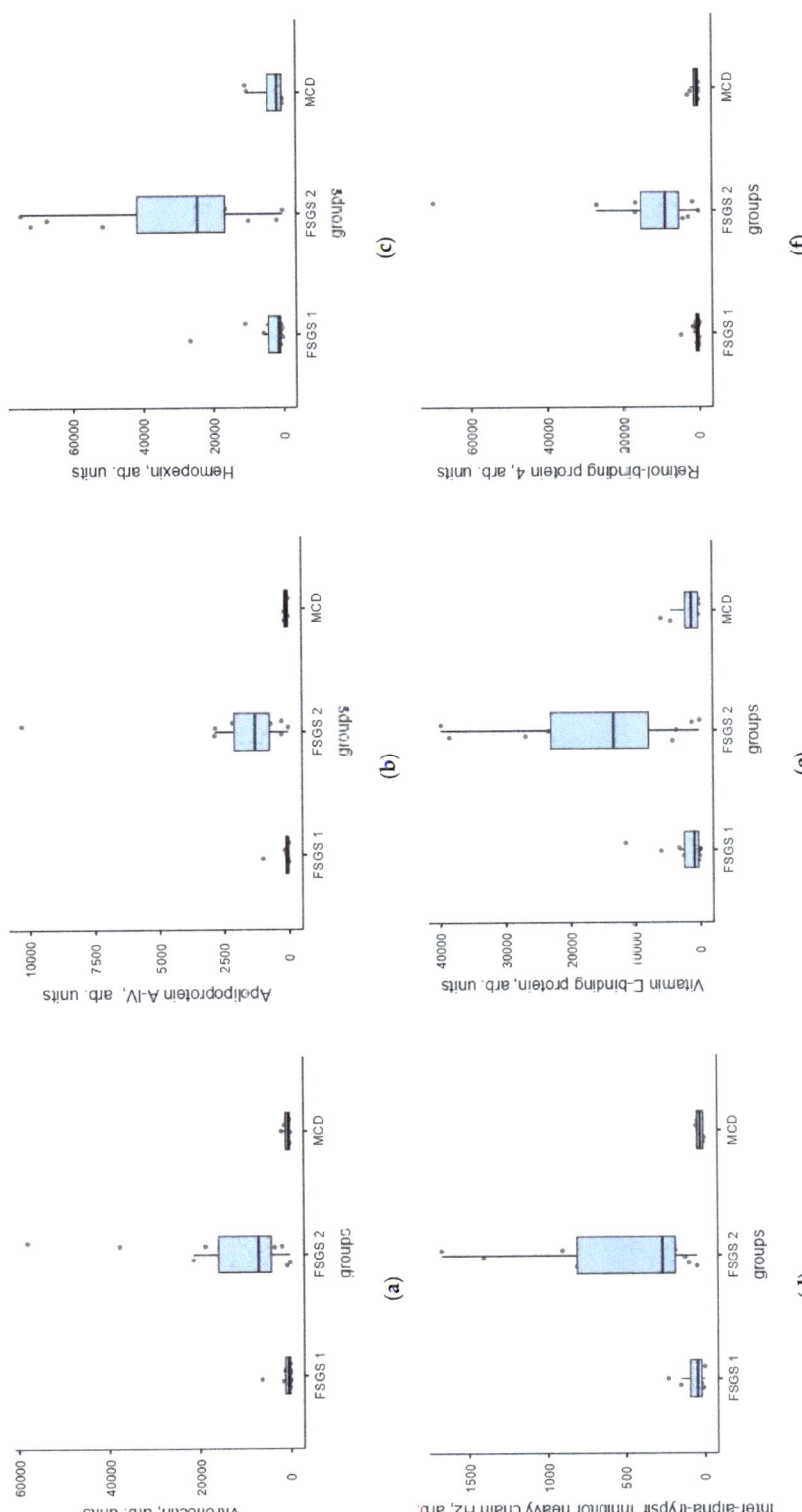

Figure 7. Protein levels in the urine of patients with FSGS (group 1—FSGS 1 and group 2—FSGS 2) and MCD in arb. units: (**a**) Vitronectin, (**b**) Apolipiprotein A-IV, (**c**) Hemopexin, (**d**) Inter-alfa-trypsin inhibitor heavy chain H2; (**e**) Vitamin-D-binding protein; (**f**) Retinol-binding protein.

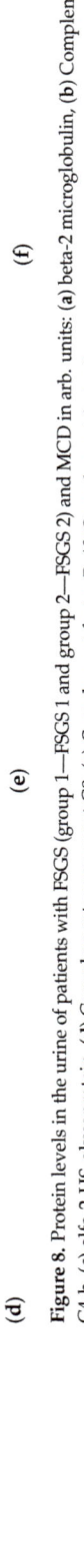

Figure 8. Protein levels in the urine of patients with FSGS (group 1—FSGS 1 and group 2—FSGS 2) and MCD in arb. units: (**a**) beta-2 microglobulin, (**b**) Complement C4-b, (**c**) alfa-2-HS-glycoprotein, (**d**) Complement component C9; (**e**) Complement factor B; (**f**) Complement factor I.

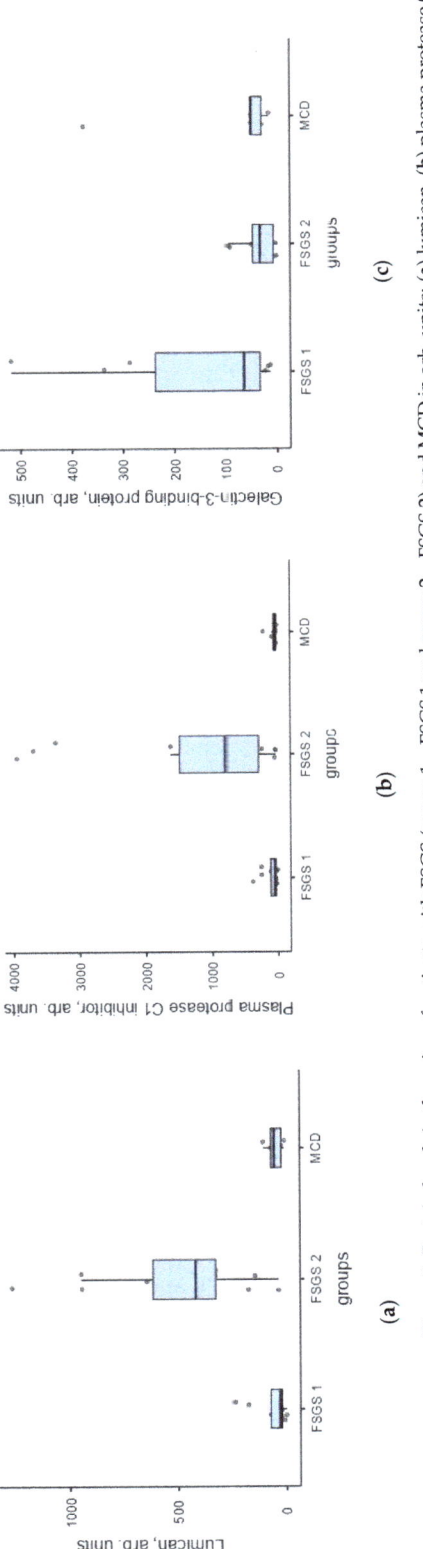

Figure 9. Protein levels in the urine of patients with FSGS (group 1—FSGS 1 and group 2—FSGS 2) and MCD in arb. units: (**a**) lumican, (**b**) plasma protease C1 inhibitor, (**c**) galectin-3-binding protein.

3. Discussion

In the present study a wide variety of proteins was identified and quantitated using two mass-spectrometric approaches in urine samples of patients with FSGS and MCD. No significant differences were found between the proteomic profiles of patients with MCD and a general FSGS group. However, we found that the differences in the urinary protein profiles in FSGS patients were highly dependent on the severity of the disease—thus the patients were subdivided into those with mild FSGS—normal kidney function and steroid-sensitive NS, and those characterized by severe proteinuria, impaired renal function and steroid-resistant NS. These two groups showed significant differences in the levels of 68 proteins. The group with a severe progressive FSGS showed a number of abundant kidney-derived proteins in urine.

Apolipoproteins, vitronectin, hemopexin and gelsolin reflect the process of active damage to podocytes [24–26,32,34,38–40,46–51]. Apolipoprotein A-1 (ApoA-1), a small 28 kDa high-density lipoprotein (HDL) component, is considered as a putative permeability factor [32,34,50]. In a study by Puig-Gay N. et al. an increase in ApoA-1b in the urine was noted immediately before the onset of proteinuria in patients with FSGS recurrence in the transplant [32]. This protein is absent in the urine of healthy individuals and in most patients with glomerular proteinuria caused by other glomerulopathies [34,50]. Our data also suggests a potential role of ApoA in the pathogenesis of primary FSGS. In terms of response to therapy, our data is consistent with that of Kalantari et al. who differentiated steroid-sensitive and steroid-resistant patients with a confirmed FSGS by urine proteome analysis. Among 21 proteins, ApoA-1 was one of the most significant marker between steroid-sensitive and steroid-resistant forms. An increase in ApoA-1 is associated with hyperlipidemia and low-density lipiprotein oxidation [51].

Like Kalantari et al. and other groups of researchers, we established the role of ApoA-1 and some other urinary proteins in diagnosis of FSGS [32,51,52], however, we took a different approach in the study and introduced a specific index that allows us to evaluate not only the response to steroid therapy, but also and the level of proteinuria and kidney function. This approach has been more effective in separating FSGS patients by urinary proteome to two groups. In addition, the group of patients with mild FSGS is comparable to those with MCD, while the proteomic profile of the FSGS group 2 is significantly different, and apparently, this model can be used to assess the severity of the disease.

Among the biomarkers of podocyte damage, we found an increase in the level of hemopexin, which is a glycoprotein with the highest affinity for hem [24]. Hemopexin is currently considered as one of the possible circulating factors of idiopathic FSGS. Hemopexin binds free methemoglobin, further recognized by CD91 on hepatocytes or macrophages in the spleen, liver, and bone marrow [25]. Cell culture studies have shown that hemopexin can induce the redistribution of the actin cytoskeleton in podocytes and development of proteinuria [24–26].

An increase in the urinary excretion of vitronectin in FSGS patients is also of interest, since vitronectin activates β3-integrins, molecules that ensure the fixation of podocytes to the GBM. In case of FSGS, the loss of vitronectin may be associated with the process of podocyte detachment from the glomerular basement membrane [38]. Elevated serum gelsolin aggravates the development of proteinuria and renal dysfunction by F-actin rearrangement, foot process effacement and cell movement [39,40]. These markers of podocyte dysfunction were elevated only in severe steroid-resistant FSGS.

In group 1, patients with mild FSGS, other factors of podocyte dysfunction are detected in the urine—galectin-3—binding protein. It is suggested that this protein is elevated in the kidney tissue in MCD and in the urine in lupus nephritis, and it appears to have a pro-inflammatory function [44,45].

Compared to other glomerulopathies, complement activation processes are not well understood in FSGS. In the second FSGS group we found a significant increase in urinary excretion of complement components C4b, C9, as well as factor B, I and a decrease in CD59, an inhibitor of the membrane attack complex, which indicates the possible role of complement activation associated with stronger damage. Our data is consistent with the results of a study by Huang J. et al., who showed the possibility of systemic complement activation in FSGS patients with increased levels of C3a, C5a, and C5b-9 in blood plasma and urine [43]. Activation of the alternative complement pathway in FSGS may be associated with a poor prognosis [30,31]. On the other hand, an increase in the level of some complement components in the urine may be the result of loss due to severe glomerular filter damage. For a more accurate asessment of complement system disorders in FSGS, the study these components in the blood of these patients is required.

The intensity of accumulation of ECM components is reflected by the excretion of fetuin A, β2 microglobulin, and immunoglobulin chains in the urine of patients with FSGS [37]. The same changes in the protein profiles indicating the damaging processes on tubular cells and accumulation of ECM in the interstitium can be noticed in patients with FSGS with impaired renal function resistant to steroid therapy in our study. An equally important component of disease progression and lack of response to steroid therapy is tubulointerstitial fibrosis and tubular damage in FSGS, which are reflected by an increase in the level in the urine of lumican and cystatin C. These processes are also evidenced by an increase in vitamin D-binding protein and retinol-binding protein 4 in the urine of FSGS patients with impaired renal function [18–21,37]. Simultaneously with the processes of interstitial inflammation, the mechanisms of accumulation of ECM components are activated [18–20]. Our data confirms the results of experimental studies [23,27–29,52]. A study of urinary proteins dynamic changes was conducted on a focal segmental glomerulosclerosis rat model (adriamycin-induced nephropathy) and showed that levels of Fetuin-A and alpha 1 microglobulin may be promising markers for early detection of FSGS. Thus, some proteins or their combinations can change with the disease progression [52]. Inter-alpha-trypsin inhibitor heavy chain H1 and H2 activate the CD44+ parietal epithelial cells, the main profibrogenic cells in the glomeruli, and thus are a powerful stimulus for glomerulosclerotic processes [27–29].

Many urine proteins are of serum origin and enter the urine through the damaged glomerular filter. However, these proteins can cause additional damage and pathology progression. For example, components of the complement system or plasminogen. The conversion of plasminogen to plasmin in urine can activate the epithelial sodium channels and cause sodium retention in the renal tubules—one of the mechanisms of renal edema [23]. Interestingly, in case of MCD and mild FSGS with a favorable prognosis, some of the proteins found in the urine seem to be of a protective nature, such as for example plasma protease C1 [35].

Perez et al. analyzed urinary peptide profiles using magnetic bead-based technology, combined with MALDI-TOF mass spectrometry, in 44 patients diagnosed with MCD and FSGS. In this work the low molecular weight fraction of urine, containing peptides of proteins were analyzed, while in our work the high-molecular protein fraction was isolated. The authors showed that FSGS patients had higher levels of uromodulin fragments and lower concentrations of fragments of A1AT [53]. In 2017 Perez V. et al. also ran a study that included 24 patients with MCD and 25 patients with FSGS and analyzed their urine proteome using two-dimensional gel electrophoresis in combination with MS to detect urinary biomarkers capable of differentiating MCD and FSGS. They showed that urine concentrations of alpha-1 antitrypsin, transferrin, histatin-3, and 39S ribosomal protein L17 were decreased in the FSGS group, and the calretinin level was increased as compared to the MCD group [54]. We did not find any significant differences between the MCD and the general FSGS groups. However, we found an increase in alpha-1 antitrypsin, and other proteins in patients with severe FSGS as compared with those with MCD and mild FSGS, who showed similar profiles of urine proteins.

Thus, we have identified a wide range of proteins that differ in patients with mild course of steroid-sensitive FSGS/MCD and FSGS patients with a progressive steroid-resistant NS. Proteins excreted in the urine reflect damage to several parts of the nephron—podocytes, tubulo-interstitium, accumulation of ECM, complement activation. Patients with MCD and FSGS with steroid-sensitivity and a favorable course of progress showed similar urine protein profiles, while severe progressive FSGS with steroid-resistant nephrotic syndrome were characterized by the early activation of the complement system and profibrogenic mechanisms and accumulation of extracellular matrix components at the onset of the disease.

4. Materials and Methods

4.1. Clinical Characteristics of the Patients

Patients with a confirmed diagnosis of FSGS (n = 30) and MCD (n = 9) were recruited for the study, 20 men and 19 women, aged 19 to 69 years, median 37 years [27,57]. The exclusion criteria were: active urinary infection, diabetes mellitus, obesity, severe arterial hypertension, liver disease, rheumatic systemic diseases, stage 5 chronic kidney disease. Impaired renal function (eGFR CKD-EPI < 60 mL/min/1.73 m^2) was detected in 16 patients, saved kidney function—in 23 (eGFR CKD-EPI > 60 mL/min/1.73 m^2).

The characteristics of the examined patients are presented in Table 5.

Table 5. Characteristics of the patients.

Parameters	FSGS [1] (n = 30)	MCD [2] (n = 9)
Age, years	40 (27.3; 57.8)	35 (28; 59)
Gender (male), n (%)	18 (60)	2 (22.2)
Arterial hypetension, n (%)	22 (73.3)	2 (22.2)
Proteinuria, g/24h	3.66 (2.50; 5.00)	3.24 (2.03; 3.5)
Serum albumin, g/L	26.55 (20.85; 33.68)	29.3 (20.00; 35.80)
Serum protein, g/L	50.8 (40.86; 58.23)	61.4 (46.5; 65.3)
Nephrotic syndrome, n (%)	21 (70)	9 (100)
Creatinine, mkmol/L	109.31 (77.57; 152.65)	85.9 (71.8; 115.9)
eGFR[2] CKD-EPI [3], mL/min/1.73 m^2	64.68 (41.4; 97.09)	73 (55.58; 105.00)
eGFR< 60 mL/min/1.73 m^2, n (%)	12 (40.0)	4 (44.4)
Steroid-resistant NS, n (%)	14 (46.7)	0

[1] Focal segmental glomerulosclerosis, [2] Minimal change disease, [3] Estimated glomerular filtration rate using the CKD-EPI formula. The table shows the median, in brackets—the 1st and 3rd quartiles.

4.2. Urine Sample Preparation for LC-MS/MS

First morning urine samples were collected from all examined patients. The middle portion of freshly passed morning urine was collected in 10 mL test tubes, centrifuged at 3000 rpm for 15 min, the supernatant was frozen in 1 mL aliquots and stored at −20 °C.

Urine aliquots with a volume of 0.1 mL were quickly thawed and 0.5 mL of cold acetone was added to precipitate proteins overnight at −20 °C. Then the samples were centrifuged at 20,000× g for 10 min, the supernatant was removed, the precipitate was dissolved in 50 μL of 8 M urea/200 mM Tris-HCL, pH 8.5. The proteins were restored with 5 mM dithiotreitol for 30 min at 37 °C, alkylated with 20 mM iodoacetamide in the dark for 30 min. Before hydrolysis, 200 μL of deionized water was diluted, trypsin (Trypsin Gold, Promega, Madison, WI, USA) was added in an enzyme-protein ratio of 1:25, incubated overnight at 37 °C. The reaction was stopped by adding formic acid to the final concentration of 1%. Peptides were centrifuged at 18,000× g, the supernatant was left for desalting. Desalting was carried out by solid-phase extraction using plates (Oasis HLB 96-well Microelution Plate, Waters, Beverley, MA, USA). The eluate was lyophilized and dissolved in 0.1% formic acid to a concentration of 0.5mg/mL for further LC-MS/MS analysis.

4.3. Label-Free Untargeted LC-MS/MS Urine Proteomic Analysis

The resulting tryptic peptide mixture was analyzed using liquid chromatography coupled with tandem mass spectrometry (LC-MS/MS) method based on a nano-HPLC Dionex Ultimate3000 system (Thermo Fisher Scientific, Madison, WI, USA) and a timsTOF Pro (Bruker Daltonics, Billerica, MA, USA) mass spectrometer. A packed emitter column (C18, 25 cm × 75 μm 1.6 μm) (Ion Optics, Parkville, Australia) was used to separate peptides at a flow rate of 400 nL/min by gradient elution from 4% to 90% of phase B during 40 min. Mobile phase A consisted of 0.1% formic acid in water and mobile phase B consisted of 0.1% formic acid in acetonitrile.

Mass spectrometric analysis was performed using the parallel accumulation serial fragmentation (PASEF) acquisition method. An electrospray ionization (ESI) source was operated at 1500 V capillary voltage, 500 V end plate offset and 3.0 L/min of dry gas at temperature of 180 °C. The measurements were carried out in the m/z range from 100 to 1700 Th. The ion mobility was in the range from 0.60 to 1.60 V s/cm^2. The total cycle time was 1.88 s and the number of PASEF MS/MS scans was set to 10.

Targeted quantitative LC-MS/MS using multiple reaction monitoring (MRM) with stable isotope labelled peptide standards (SIS).

Targeted quantitative LC-MS analysis was carried out using synthetic stable-isotope labeled internal standard (SIS) and natural (NAT) synthetic proteotypic peptides for measurements of the corresponding proteins in urine. The selected 22 SIS and NAT synthetic peptides had been previously validated for use in LC/MRM-MS experiments [55]. LC-MS parameters, such as the LC gradient and the MRM parameters (Q1 and MRM scans) were adapted and optimized based on the previous studies [56]. The SIS peptide mixture was spiked in each urine sample at a balanced concentration which was optimized in experiments with dilution series of urine samples with proteinuria. Standard curves were generated using NAT and SIS peptide standards with a pooled urine sample as matrix.

All samples were analyzed in duplicate by HPLC-MS system consisting of an ExionLC™ (UHPLC system (ThermoFisher Scientific, Waltham, MA, USA) coupled online to a SCIEX QTRAP 6500+ triple quadrupole mass spectrometer (SCIEX, Toronto, ON, Canada). The loaded sample volume was 10 µL per injection. HPLC separation was carried out using Zorbax Eclipse Plus C18 RRHD column (150 × 2.1 mm, 1.8 µm) (Agilent, Santa Clara, CA, USA) with gradient elution. Mobile phase A was 0.1% FA in water; mobile phase B was 0.1% FA in acetonitrile. LC separation was performed at a flow rate of 0.4 mL/min using a 53 min gradient from 2 to 45% of mobile phase B. Mass-spectrometric measurements were carried out using the MRM acquisition method. The electrospray ionization (ESI) source settings were as follows: ion spray voltage 4000 V, temperature 450 °C, ion source gas 40 L/min. The corresponding transition list for MRM experiments with retention times values and Q1/Q3 masses for each peptide were adapted from the previous studies [56].

Skyline Quantitative Analysis software (version 20.2.0.343, University of Washington) was used for quantitative analysis.

4.4. Data Analysis

The data obtained were analyzed using PEAKS XPro software (BSI, North Waterloo, ON, Canada) according to the following parameters: parent mass error tolerance −20 ppm; fragment mass error tolerance −0.03 Da; enzyme—trypsin; missed cleavages—3; fixed modifications—Carbamidomethyl (C); variable modifications—Oxidation (M), Acetylation (N-term). The search was carried out using the SwissProt Human database. False discovery rate threshold was set to 0.01. Scripts written in R version 3.3.3 [58] and RStudio 1.383 [57] were used for statistical processing of the results.

5. Conclusions

Thus, the proteomic profile of urine from patients with FSGS and MCD is characterized by a large number of excreted proteins, but no significant differences between these two forms were revealed. However, the FSGS patients showed high variability inside the group and clustered into two subgroups, which could be reliably distinguished basing on the proteomic profile. Results of the label free analysis were validated using targeted LC-MS based on multiple reaction monitoring (MRM) with stable isotope labelled peptide standards (SIS) available for 47 of the 76 proteins identified as differentiating between at least one pair of groups. Quantitative MRM SIS validation measurements for these 47 proteins revealed 22 proteins with significant differences between at least one of the two group pairs and 14 proteins were validated for both comparisons. In addition, all of the 22 proteins validated by MRM SIS analysis showed the same direction of change as at the discovery stage with label-free LC-MS analysis, i.e., up or down regulation in MCD and FSGS1 against FSGS2. In patients with severe FSGS 2, the urine proteome panel reflects damage to podocytes (Vitronectin, Hemopexin, Gelsolin, Apolipiprotein A), complement activation (Complement component C4b, C9, Complement factor B and I), and accumulation of the extracellular matrix and tubular damage (Cystatin C, Vitamin D-binding protein, Retinol-binding protein 4, Alpha-2-HS-glycoprotein, Plasma protease C1 inhibitor, Lumican, Clusterin).

Supplementary Materials: The following supporting information can be downloaded at: https://www.mdpi.com/article/10.3390/ijms232012607/s1.

Author Contributions: Conceptualization, N.V.C. and A.S.K.; methodology, D.N.K.; software, A.G.B.; formal analysis, A.G.B. and D.N.K.; investigation, A.V., A.E.B., M.I.I. and N.V.C.; data curation, M.L. and S.M.; writing—original draft preparation, N.V.C. and A.S.K.; writing—review and editing, E.N.N. All authors have read and agreed to the published version of the manuscript.

Funding: This research was funded by the Russian Science Foundation, grant #21-74-20173.

Institutional Review Board Statement: The study was conducted in accordance with the Declaration of Helsinki, and approved by Ethical Committee of the Medical Research and Educational Center of Lomonosov University, Approval Code: Protocol 12/21, Approval Date: 13 December 2021.

Informed Consent Statement: Informed consent was obtained from all subjects involved in the study.

Conflicts of Interest: The authors declare no conflict of interest.

Abbreviations

A1AT	Alpha-1 antitrypsin
ApoA-1	Apolipoprotein A-1
CD2AP	CD2 Associated Protein
CFP	Complement factor P (properdin)
CKD-EPI	Chronic Kidney Disease Epidemiology Collaboration formula
ECM	Extracellular matrix
ESI	Electrospray ionization
eGFR	Estimated glomerular filtration rate
FASP	Filter-aided sample preparation
FSGS	Focal segmental glomerulosclerosis
GBM	Glomerular basement membrane
HDL	High-density lipoprotein
HPLC	High-performance liquid chromatography
LC-MS	Liquid chromatography—mass spectrometry
LC-MS/MS	Liquid chromatography with tandem mass spectrometry
LC/MRM-MS	Liquid chromatography/Multiple reaction monitoring—mass spectrometry
LDL	Low density lipoproteins
MALDI-TOF MS	Matrix-Assisted Laser Desorption—Ionisation-Time of Flight Mass Spectrometry
MCD	Minimal change disease
MRM	Multiple reaction monitoring
MS	Mass spectrometry
NAT	Natural synthetic proteotypic peptides
NS	Nephrotic syndrome
PASEF	Parallel Accumulation—Serial Fragmentation method
PEDF	Pigment epithelium-derived factor
SIS	Stable isotope labelled peptide standards
TIF	Tubulointerstitial fibrosis

References

1. Praga, M.; Morales, E.; Herrero, J.C.; Campos A.P.; Domínguez-Gil, B.; Alegre, R.; Vara, J.; Martínez, M.A. Absence of hypoalbuminemia despite massive proteinuria in focal segmental glomerulosclerosis secondary to hyperfiltration. *Am. J. Kidney Dis.* **1999**, *33*, 52–58. [CrossRef]
2. Rydel, J.J.; Korbet, S.M.; Borok, R.Z.; Schwartz, M.M. Focal segmental glomerular sclerosis in adults: Presentation, course and response to treatment. *Am. J. Kidney Dis.* **1995**, *25*, 534–542. [CrossRef]
3. Vivarelli, M.; Massella, L.; Ruggiero, B.; Emma, F. Minimal Change Disease. *Clin. J. Am. Soc. Nephrol.* **2016**, *12*, 332–345. [CrossRef] [PubMed]
4. Chun, M.J.; Korbet, S.M.; Schwartz, M.M.; Lewis, E.J. Focal Segmental Glomerulosclerosis in Nephrotic Adults: Presentation, Prognosis, and Response to Therapy of the Histologic Variants. *J. Am. Soc. Nephrol.* **2004**, *15*, 2169–2177. [CrossRef]
5. Nakayama, M.; Katafuchi, R.; Yanase, T.; Ikeda, K.; Tanaka, H.; Fujimi, S. Steroid responsiveness and frequency of relapse in adult-onset minimal change nephrotic syndrome. *Am. J. Kidney Dis.* **2002**, *39*, 503–512. [CrossRef]
6. Korbet, S.M.; Schwartz, M.M.; Lewis, E.J. Primary Focal Segmental Glomerulosclerosis: Clinical Course and Response to Therapy. *Am. J. Kidney Dis.* **1994**, *23*, 773–783. [CrossRef]
7. Wehrmann, M.; Bohle, A.; Held, H.; Schumm, G.; Kendziorra, H.; Pressler, H. Long-term prognosis of focal sclerosing glomerulonephritis. An analysis of 250 cases with particular regard to tubulointerstitial changes. *Clin. Nephrol.* **1990**, *33*, 115–122.
8. Sethi, S.; Zand, L.; Nasr, S.H.; Glassock, R.J.; Fervenza, F.C. Focal and segmental glomerulosclerosis: Clinical and kidney biopsy correlations. *Clin. Kidney J.* **2014**, *7*, 531–537. [CrossRef]
9. Cunningham, R.; Ma, D.; Li, L. Mass spectrometry-based proteomics and peptidomics for systems biology and biomarker discovery. *Front. Biol.* **2012**, *7*, 313–335. [CrossRef]
10. Di Meo, A.; Pasic, M.D.; Yousef, G.M. Proteomics and peptidomics: Moving toward precision medicine in urological malignancies. *Oncotarget* **2016**, *7*, 52460–52474. [CrossRef]
11. Feist, P.; Hummon, A.B. Proteomic Challenges: Sample Preparation Techniques for Microgram-Quantity Protein Analysis from Biological Samples. *Int. J. Mol. Sci.* **2015**, *16*, 3537–3563. [CrossRef]
12. Filip, S.; Pontillo, C.; Schanstra, J.P.; Vlahou, A.; Mischak, H.; Klein, J. Urinary proteomics and molecular determinants of chronic kidney disease: Possible link to proteases. *Expert Rev. Proteom.* **2014**, *11*, 535–548. [CrossRef]
13. Mischak, H.; Delles, C.; Vlahou, A.; Vanholder, R. Proteomic biomarkers in kidney disease: Issues in development and implementation. *Nat. Rev. Nephrol.* **2015**, *11*, 221–232. [CrossRef]
14. Decramer, S.; de Peredo, A.G.; Breuil, B.; Mischak, H.; Monsarrat, B.; Bascands, J.-L.; Schanstra, J.P. Urine in Clinical Proteomics. *Mol. Cell. Proteom.* **2008**, *7*, 1850–1862. [CrossRef] [PubMed]
15. Ding, H.; Fazelinia, H.; Spruce, L.A.; Weiss, D.A.; Zderic, S.A.; Seeholzer, S.H. Urine Proteomics: Evaluation of Different Sample Preparation Workflows for Quantitative, Reproducible, and Improved Depth of Analysis. *J. Proteome Res.* **2020**, *19*, 1857–1862. [CrossRef] [PubMed]
16. Wiśniewski, J. Filter-Aided Sample Preparation: The Versatile and Efficient Method for Proteomic Analysis. *Methods Enzym.* **2017**, *585*, 15–27. [CrossRef]
17. Percy, A.J.; Yang, J.; Hardie, D.B.; Chambers, A.G.; Tamura-Wells, J.; Borchers, C.H. Precise quantitation of 136 urinary proteins by LC/MRM-MS using stable isotope labeled peptides as internal standards for biomarker discovery and/or verification studies. *Methods* **2015**, *81*, 24–33. [CrossRef] [PubMed]
18. Bennett, M.R.; Pordal, A.; Haffner, C.; Pleasant, L.; Ma, Q.; Devarajan, P. Urinary Vitamin D-Binding Protein as a Biomarker of Steroid-Resistant Nephrotic Syndrome. *Biomark. Insights* **2016**, *11*, 1–6. [CrossRef]
19. Mirković, K.; Doorenbos, C.R.C.; Dam, W.A.; Heerspink, H.J.L.; Slagman, M.C.J.; Nauta, F.L.; Kramer, A.B.; Gansevoort, R.T.; Borra, J.V.D.; Navis, G.; et al. Urinary Vitamin D Binding Protein: A Potential Novel Marker of Renal Interstitial Inflammation and Fibrosis. *PLoS ONE* **2013**, *8*, e55887. [CrossRef]
20. Choudhary, A.; Mohanraj, P.S.; Krishnamurthy, S.; Rajappa, M. Association of Urinary Vitamin D Binding Protein and Neutrophil Gelatinase-Associated Lipocalin with Steroid Responsiveness in Idiopathic Nephrotic Syndrome of Childhood. *Saudi J. Kidney Dis. Transpl.* **2020**, *31*, 946–956. [CrossRef]
21. Kirsztajn, G.M.; Nishida, S.K.; Silva, M.S.; Ajzen, H.; Pereira, A.B. Urinary retinol-binding protein as a prognostic marker in the treatment of nephrotic syndrome. *Nephron Exp. Nephrol.* **2000**, *86*, 109–114. [CrossRef]
22. Feng, S.; Gao, Y.; Yin, D.; Lv, L.; Wen, Y.; Li, Z.; Wang, B.; Wu, M.; Liu, B. Identification of Lumican and Fibromodulin as Hub Genes Associated with Accumulation of Extracellular Matrix in Diabetic Nephropathy. *Kidney Blood Press Res.* **2021**, *46*, 275–285. [CrossRef]
23. Svenningsen, P.; Bistrup, C.; Friis, U.G.; Bertog, M.; Haerteis, S.; Krueger, B.; Stubbe, J.; Jensen, O.N.; Thiesson, H.C.; Uhrenholt, T.R.; et al. Plasmin in Nephrotic Urine Activates the Epithelial Sodium Channel. *J. Am. Soc. Nephrol.* **2009**, *20*, 299–310. [CrossRef]
24. Lennon, R.; Singh, A.; Welsh, G.I.; Coward, R.J.; Satchell, S.; Ni, L.; Mathieson, P.W.; Bakker, W.W.; Saleem, M.A. Hemopexin Induces Nephrin-Dependent Reorganization of the Actin Cytoskeleton in Podocytes. *J. Am. Soc. Nephrol.* **2008**, *19*, 2140–2149. [CrossRef]
25. Pukajło-Marczyk, A.; Zwolińska, D. Involvement of Hemopexin in the Pathogenesis of Proteinuria in Children with Idiopathic Nephrotic Syndrome. *J. Clin. Med.* **2021**, *10*, 3160. [CrossRef]

26. Kapojos, J.J.; Poelstra, K.; Borghuis, T.; Banas, B.; Bakker, W.W. Regulation of Plasma Hemopexin Activity by Stimulated Endothelial or Mesangial Cells. *Nephron Exp. Nephrol.* **2004**, *96*, p1–p10. [CrossRef]
27. Mambetsariev, N.; Mirzapoiazova, T.; Mambetsariev, B.; Sammani, S.; Lennon, F.E.; Garcia, J.G.; Singleton, P.A. Hyaluronic Acid Binding Protein 2 Is a Novel Regulator of Vascular Integrity. *Arter. Thromb. Vasc. Biol.* **2010**, *30*, 483–490. [CrossRef]
28. Kaul, A.; Singampalli, K.L.; Parikh, U.M.; Yu, L.; Keswani, S.G.; Wang, X. Hyaluronan, a double-edged sword in kidney diseases. *Pediatr. Nephrol.* **2021**, *37*, 735–744. [CrossRef]
29. Merchant, M.L.; Barati, M.T.; Caster, D.J.; Hata, J.L.; Hobeika, L.; Coventry, S.; Brier, M.E.; Wilkey, D.W.; Li, M.; Rood, I.M.; et al. Proteomic Analysis Identifies Distinct Glomerular Extracellular Matrix in Collapsing Focal Segmental Glomerulosclerosis. *J. Am. Soc. Nephrol.* **2020**, *31*, 1883–1904. [CrossRef]
30. Thurman, J.M.; Wong, M.; Renner, B.; Frazer-Abel, A.; Giclas, P.C.; Joy, M.S.; Jalal, D.; Radeva, M.K.; Gassman, J.; Gipson, D.S.; et al. Complement Activation in Patients with Focal Segmental Glomerulosclerosis. *PLoS ONE* **2015**, *10*, e0136558. [CrossRef]
31. Zoshima, T.; Hara, S.; Yamagishi, M.; Pastan, I.; Matsusaka, T.; Kawano, M.; Nagata, M. Possible role of complement factor H in podocytes in clearing glomerular subendothelial immune complex deposits. *Sci. Rep.* **2019**, *9*, 7857. [CrossRef]
32. Puig-Gay, N.; Jacobs-Cacha, C.; Sellarès, J.; Guirado, L.; Roncero, F.G.; Jiménez, C.; Zárraga, S.; Paul, J.; Lauzurica, R.; Alonso, Á.; et al. Apolipoprotein A-Ib as a biomarker of focal segmental glomerulosclerosis recurrence after kidney transplantation: Diagnostic performance and assessment of its prognostic value—A multi-centre cohort study. *Transpl. Int.* **2018**, *32*, 313–322. [CrossRef]
33. Kopp, J.B.; Winkler, C.A.; Zhao, X.; Radeva, M.K.; Gassman, J.J.; D'Agati, V.D.; Nast, C.C.; Wei, C.; Reiser, J.; Guay-Woodford, L.M.; et al. Clinical Features and Histology of Apolipoprotein L1-Associated Nephropathy in the FSGS Clinical Trial. *J. Am. Soc. Nephrol.* **2015**, *26*, 1443–1448. [CrossRef]
34. Jacobs-Cachá, C.; Puig-Gay, N.; Helm, D.; Rettel, M.; Sellarès, J.; Meseguer, A.; Savitski, M.M.; Moreso, F.J.; Soler, M.J.; Seron, D.; et al. A misprocessed form of Apolipoprotein A-I is specifically associated with recurrent Focal Segmental Glomerulosclerosis. *Sci. Rep.* **2020**, *10*, 1159. [CrossRef]
35. Bukosza, E.N.; Kornauth, C.; Hummel, K.; Schachner, H.; Huttary, N.; Krieger, S.; Nöbauer, K.; Oszwald, A.; Fazeli, E.R.; Kratochwill, K.; et al. ECM Characterization Reveals a Massive Activation of Acute Phase Response during FSGS. *Int. J. Mol. Sci.* **2020**, *21*, 2095. [CrossRef]
36. Catanese, L.; Siwy, J.; Mavrogeorgis, E.; Amann, K.; Mischak, H.; Beige, J.; Rupprecht, H. A Novel Urinary Proteomics Classifier for Non-Invasive Evaluation of Interstitial Fibrosis and Tubular Atrophy in Chronic Kidney Disease. *Proteomes* **2021**, *9*, 32. [CrossRef]
37. Fischer, D.-C.; Schaible, J.; Wigger, M.; Staude, H.; Drueckler, E.; Kundt, G.; Haffner, D. Reduced Serum Fetuin-A in Nephrotic Children: A Consequence of Proteinuria? *Am. J. Nephrol.* **2011**, *34*, 373–380. [CrossRef]
38. Shen, J.; Zhu, Y.; Zhang, S.; Lyu, S.; Lyu, C.; Feng, Z.; Hoyle, D.L.; Wang, Z.Z.; Cheng, T. Vitronectin-activated $\alpha v \beta 3$ and $\alpha v \beta 5$ integrin signalling specifies haematopoietic fate in human pluripotent stem cells. *Cell Prolif.* **2021**, *54*, e13012. [CrossRef]
39. Urosev, D.; Ma, Q.; Tan, A.L.C.; Robinson, R.C.; Burtnick, L.D. The Structure of Gelsolin Bound to ATP. *J. Mol. Biol.* **2006**, *357*, 765–772. [CrossRef]
40. Prochniewicz, E.; Zhang, Q.; Janmey, P.A.; Thomas, D.D. Cooperativity in F-Actin: Binding of Gelsolin at the Barbed End Affects Structure and Dynamics of the Whole Filament. *J. Mol. Biol.* **1996**, *260*, 756–766. [CrossRef]
41. Conti, M.; Moutereau, S.; Zater, M.; Lallali, K.; Durrbach, A.; Manivet, P.; Eschwège, P.; Loric, S. Urinary cystatin C as a specific marker of tubular dysfunction. *Clin. Chem Lab. Med.* **2006**, *44*, 288–291. [CrossRef] [PubMed]
42. Wyatt, A.R.; Yerbury, J.J.; Berghofer, P.; Greguric, I.; Katsifis, A.; Dobson, C.M.; Wilson, M.R. Clusterin facilitates in vivo clearance of extracellular misfolded proteins. *Cell. Mol. Life Sci.* **2011**, *68*, 3919–3931. [CrossRef] [PubMed]
43. Huang, J.; Cui, Z.; Gu, Q.-H.; Zhang, Y.-M.; Qu, Z.; Wang, X.; Wang, F.; Cheng, X.-Y.; Meng, L.-Q.; Liu, G.; et al. Complement activation profile of patients with primary focal segmental glomerulosclerosis. *PLoS ONE* **2020**, *15*, e0234934. [CrossRef] [PubMed]
44. Ding, H.; Shen, Y.; Lin, C.; Qin, L.; He, S.; Dai, M.; Okitsu, S.L.; DeMartino, J.A.; Guo, Q.; Shen, N. Urinary galectin-3 binding protein (G3BP) as a biomarker for disease activity and renal pathology characteristics in lupus nephritis. *Arthritis Res. Ther.* **2022**, *24*, 77. [CrossRef]
45. Ostalska-Nowicka, D.; Nowicki, M.; Kondraciuk, B.; Partyka, M.; Samulak, D.; Witt, M. Expression of galectin-3 in nephrotic syndrome glomerulopaties in children. *Folia Histochem. Cytobiol.* **2009**, *47*, 315–322. [CrossRef]
46. Sidenius, N.; Andolfo, A.; Fesce, R.; Blasi, F. Urokinase regulates vitronectin binding by controlling urokinase receptor oligomerization. *J. Biol. Chem.* **2002**, *277*, 27982–27990. [CrossRef]
47. Chavakis, T.; Kanse, S.N.; Yutzy, B.; Lijnen, H.R.; Preissner, K.T. Vitronectin Concentrates Proteolytic Activity on the Cell Surface and Extracellular Matrix by Trapping Soluble Urokinase Receptor-Urokinase Complexes. *Blood* **1998**, *91*, 2305–2312. [CrossRef]
48. Nafar, M.; Kalantari, S.; Samavat, S.; Rezaei-Tavirani, M.; Rutishuser, D.; Zubarev, R.A. The Novel Diagnostic Biomarkers for Focal Segmental Glomerulosclerosis. *Int. J. Nephrol.* **2014**, *2014*, 574261. [CrossRef]
49. Medyńska, A.; Chrzanowska, J.; Kościelska-Kasprzak, K.; Bartoszek, D.; Żabińska, M.; Zwolińska, D. Alpha-1 Acid Glycoprotein and Podocin mRNA as Novel Biomarkers for Early Glomerular Injury in Obese Children. *J. Clin. Med.* **2021**, *10*, 4129. [CrossRef]
50. Gomo, Z.A.; Henderson, L.O.; Myrick, J.E. High-density lipoprotein apolipoproteins in urine: I. Characterization in normal subjects and in patients with proteinuria. *Clin. Chem.* **1988**, *34*, 1775–1780. [CrossRef]

51. Kalantari, S.; Nafar, M.; Rutishauser, D.; Samavat, S.; Rezaei-Tavirani, M.; Yang, H.; Zubarev, R.A. Predictive urinary biomarkers for steroid-resistant and steroid-sensitive focal segmental glomerulosclerosis using high resolution mass spectrometry and multivariate statistical analysis. *BMC Nephrol.* **2014**, *15*, 141. [CrossRef]
52. Zhao, M.; Li, M.; Li, X.; Shao, C.; Yin, J.; Gao, Y. Dynamic changes of urinary proteins in a focal segmental glomerulosclerosis rat model. *Proteome Sci.* **2014**, *12*, 42. [CrossRef]
53. Pérez, V.; Ibernón, M.; López, D.; Pastor, M.C.; Navarro, M.; Navarro-Muñoz, M.; Bonet, J.; Romero, R. Urinary Peptide Profiling to Differentiate between Minimal Change Disease and Focal Segmental Glomerulosclerosis. *PLoS ONE* **2014**, *9*, e87731. [CrossRef]
54. Pérez, V.; López, D.; Boixadera, E.; Ibernón, M.; Espinal, A.; Bonet, J.; Romero, R. Comparative differential proteomic analysis of minimal change disease and focal segmental glomerulosclerosis. *BMC Nephrol.* **2017**, *18*, 49. [CrossRef]
55. Kuzyk, M.A.; Parker, C.E.; Domanski, D.; Borchers, C.H. Development of MRM-based assays for the absolute quantitation of plasma proteins. *Methods Mol. Biol.* **2013**, *1023*, 53–82. [CrossRef]
56. Kononikhin, A.S.; Zakharova, N.V.; Semenov, S.D.; Bugrova, A.E.; Brzhozovskiy, A.G.; Indeykina, M.I.; Fedorova, Y.B.; Kolykhalov, I.V.; Strelnikova, P.A.; Ikonnikova, A.Y.; et al. Prognosis of Alzheimer's Disease Using Quantitative Mass Spectrometry of Human Blood Plasma Proteins and Machine Learning. *Int. J. Mol. Sci.* **2022**, *23*, 7907. [CrossRef]
57. R Studio Team. *RStudio: Integrated Development for R*; RStudio, PBC: Boston, MA, USA, 2020. Available online: http://www.rstudio.com/ (accessed on 6 July 2022).
58. R Core Team. *R: A Language and Environment for Statistical Computing*; R Foundation for Statistical Computing: Vienna, Austria, 2021. Available online: https://www.R-project.org/ (accessed on 6 July 2022).

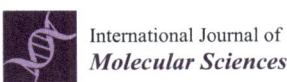

Review

Short-Chain Fatty Acids in Chronic Kidney Disease: Focus on Inflammation and Oxidative Stress Regulation

Giorgia Magliocca [1,2], Pasquale Mone [3,4,5], Biagio Raffaele Di Iorio [6], August Heidland [7] and Stefania Marzocco [1,*]

1. Department of Pharmacy, University of Salerno, 84084 Fisciano, Italy; gmagliocca@unisa.it
2. PhD Program in Drug Discovery & Development at University of Salerno, 84084 Fisciano, Italy
3. Department of Medicine, Division of Cardiology, Albert Einstein College of Medicine, 1300 Morris Park Avenue, New York NY 10461, USA; pasquale.mone@einsteinmed.edu
4. ASL Avellino, 83100 Avellino, Italy
5. Department of Mental and Physical Health and Preventive Medicine, University of Campania "Luigi Vanvitelli", 80138 Naples, Italy
6. UOC Nephrology AORN "San Giuseppe Moscati", C.da Amoretta, 83100 Avellino, Italy; br.diiorio@gmail.com
7. Department of Internal Medicine and KfH Kidney Center University of Würzburg, KfH Kidney Center Würzburg, 97080 Würzburg, Germany; august.heidland@t-online.de
* Correspondence: smarzocco@unisa.it; Tel.: +39-089-969250

Abstract: Chronic Kidney Disease (CKD) is a debilitating disease associated with several secondary complications that increase comorbidity and mortality. In patients with CKD, there is a significant qualitative and quantitative alteration in the gut microbiota, which, consequently, also leads to reduced production of beneficial bacterial metabolites, such as short-chain fatty acids. Evidence supports the beneficial effects of short-chain fatty acids in modulating inflammation and oxidative stress, which are implicated in CKD pathogenesis and progression. Therefore, this review will provide an overview of the current knowledge, based on pre-clinical and clinical evidence, on the effect of SCFAs on CKD-associated inflammation and oxidative stress.

Keywords: chronic kidney disease; short-chain fatty acids; oxidative stress; inflammation; uremic toxins

1. Introduction

The human intestinal tract hosts different microbial communities playing a pivotal role in maintaining health conditions. Gut microbiota imbalance can also exacerbate some actions promoting a cascade of metabolic abnormalities and vice versa. In numerous diseases, such as obesity, type 2 diabetes, as well as cardiovascular and auto-immune diseases, a marked alteration in microbiota composition and functions occurs [1,2]. Moreover, in Chronic Kidney Disease (CKD) patients, the gut microbiota is quantitatively and qualitatively changed with respect to healthy subjects contributing to uremic syndrome and CKD-related complications [3–5]. In CKD patients, microbiota metabolite changes exert major consequences. In fact, metabolites generally proven to promote health—particularly short-chain fatty acids (SCFAs)—are reduced while uremic toxins, such as indoles, ammonia, and trimethylamine N-oxide, produced by gut microbiota, accumulate—both for their overproduction and for the reduced excretion by impaired kidney function—thus enhancing CKD development and progression [6–9]. Lowered SCFAs production results in impaired CKD due to gut dysbiosis and also a decreased consumption of dietary fibre that, on the one hand, reduces SCFAs production and on the other are, involved in increased amino nitrogen, which can be transformed into uremic toxins by gut microbiota [10]. The accumulation of these gut-derived compounds correlates with systemic inflammation and protein wasting and enhances cardiovascular complications in these patients [11]. The dysbiotic gut microbiome in CKD is associated with immune dysregulation, insulin resistance, cardiovascular disease, as well as local (gut) and systemic inflammation and oxidative stress conditions [12–15]. Thus, there has been a great interest in potentially healthy microbiota metabolites such as SCFAs, which levels result in impaired CKD.

SCFAs are produced in the distal small intestine and the colon by anaerobic bacteria and are the end products of fermentation from complex carbohydrates that are indigestible by the human host [16]. The three major SCFAs, consisting of one to six carbon atoms, produced by gut bacteria are acetic (two carbons), propionic (three carbons), and butyric acids (four carbons). SCFAs contribute to the health of the gut (microbiome and mucosa) and the overall health of the host, with properties including anti-diabetic, anti-cancer, antibacterial, anti-inflammatory, and anti-oxidative effects [17,18]. On the other hand, lower SCFA levels contribute to different diseases such as inflammatory bowel disease [19,20], rheumatoid arthritis, and multiple sclerosis [21,22]. Moreover, SCFAs supplementation exerts anti-inflammatory actions, both at the intestinal and cardiovascular levels [23,24], and influences immune reactions [25–27]. Considering the anti-inflammatory potential of SCFAs, their reduced levels in CKD, and that the CKD is associated with systemic, chronic microinflammation and oxidative stress conditions that contribute to both the disease progression and to its related complications, SCFAs and SCFAs producing microorganisms could be one of the missing pieces of the puzzle in CKD-associated inflammation and oxidative stress. This review will provide an overview of the current knowledge on the effect of SCFAs on CKD-associated inflammation and oxidative stress.

2. Short-Chain Fatty Acids (SCFAs)

Short-chain fatty acids (SCFA) are the end products of microbial fermentation activity. Dietary fibre escapes digestion and absorption in the small intestine and is metabolised in the colon and cecum, from which mainly acetate, propionate, butyrate, and formate are generated; while lactate is obtained from the fermentation of selected non-digestible carbohydrates, which are often also rapidly metabolised into acetate, propionate, and butyrate [28,29]. Within the intestinal microbial flora, the bacterial species most involved in SCFAs production are *Butyricicoccus* spp., *Faecalibacterium prausnitzii*, *Roseburia* spp., *Bacterioides* spp. and *Bifidobacterium*, converting dietary fibre in the gut into monosaccharides through a series of reactions mediated by specific enzymes. Acetate can be produced via acetyl–CoA or the Wood–Ljungdahl pathway; propionate is produced by the conversion of succinate to methylmalonyl-CoA via the succinate pathway or can be synthesised from acrylate with lactate as a precursor via the acrylate pathway and via the propanediol pathway; butyrate is formed either via the classical pathway by reduction by phosphotransbutyl kinase and butyrate kinase, or via the butyryl-CoA/acetate CoA-transferase pathway. In addition, some microbes in the gut can use both lactate and acetate to synthesise butyrate [30,31]. However, when fermentable fibres are scarce, microbes exploit less favourable energy sources for SCFAs production, such as amino acids from dietary or endogenous proteins, or dietary fat, also producing branched-chain fatty acids [32,33]. Although the intestinal lumen is the main site of SCFA production, their concentration varies both throughout the intestinal tract and systemically [34]. Butyrate is absorbed by the intestinal epithelium and consumed locally because it is the main energy source of colonocytes [35], while propionate and acetate cross the portal vein so that the former is metabolised in the liver [36], and the latter remains the most abundant SCFAs in the peripheral circulation, reaching organs such as the brain, pancreas, muscle, and adipose tissue, where it regulates several physiological functions [37]. In fact, SCFAs also play a key role in organs outside the digestive tract because numerous transmembrane proteins, receptors and transporters that specifically bind SCFAs and other monocarboxylic acids are expressed in a wide variety of cells [38,39]. Thus, SCFAs are associated with human health benefits for both their metabolic and/or structural properties and their signalling properties.

Mechanism, Role and Functions of SCFAs

SCFAs are versatile molecules involved in cell signalling in a wide range of physiological and pathological conditions [40]. Numerous pieces of evidence report that the disruption of SCFAs generated by the gut microbiota is associated with diseases, including inflammatory bowel disease, obesity, diabetes mellitus type 1 and 2, autism, major depression, colon cancer, and renal diseases [41,42]. The functions of SCFAs are mainly related to their activation of free fatty acid receptors (FFARs) belonging to the family of orphan G-protein-coupled receptors (GPCRs) and olfactory receptors (Olfr) or as histone deacetylase inhibitors (HDACs). FFARs are G-protein-coupled transmembrane receptors that bind fatty acids with carbon chains of different lengths. In particular, SCFAs are ligands of the GPR41 and GPR109A receptors coupled to the Gi/0 protein and the GPR43 receptor coupled to both Gi/0 and Gq proteins. GPR109A responds predominantly to butyrate, which also has a high affinity for the GPR43 receptor, while propionate is a potent agonist for both GPR41 and GPR43; acetate is more selective for the GPR43 receptor. Furthermore, both acetate, propionate, and butyrate also bind to the Olfr78 receptor [39,43]. In addition to their metabolic and structural roles, SCFAs possess several metabolic and signalling properties. Indeed, after intestinal microbial fermentation, they can act locally (Table 1; [44–46]). In the intestine, butyrate is used more as an energy source for colonocytes and can be converted into glucose by intestinal gluconeogenesis, leading to satiety and a decrease in hepatic glucose production. Butyrate binds to the GPR109A receptor, which is mainly expressed intestinally on the apical membrane of colonic and small intestinal epithelial cells, and whose activation is responsible for both the activation of the NLRP3 inflammasome, which is essential for intestinal homeostasis, and anti-inflammatory effects through increased IL (Interleukin)-18. Butyrate also binds to the GPR109A expressed on dendritic cells (DCs) and induces the differentiation of naive T cells into Th1 and Th17 cells and the increase in IL-10 in T-Reg cells providing an anti-inflammatory function and enhancing the intestinal immune response. Moreover, in the intestine, but to a lesser extent, acetate and propionate bind to the GPR43 receptor, whose signalling functions are mediated by the Gq protein to induce the release of pancreatic peptide YY (PYY) and Glucagon-like peptide 1 (GLP-1) and influence satiety and intestinal transit. The binding of propionate and acetate to the intestinal receptor GPR43 also induces the activation of the transcription factor forkhead box P3 (FOXP3) by regulatory T lymphocytes, resulting in cell expansion and differentiation into mast cells, neutrophils, and eosinophils, respectively, implementing intestinal immunity. Then, SCFAs bind to the receptors on the immune cells of the lamina propria and enteric nervous system cells, where propionate activates the GPR41 receptor and stimulates motility and secretory activity in the colon and intestine [24,47–50]. In addition to acting locally, SCFAs from the gut can also be absorbed into the bloodstream either through anion exchange between SCFAs and HCO_3 or through the membrane by a diffusive process promoted by the pH gradient during the diffusion of protonated SCFAs [51]. Systemically, however, acetate concentrations are higher than propionate and butyrate, and the functions of SCFAs mainly depend on the binding to the GPR43 and GPR41 receptors, inducing beneficial effects throughout the body. The GPR43 receptor has a potential role in inflammation and is most highly expressed in immune cells, adipose tissue and the subset of large renal vessels, renal afferent arteriole and juxtaglomerular apparatus, where it is involved in the regulation of renin secretion. The GPR41 receptor is expressed in the peripheral nervous system and adipose tissue and at low levels in the spleen, lymph nodes, bone marrow, peripheral blood mononuclear cells, and blood vessel endothelial cells. In the bone marrow, the activation of GPR41 induces the hematopoiesis of DCs, and in the brain, it reduces the permeability of the blood-brain barrier, increases neurogenesis, and stimulates microglia activity. In the peripheral nervous system, it induces sympathetic activation through the release of norepinephrine, leading to an increase in heart rate, energy expenditure, and satiety. However, these events are also associated with a number of hepatic events, such as increased hepatic insulin sensitivity and the activation of AMPK-dependent signalling, reduced gluconeogenesis, and reduced lipid accumulation. GPR43, GPR41, and GPR109A promote anti-lipolytic activity through increased glucose and lipid metabolism. SCFAs are also inhibitors of intracellular HDAC [48,52,53]. SCFAs enter the cell by diffusion and/or the transport mediated by sodium channel-coupled transporter protein SLC5A8 and, through HDAC inhibition, act on epigenetic modulation. In particular, butyrate and propionate as HDAC inhibitors in the intestine and colon protect against colorectal cancer and inflammation. Systemically, however, HDAC inhibition influences gene expression to exhibit anti-tumour, anti-fibrotic, and anti-inflammatory activities. In the lungs, for example, acetate reduces asthma symptoms and increases T-reg cells through HDAC9 inhibition [54,55].

Table 1. Acetate, propionate, and butyrate are formed in the human colon in an estimated ratio of approximately 3:1:1. Different bacteria are involved in SCFAs production, and once produced, SCFAs are able to bind to different receptors. In the table are indicated the receptors for which each SCFA has a major affinity and their intestinal and non-intestinal expression.

SCFAs	Producers	Binding	Intestinal Expression	Non Intestinal Expression
Acetate	*Akkermansia muciniphila*, *Bacteroides* spp., *Bifidobacterium* spp., *Prevotella* spp., *Ruminococcus* spp., *Blautia hydrogenotrophica*, *Clostridium* spp., *Streptococcus* spp.	GPR43 / Olfr78	Colonic, Small intestinal epithelium, Colonic lamina propria cells, Leukocytes in small intestinal	Polymorphonuclear cells, Adipocytes, Skeletal muscle, Heart, Spleen
Propionate	*Bacteroides* spp., *Phascolarctobacterium succinatutens*, *Dialister* spp., *Veilonella* spp., *Megasphera elsdenii*, *Coprococcus catus*, *Ruminococcus obeum*, *Salmonella* spp., *Roseburia inulinivorans*	GPR43 / GPR41 / Olfr78	Colonic, Small intestinal epithelium, Colonic lamina propria cells (mast cells), Pancreas, Gut enteroendocrine cells located in the crypts and lower part of the villi	Spleen, Bone marrow, Lymph nodes, Adipose tissue, Periportal afferent system, Peripheral nervous system, Peripheral blood mononuclear cells
Butyrate	*Coprococcus viene*, *Coprococcus eutacus*, *Anaerostipes* spp., *Coprococcus catus*, *Eubacterium rectale*, *Eubacterium hallii*, *Faecalibacterium prausnitzii*, *Roseburia* spp.	GPR109A / GPR41 / GPR43	Apical membrane of colonic/small intestinal epithelium, Macrophages, Monocytes, Neutrophils, Dendritic cells	Adipocytes (white and brown), Epidermal Langerhans cells, Retinal pigment epithelium

3. Chronic Kidney Disease (CKD)

Chronic kidney disease (CKD) is a growing global problem associated with a high risk of morbidity and mortality. This condition adversely affects both human health and the expenditure of healthcare systems worldwide [56,57]. The international guidelines provided by KDIGO define CKD as an abnormality in kidney structure or function, present for >3 months, with health implications. CKD is an irreversible clinical condition associated with a definitive alteration of renal function and structure, with a slow and progressive evolution. In addition, due to the long course of CKD, one or more episodes of Acute Kidney Disease are observed, superimposed on CKD [58,59]. The loss of renal function and the progression to end-stage renal failure are evidenced by the loss of tubular cells and their replacement by collagen scars, as well as the high density of infiltrating macrophages [59–61]. In addition, in kidneys with CKD, the activation of the renin-angiotensin system and a reduced number of glomeruli also induce hyperfiltration and increased tubular oxygen consumption, worsening the imbalances between oxygen demand and release [62]. However, the progressive loss of renal function is linked to inflammation, the overproduction of reactive species, decreased antioxidant defences in endothelial cells (EC), the stimulation of cross-talk between EC and macrophages, and the increased expression of adhesion molecules (E-selectin, P-selectin,

ICAM-1 and VCAM-1) with infiltration by monocytes and macrophages into the activated endothelium. Neutrophils are the first cells to accumulate in the renal parenchyma, further releasing reactive molecules, proteinases, elastases, myeloperoxidases, cationic peptides, cytokines, and pro-inflammatory chemokines to recruit and activate other neutrophils but also natural killer cells, monocytes, and macrophages, exacerbating renal damage through a synergistic interaction [63–65]. These events, which can occur in both the renal cortex and medulla, are therefore associated with a wide range of detrimental effects such as altered renal blood flow, sodium/fluid retention, inflammation, fibrotic changes, and proteinuria [66]. An event that frequently occurs with declining kidney function is the retention of toxic metabolites that are not excreted and subsequently accumulate in the systemic circulation. These metabolites are called uremic toxins, and they lead to uremic syndrome, which, in addition to the progressive loss of kidney function, is associated with symptoms such as nausea, vomiting, fatigue, anorexia, muscle cramps, itching, altered mental status and others, leading to a reduced quality of life, morbidity, and mortality [67]. Uremic toxins can be classified according to their physico-chemical characteristics, such as water-soluble free solutes with a low molecular weight (<500 Da; e.g., Guanidine, Creatinine, Urea, Trimethylamine N-oxide, Inorganic phosphorus), protein-bound uremic toxins (<200 Da; e.g., Indoxyl Sulfate (IS), p-Cresyl Sulfate (pCS), Indole-3-acetic acid, Phenol Quinolinic acid, Putrescine), and medium molecules ($\geq$500 Da; e.g., β2- microglobulin, Leptin, IL-6, β-trace protein, Parathyroid hormone). Despite the fact that most of these metabolites are eliminated by dialysis, except the plasma protein-bound [68], the resulting accumulation of uremic toxins is associated with CKD progression and related complications, such as cardiovascular, central nervous system, gastrointestinal, and other areas, also trigger inflammation and oxidative stress and impaired immune response [59–78].

Gut Microbiota and SCFAs in CKD

The complex functions of the gut microbiota are related to other organs and result in the formation of an '-axis' between them [79]. The gut microbiota plays an important role in kidney homeostasis, regulating the gut-kidney axis [80], and intestinal dysbiosis is implicated in the pathogenesis of various renal disorders, including urinary tract infections (UTIs) that are also related to the "intestinal bloom of uropathogens" with a prevalence of the uropathogenic *Escherichia coli* [81,82]. These infections can also evolve into pyelonephritis as a complication of an ascending urinary tract infection that spreads from the bladder to the kidneys and their collecting systems, which still results in the significant morbidity and mortality associated with the severe cases of this disease [83]. A marked gut dysbiosis is also commonly observed in CKD patients and results from qualitative and quantitative changes in the composition and metabolic activities of the gut microbiota [84]. This may be due to both the use of antibiotics and drugs (e.g., iron-containing or resin-based phosphate binders) and changes in diet, including a decrease in resistant starch and/or fibre content or restriction of fruits and vegetables, as well as a decrease in colonic transit time in patients with uremia [85,86]. Furthermore, during CKD, the colon becomes the main route for uric acid and oxalate secretion. The influx of urea, uric acid, and oxalate into the colon affects the composition and metabolism of the gut microbiota, promoting the overgrowth of urease-producing bacteria and changes in the growth of the bacterial communities themselves [23]. Thus, an increase in Phyla *Actinobacteria, Firmicutes* and *Proteobacteria* microbes and a decrease in *Bifidobacteria* and *Lactobacilli* and SCFA levels have been reported in the course of CKD and in patients with end-stage renal disease [4,87]. These aspects reflect the evidence that SCFA levels progressively decrease during the different stages of CKD and, ultimately, in dialysis patients [88]. SCFAs produced by bacteria in the kidney protect tubular cells from oxidative stress and mitochondria biogenesis, reduce renal ischaemia-reperfusion injury, inflammation, reactive molecules, and immune and apoptotic cell infiltration in damaged kidneys [89]. Thus, the dysbiotic microbiota produces both a large amount of NH_3/NH_4OH that influences the pH of the intestinal lumen and toxic metabolites such as indoles and phenols that are further metabolised in the liver and intestine into pCS, IS, and

TMO. Generally, pCS accumulates in tubular cells and binds to OAT receptors located on the basolateral membrane of renal proximal tubular cells and generates reactive oxygen species, whereas IS binds to OAT receptors and activates NF-κB and AP-1-dependent gene transcription, inducing inflammation and nephrotoxicity [90]. Thus, these toxic metabolites may lead to accelerated renal damage by both promoting the progression of oxidative stress and inflammation and by promoting the alteration of the gut microbiota, which, by further producing gut-derived toxins, also alters the function of the intestinal epithelial barrier. At the same time, these toxic metabolites are absorbed through the damaged intestinal barrier and released into the systemic circulation. Indeed, there is considerable evidence to suggest that gut dysbiosis may contribute to the progression of some of the events that occur over the course of CKD, such as oxidative stress, endotoxemia, inflammation, and an increased prevalence of comorbidities [91–94]. Thus, it seems clear that there is a close relationship between the gut microbiota and renal function that is implicated in renal physiology and disease conditions.

4. Inflammation and Oxidative Stress in CKD

Chronic inflammation is a common comorbid condition in CKD. The increased production and reduced clearance of pro-inflammatory cytokines, oxidative stress, and acidosis contribute to the chronic inflammatory state but also to metabolic alterations and chronic and recurrent infections, especially in dialysis patients. Furthermore, metabolic alterations and intestinal dysbiosis create additional inflammatory stimulation with the involvement of the cells of the innate immune response system [95–97]. Among the inflammatory markers in CKD, IL-1, IL-6, TNF (Tumor Necrosis Factor)-α, C-reactive protein (CRP), adipokines, adhesion molecules, and the CD40 ligand are particularly important and associated with many complications (e.g., malnutrition, coronary calcification, atherosclerosis, atrial fibrillation, left ventricular hypertrophy, heart failure, insulin resistance, oxidative stress, endothelial dysfunction, mineral and bone diseases, anaemia, and erythropoietin resistance). In addition to being produced by lymphocytes, these pro-inflammatory factors are produced by visceral adipose tissue, which becomes dysfunctional during CKD by expressing a high level of pro-inflammatory cytokine mRNA [98]. Alongside the levels of these cytokines, there is also an increase in pro-inflammatory enzymes such as cyclooxygenase-2 (COX-2) and inducible nitric oxide synthase (iNOS), which are positively regulated by the activation of NF-κB in CKD [99,100]. Several studies have also demonstrated that uremic toxins, such as IS, are able to increase the levels of TNF-α and IL-6, causing an exacerbation of the inflammatory state and favouring oxidative stress [101,102]. Indeed, oxidative stress is also frequently observed in the early stages of chronic renal failure onwards and, in addition to being a non-traditional risk factor for all causes of mortality, tends to exacerbate during the course of the disease and can sometimes persist to a certain degree after kidney transplant [103,104]. Oxidative stress is responsible for several pathological conditions that are considered risk factors for CKD, such as diabetes, hypertension, and atherosclerosis, and is also responsible for the progression of kidney damage, which leads to renal ischemia, glomerular damage, cell death, and apoptosis, which also exacerbate the severe inflammatory processes already underway [105,106]. Oxidative stress is a condition of imbalance between the excessive production of oxidants and the reduced capacity of antioxidant systems, which leads to metabolic dysregulation and the oxidation of lipids, DNA, and proteins, as well as affecting the cellular activity and inhibiting the activity of cytoprotective enzymes [102,107]. Oxidative stress is linked to the production of highly reactive intermediates, reactive oxygen (ROS), and nitrogen (RNS) species, whose excessive generation is associated with impaired electron transport chains, reduced ATP synthesis, mitochondrial dysfunction, cell damage, apoptosis, and even damage to all of the cellular constituents [108]. Mitochondria are mainly responsible for the production of reactive molecules through the electron transport chain, especially ROS, which are also able to improve the inflammatory response. Indeed, during the pathogenesis of kidney disease, mitochondria in damaged cells become one of the main sources of excess ROS, which in turn implements the activation of transcription factors NF-κB, AP-1, and p53, exacerbating the production of pro-inflammatory cytokines and chemokines such as IL-1β, IL-6, IL-8, IL-1, and TNF-α, monocyte chemoattractant protein-1 (MCP-1), interferon-invasive protein-10 (IP-10), molecules of adhesion such as selectin, ICAM, VCAM, ELAM, inflammatory enzymes, such as iNOS and COX-2, and further ROS/RNS [109–113]. The main markers of oxidative stress that have significantly elevated levels in the blood and/or circulating tissues in patients with CKD are malondialdehyde (MDA), a low-density oxidized lipoprotein, advanced glycation end products, and l'8-hydroxide-oxyguanosine. For example the interaction between AGE and the RAGE receptor induces the activation of the MAP kinase transduction pathway, leading to the nuclear translocation of NF-κB and the activation of second messengers, resulting in an increase in cytokines, pro-inflammatory enzymes, and adhesion molecules [114–116]. Thus, as oxidative stress can further exacerbate inflammation, inflammation and oxidative stress are important mediators in the development and progression of kidney disease and associated complications, where one generates and amplifies the other, and the antioxidant systems are severely compromised [94]. In fact, this condition also depends on the reduced activation of antioxidant responses, such as the transcription factor Nrf2 (Erythroid-related nuclear factor 2), the main cellular defence factor that regulates the genes coding for antioxidant and detoxifying proteins and enzymes. Generally, Nrf2 is in a quiescent state sequestered by the cytosolic repressor Keap1 (Kelch-like ECH-associated protein 1), which also promotes its rapid proteasomal degradation; in contrast, under oxidative and electrophilic stress conditions, Nrf2 is released by Keap1, which in this case acts as an electrophilic sensor and, together with the small Maf protein (sMAF), binds to the antioxidant response element (ARE) in the promoter region of genes coding for phase II and antioxidant enzymes to counteract oxidative stress [117–119]. In addition, Nrf2 also directly suppresses the expression of pro-inflammatory NF-κB target genes by binding to their promoters and inhibiting their transcription [120]. However, in the course of CKD, the excessive production of ROS reduces the activation of Nrf2, and its deficiency increases the susceptibility to kidney damage. Indeed, several studies have shown that during CKD, Nrf2 has a renoprotective effect by controlling uremic inflammation and improving antioxidant defences, leading to a reduction in renal fibrosis, tubular damage, and renal hypoxia [121].

SCFAs, Inflammation and Oxidative Stress

SCFAs produced by the intestinal microbiome are able to act on inflammation and oxidative stress through complex mechanisms of regulation, and, moreover, they also regulate the immune response. SCFAs suppress inflammation in many organs by reducing the migration and proliferation of immune cells and cytokine levels and by inducing apoptosis [122]. Through the inhibition of HDAC, they influence the inhibition of the nuclear factor, NF-κB, and the transcription of genes that code for pro-inflammatory cytokines. Furthermore, they are also able to reduce the inflammatory response through the reduction in neutrophil recruitment, with increased levels of TGF-β and IL-10 and reduced levels of IL-6, IL-1β, NO, and TNF-α. At the same time, SCFAs promote the production of T cells that release IL-10 and T-reg to prevent inflammatory responses and act on DCs to limit the expression of T cell activating molecules, resulting in the generation of tolerogenic rather than inflammatory T cells, thus reducing inflammatory responses. SCFAs can also modulate the immune response due to a direct effect on T cells, binding to GPR41, GPR43, and GPR109A receptors and activating Olfr78 receptor signalling to regulate T lymphocyte function by increasing the generation of Th1 and Th17 cells to improve immunity (Figure 1). Butyrate, for example, has shown both an inhibitory effect on the formation of NLRP3 inflammasomes and an improvement in tight junction function in intestinal and vascular endothelial cells [123,124]. Moreover, butyrate, through HDAC inhibition, was able to modulate the immune response by reducing iNOS levels and NF-κB activation [125].

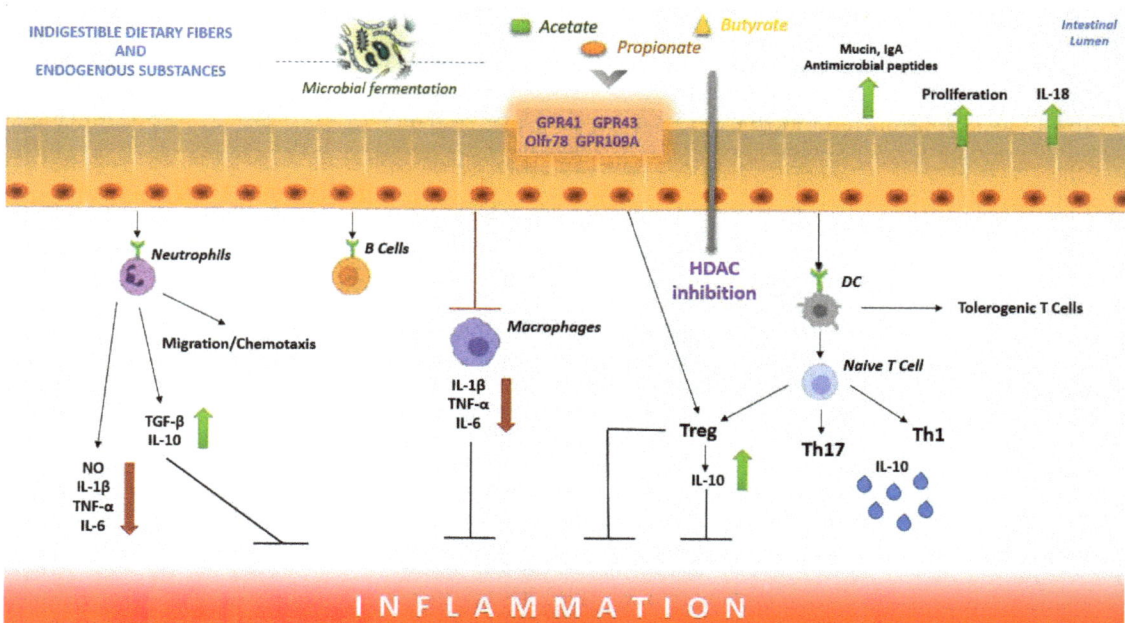

Figure 1. Overview of the effect of the SCFAs on inflammation. In the intestinal lumen, SCFAs induce the secretion of IL-18, MUC2 and antimicrobial peptides from intestinal epithelial cells, induce IgA secretion from B lymphocytes and regulate tight junction expression. SCFAs bind to GPR41, GPR43, GPR109A receptors and activate Olfr78 receptor signalling to regulate T cell function increasing the generation of Th1 and Th17 cells and promoting the production of T cells that release IL-10 and T regs. SCFAs act on DCs to limit the expression of T cells activating molecules, resulting in the generation of tolerogenic T cells rather than inflammatory T-cells. SCFAs also reduce neutrophil recruitment, with increased levels of TGF-β, IL-10 and decreased levels of IL-6, IL-1β, NO, and TNF-α. Instead, through HDAC inhibition, they influence the inhibition of nuclear factor NF-κB, to inhibit inflammation. Abbreviations: DCs, Dendritic Cells; SCFAs, Short-chain Fatty Acids; GPCRs, G-Protein-coupled Receptors; HDAC, Histone Decetylase; NO, Nitric Oxide; TGF-β, Transforming Growth Factor beta; TNF-α, Tumor Necrosis Factor alpha; IL, Interleukin; Mucin, MUC2; NF-κB, Nuclear Factor Kappa-light-chain-enhancer of Activated B cells.

Furthermore, numerous studies have shown that SCFAs, particularly butyrate and propionate, were also able to modulate the Keap1-Nrf2-dependent cellular signalling pathway to maintain redox homeostasis through both direct and indirect mechanisms (Figure 2; [125–130]). Butyrate, through the recognition of the GPR109A receptor, induces the activation of the nuclear factor Nrf2, which encodes antioxidant enzymes for the inactivation of ROS [108]. Furthermore, butyrate has a synergistic action on the activation of Nrf2 because, by spreading in the cell lumen, it inactivates HDAC and consequently increases the production of histone H3K9ac thus inducing an epigenetic modification on the Nrf2 promoter, as demonstrated through various studies [125,126,131–133]. Acetate, propionate, and butyrate can synergistically activate the translocation of Nrf2 through the recognition of GPR41 and GPR43 receptors [134–136].

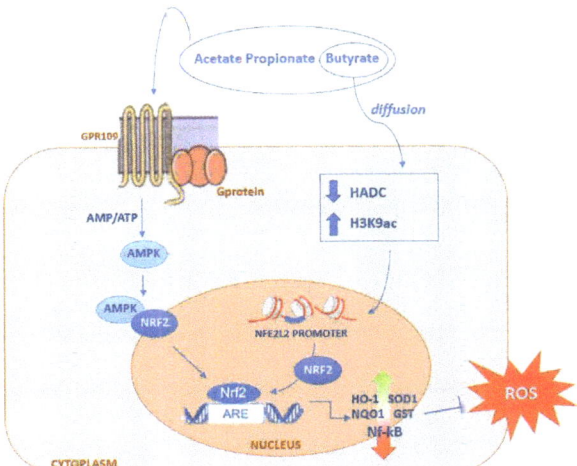

Figure 2. Direct and indirect mechanism of SCFAs on Nrf2 activation for modulation of oxidative stress. Binding of SCFAs to GPRC receptors induces direct activation of the nuclear factor Nrf2. Butyrate, on the other hand, also has a synergistic effect on Nrf2 activation because it diffuses into the cell lumen and, through HDAC inhibition, increases the production of histone H3K9ac, thus inducing an epigenetic modification on the Nrf2 promoter, indirectly activating Nrf2-dependent gene translocation and transcription. Abbreviations: AMPK, Activated Protein Kinase; HDAC, Histone Deacetylase; Nrf2, Nuclear Erythroid-Related Factor 2; ARE, Antioxidant Response element; HO-1, Heme Oxygenase-1; NQO1, NAD(P)H Quinone Dehydrogenase-1; NF-κB, Nuclear Factor Kappa-light-chain-enhancer of Activated B cells; SOD1, Superoxide Dismutase 1; GST, Glutathione S-transferase.

5. Effects of SCFAs in CKD

CKD is linked to inflammation, oxidative stress, and dysbiosis of the immune system. These factors contribute to the progressive deterioration of renal function, loss of blood pressure control, metabolic dysfunction, and a loss of functional integrity of the intestinal epithelial barrier. Furthermore, the perpetuation of systemic inflammation and oxidative stress, together with the accumulation of toxic metabolites, are responsible for the onset of all comorbidities associated with CKD, such as changes in the cardiovascular, pulmonary, ocular, central nervous, musculoskeletal, gastrointestinal, mitochondrial, and immune systems [73,137–142]. However, in recent years, the gut microbiota has been assumed to play a central role in renal disease through the production of SCFAs, which have been shown to ameliorate renal damage by modulating inflammatory and immune responses [140–142]. Numerous studies, both pre-clinical and clinical, have already demonstrated the potential beneficial effect that SCFAs could have in the course of CKD, even improving some of the secondary complications that occur.

5.1. Pre-Clinical Observations

In vitro studies in cellular models were used to assess the relationship between SCFAs and inflammation and oxidative stress. Huang et al. evaluated the effect of SCFAs on oxidative stress and inflammation induced by high levels of glucose and lipopolysaccharide (LPS) in mouse glomerular mesangial cells (CMG) SV-40 MES 13) in the presence of acetate and butyrate or GPR43 agonist. The results indicated that both the treatment with SCFA and the treatment with the GPR43 agonist reduced MCP-1, IL-1β, and ICAM-1 levels. Moreover, both acetate and butyrate and the agonist GPR43 inhibited the generation of ROS and MDA and reversed the decrease in SOD induced by high levels of glucose and LPS. These pieces of evidence support the hypothesis that both SCFAs and the GPR43 signalling pathway may act as potential therapeutic targets in inflammation and oxidative stress in glomerular mesangial cells [143]. Andrade-Olivera and colleagues also confirmed that SCFAs modulated the inflammatory process. In renal tubular epithelial cells (TECs) stimulated with an inflammatory cocktail (LPS, zymosan, and TNF-α) and treated with butyrate, propionate, and acetate indicated that SCFAs reduce NF-κB activation, nitric oxide production, and ROS production in TECs. Furthermore, the translocation of hypoxia-inducible factor (HIF)-1 α transcription factor to the nucleus, a hallmark of hypoxia, was also reduced due to the role of SCFA. Therefore, treatment with SCFAs seems to counteract the inflammatory response and hypoxia in renal tubular epithelial cells. SCFAs could also modulate the inflammatory response, regulating immune cells and reducing the expression of the costimulatory molecules, CD80 and CD40, in bone marrow dendritic cells (DCs), and reducing CD8+ and CD4+ cell proliferation after treating antigen-presenting cells (APCs) from RAGKO mice with LPS, with or without SCFAs, for 24 h. Other studies performed in animal models of renal disease evaluated the effects of SCFA. In particular, acetate showed to have beneficial effects in preserving the structure of the kidney, reducing ROS, cytokines, and chemokines. Then, low mRNA levels of toll-like receptor 4, and its endogenous ligand, lower the activation of the NF-κB pathway, wherein low levels of activated neutrophils and macrophages, a low frequency of infiltrating macrophages, and a low frequency of activated DCs were observed. Acetate also increased the expression of GPR43 by modulating the expression of genes encoding for enzymes involved in epigenetic modifications and inhibited the activity of HDACs [144]. Butyrate appears to modulate the inflammatory response in vitro, also modifying the profibrotic cytokine transforming growth factor beta (TGF- β1) generation on immortalised human renal proximal tubular epithelial cells (HK-2 cells). There is strong evidence that this cytokine is involved in renal fibrosis in all renal diseases, and butyrate reduces the basal generation of TGF-β1 in renal tubular epithelial cells; in addition, butyrate mediates its effect through the inhibition of ERK/MAP kinase. This evidence was useful in confirming the role of butyrate in preventing renal fibrosis through the reduction of TGF-β1 and provided a useful basis for subsequent studies on dietary supplementation with Acacia(sen) SUPERGUM™ (gum arabic) that, increasing systemic levels of butyrate, may therefore have a potential beneficial effect in renal disease through the suppression of TGF-β1 activity [145–148]. SCFAs are, therefore, able to directly modulate some of the pro-inflammatory and oxidative stress parameters, as also demonstrated by other studies [149,150].

The effect of SCFAs in modulating inflammation and oxidative stress response was also reported in in vivo studies in animal models of chronic renal failure, which also correlated with a number of secondary complications.

Acute Kidney Injury (AKI) is an important risk factor for CKD. Therefore, Liu et al. used a mouse model of folic acid nephropathy to examine the effect of dietary fibre, from which SCFAs are derived after microbial fermentation, on the development of AKI and, consequently, on the progression of CKD. Wild-type and knockout mice for GPR41, GPR43, or GPR109A receptors in which folic acid nephropathy had been induced were fed fibre-rich diets or treated with SCFAs. The gut microbiota was examined by RNA sequencing, and an increase in *Bifidobacterium* and *Prevotella* was observed, which also increased the concentration of SCFAs in both faeces and serum. After 28 days, the animals showed improved kidney function, fewer tubular lesions, and fewer interstitial fibrosis; chronic inflammation was evaluated by the gene expression analysis of various inflammatory parameters, such as TLR-2, TLR-4, pro-inflammatory cytokines (e.g., TNF-α, IL-6, IL-18, IL-1β, IL-4, IL-10, and IFNγ), and anti-inflammatory cytokine IL-10, the activation of NLRP3 inflammasome, chemokines (e.g., CXCL2, CCL2, and CXCL10), TGF-β1 expression and pro-inflammatory enzymes (e.g., iNOS). The SCFAs treatment led to similar protection through the inhibition of HDAC and GPR41-, GPR43-, and GPR109A-dependent signalling. Thus, both dietary manipulation and SCFAs have been shown to significantly reduce the damage of AKI and, thus, the risk of CKD progression [151]. Diabetic nephropathy is a chronic inflammatory condition that often overlaps with CKD, in the pathogenesis of which oxidative stress and NF-κB signalling are mainly observed. Huang et al. evaluated the role of acetate, propionate, and butyrate both in vitro on GMC cells (SV-40 MES 13) and in different animal models such as mice with type 2 diabetes (T2D) induced by streptozotocin (STZ), diabetic nephropathy (DN), and GMC cells of high-glucose mice, but also in a high-fat diet (HFD). In GMCs, SCFAs inhibited oxidative stress by reducing ROS and MDA and increased SOD, reduced NF-κB activation, enhanced the interaction between β-arrestin-2 and I-κBα, and reduced the release of MCP-1 and IL-1 β. For in vivo studies, however, the kidneys were used for the pathology assessment, and biochemical analyses were performed. The results showed that SCFAs, particularly butyrate, improved hyperglycaemia and insulin resistance, reduced proteinuria, serum creatinine, urea nitrogen and cystatin C, inhibited mesangial matrix accumulation and renal fibrosis, and blocked NF-κB activation in mice by GPR43-mediated signalling. SCFAs ameliorated the renal damage of DT2 and demonstrated antioxidant and anti-inflammatory effects mediated by the overexpression of GPR43 [152]. These results were also confirmed by another study. Diabetes was induced by STZ in wild-type C57BL/6 and GPR43 or GPR109A knockout mice, and then they were fed fibre-rich diets followed by sodium acetate, sodium propionate, and sodium butyrate. After 12 weeks, stool, urine, and plasma samples were collected and examined. The results indicated that diabetic mice fed a high-fibre diet had less albuminuria, glomerular hypertrophy, podocyte lesions, and fibrosis and were less likely to develop diabetic nephropathy and, consequently, CKD. The fibre also promoted the expansion of SCFA-producing bacteria such as *Prevotella* and *Bifidobacterium*, which increased the faecal and systemic SCFA concentrations, and reduced the expression of genes encoding for inflammatory cytokines, chemokines, and fibrosis-promoting proteins in diabetic kidneys. In vitro studies used TEC cells and podocytes isolated from C57BL/6 mice, both treated with either acetate, propionate, or butyrate. The results indicated that SCFAs modulated inflammation by reducing the chemokines CCL2 and CXCL10 and the cytokines IL-6 and TNF-α. In addition, the expression of the fibrosis-related genes TGF-β and fibronectin was also reduced [153]. These effects depended on the modulation of inflammation by SCFAs through the GPR41 and GPR43 receptors, as also shown in other studies. Indeed, butyrate, through the activation of the GPR109A receptor in renal podocytes, influences the gene transcription of pro-inflammatory cytokines and controls inflammatory responses. This GPR109A receptor phenotype in renal podocytes was associated with an increase in podocyte-related proteins and a normalised pattern of acetylation and methylation at the promoter sites of genes that are essential for podocyte function. Thus, the protective effect of butyrate-dependent GPR109A signalling ameliorated proteinuria by preserving the podocytes on the glomerular basement membrane and attenuating glomerulosclerosis and tissue inflammation [154,155]. There is a large body of evidence that CKD is associated with impaired function and decreased integrity of the intestinal epithelial barrier. Indeed, chronic low-grade inflammation and marked alteration of the intestinal microbiota can be observed in the intestine, which, by further producing toxic metabolites, promotes increased inflammation and its progression to the systemic level. Hung et Suzuki conducted a study in which they evaluated whether fermentable dietary fibre (DF), such as unmodified guar gum (GG) and partially hydrolysed GG (PHGG), could cause an increase in SCFA concentrations and, consequently, restore intestinal barrier permeability and function, thereby also improving inflammation in cases of CKD. Thirty-three seven-week-old male mice were fed a diet supplemented with adenine for 14 days to induce CKD and were subsequently examined. Twenty-seven of these mice were then divided into three groups (CKD, CKD+GG, and CKD+PHGG), while six mice received a control diet. Pro-inflammatory parameters, such as TNF-α and IL-1β, tight junction proteins, such as zonula occludens (ZO)-1, ZO-2 and occludin, serum urea and creatinine, intestinal barrier permeability, SCFA levels, and bacterial populations were examined. The results indicated that in the mice fed with GG and PGHH, not only was inflammation reduced, but high caecal levels of SCFAs, intestinal barrier function, and bacterial population composition, in particular *Lactobacillus*, were also improved. Thus, SCFAs, produced through the intestinal fermentation of PHGG and GG and transported into the circulatory system, have been shown to suppress inflammation and renal fibrosis directly [156]. In another study, the effects of the prebiotic fibre, xylooligosaccharide (XOS), on renal function and gut microbiota in mice with adenine-induced CKD were evaluated. The mice were fed adenine for 3 weeks to induce CKD and then fed XOS for a further 3 weeks. The results indicated that XOS reduced the renal damage in CKD mice, improved intestinal bacterial populations, increased the caecal production of SCFAs and reduced the levels of the uremic toxin IS [157].

The study sections and results are summarised in Table 2.

Table 2. Pre-clinical studies report a related improvement in SCFA levels both in in vitro and animal models.

Pre-Clinical Studies	Treatment	Parameters Evaluated	Effect	References
Mouse glomerular mesangial cells (SV-40 MES 13)	Acetate, Butyrate, GPR43 agonist	Cell viability assays, detection of ROS, MDA and SOD, MCP-1, IL-1β and ICAM-1	Butyrate, Acetate, and GPR43 agonist reduced inflammatory markers	Huang et al., 2017 [132]
Renal tubular epithelial cells		NF-κB activation, NO production, ROS production	SCFAs reduced inflammation and hypoxia and also modulated immune response	
Bone marrow dendritic cells		Molecules CD80 and CD40		
Antigen-presenting cells from RAGKO mice		Proliferation of CD8+ and CD4+ cells		
Male C57BL/6 mice with AKI	Butyrate, Propionate, Acetate	Apoptosis assessment, immunohistochemical analysis, mitochondrial DNA, DNA methylation, NF-κB levels, TLR-4, IL-6, IFN-γ, TNF-α, TGF-β1, MCP-1, IL-1β, GSS/GSSH ratio	Acetate reducing ROS, cytokines and chemokines; Low mRNA levels of TLR-4, lower activation of the NF-κB pathway, low levels of activated neutrophils and macrophages, a low frequency of infiltrating macrophages and a low frequency of activated DCs were observed. Acetate also increased the expression of GPR43 and inhibited the activity of HDACs	Andrade-Olivera et al., 2015 [133]
Immortalised human renal proximal tubular epithelial cells (HK-2 cells)	Butyrate	TGF-β1 levels and expression	Butyrate reduces the basal generation of TGF-β1 through inhibition of the ERK/MAP kinase	Matsumoto et al., 2006 [137]

Table 2. Cont.

Pre-Clinical Studies	Treatment	Parameters Evaluated	Effect	References
Wild-type and knockout C57BL/6 mice for GPR41, GPR43, or GPR109A receptors with diabetic nephropathy	Propionate, Butyrate	Assessment of serum creatinine, histological examination of renal tissues, evaluation of microbial composition, and SCFA levels, gene expression analysis of TLR-2, TLR-4, NLRP3, TNF-α, IL-6, IL-18, IL-1β, IL-4, IL-10, IFNγ, CXCL2, CCL2, CXCL10, iNOS, KIM1, MMP2, MMP9, TGFβ1, HDAC1-11, and GAPDH	Reduced inflammation and kidney injury, increased Bifidobacterium and Prevotella that increased faecal and serum SCFA concentrations	Liu et al., 2021 [140]
Mouse glomerular mesangial cells (SV-40 MES 13)	Acetate, Propionate, Butyrate	Cell viability assays, detection of ROS, MDA and SOD, Western blot analysis or ELISA for GPR43, β-arrestin-2, NF-κB, p65, MCP-1, IL-1β, I-κBα, GAPDH	Butyrate restored high glucose concentrations, oxidative stress, NF-κB signalling, and interaction between β-arrestin-2 and I-κB α-induced GPR43	Huang et al., 2020 [141]
Eight-week-old male C57BL/6 mice with type 2 diabetes induced by streptozotocin, diabetic nephropathy	Acetate, Propionate, Butyrate	FBG levels, ACR, FINS, BUN, SCr, serum cystatin C, TC, TG, LDL and LDL-C, renal glomerular histology, immunohistochemical staining for GPR43, β-arrestin-2, NF-κB, p65, MCP-1	Butyrate improved hyperglycemia, improved insulin resistance of T2D, prevented renal dysfunction in T2D, inhibited DT2-induced renal NF-κB activation and regulated GPR43-β-Arrestin2-signalling	
Renal tubular epithelial cells and podocytes were isolated from C57BL/6 mice	Acetate, Propionate, Butyrate	mRNA expression of IL-6, IFN-γ, TNF-α, CCL2, CXCL10	Butyrate and propionate significantly inhibited inflammation	
Wild-type and knockout C57BL/6 mice lacking genes for GPR43 or GPR109A with diabetic nephropathy	Fibre-rich diets, Sodium Acetate, Sodium Propionate, and Sodium Butyrate	Immunohistochemical analysis, histological analysis, real-time PCR for TLR-2, TLR-4, IL-6, IFN-γ, TNF-α, CCL2, CXCL10, TGF-β1, fibronectin, and GAPDH, bacterial DNA sequencing analysis, analysis of SCFA levels	Increased Prevotella and Bifidobacterium, increased SCFA, modulation of inflammation in renal tubular cells and podocytes under hyperglycemic conditions	Li et al., 2020 [142]

Table 2. Cont.

Pre-Clinical Studies	Treatment	Parameters Evaluated	Effect	References
33 7-week-old male ICR with CKD adenine-induced	DF, GG, PHGG	Evaluation of TNF-α, MCP-1, IL-1β, IL-6, Tgfb1, Col1A1, Acta2, TLR-4 and Myd88 mRNA levels, expression levels of ZO-1, ZO-2, occludin, JAMA, claudin 3, claudin 4, and claudin 7, serum creatinine and urea analysis, immunohistochemistry analysis, microbiota composition analysis, SCFA levels, IgA of the mucosa and the mucus itself	Colonic barrier protection and reduced endotoxemia, restoration of tight junction protein expression and localisation, increased Bifidobacterium, increased propionic and butyric acid production correlated with a reduction in pro-inflammatory parameters	Hung et Suzuki, 2018 [145]
Seven-week-old male C57BL/6J mice with CKD adenine-induced	XOS	Col1A1, Cgtf, IL-6, TNF-α, Arg, Ym1, Defa, Pla2g2a, Reg3γ, caecal SCFAs, histological analysis of renal tissue	Reduced gene expression of markers observed in CKD, including lColA1 and Cgtf, IL-6 and the M2 macrophage marker, Defa5, reduced IS and pCS and increased SCFA-producing bacteria, and improved renal function	Yang et al., 2018 [144]
Male isogenic Balb/c mice and C57BL/6 with nephropathy	Diet of high amylose butyrate-releasing corn starch	Immunohistochemical analysis, DNA expression, analysis TGF-β1, Fsp1, ActaII, Col4α1, Mmp9, Timp1, urinary albumin analysis, monoclonal antibody generation for GPR109A and GPR43, analysis of SCFAs concentrations, measurement of pro-inflammatory cytokines, isolation and polarisation of bone marrow-derived macrophages, HDAC activity, DNA methylation	Butyrate attenuates inflammation and renal fibrosis through its receptors GPR109A, GPR43, and GPR41	Felizardo et al., 2019 [143]

Abbreviations: ROS, Reactive Oxygen Species; SOD, Super Oxide Dismutase; MDA, Malondialdehyde; IL, Interleukin; MCP-1, Monocyte Chemoattractant Protein-1; ICAM-1, Intracellular Adhesion Molecule-1; NF-κB, Nuclear Factor Kappa-light-chain-enhancer of Activated B cells; NO, Nitric Oxide; TLR, Toll-Like Receptor; TNF-α, Tumor Necrosis Factor alpha; *TGF-β*, Transforming Growth Factor beta; INF-γ, Interferon gamma; MMP, Matrix Metallopeptidase; KIM-1, Kidney Injury Molecule; HDAC, Histone Deacetylase; GAPDH, Glyceraldehyde 3-Phosphate Dehydrogenase; GPR, G-Protein-coupled Receptor; FBG, Fasting Blood Glucose; ACR, Random Urine Albumin-Creatinine ratios; FINS, Fasting Insulin Levels; BUN, Urea Nitrogen Levels; SCr, Serum Creatinine; TC, Total Cholesterol; TG, Triglycerides; LDL, Low-Density Lipoprotein; LDL-C, Low-Density Lipoprotein Cholesterol; CCL2, C-C Motif Chemokine Ligand 2; CXCL10, C-X-C motif chemokine ligand 10; SCFAs, Short-chain Fatty Acids; Fsp1, Fibroblast-Specific Protein 1; Col4α1, Kidney Collagen type IV alpha 1; ActaII, Actin alpha 2, Smooth Muscle; Col1A1, Kidney Collagen type I; IgA, Immunoglobulin A; ZO, JAMA; Defa5, Ileal Defensins alpha; Pla2g2a, Phospholipase A2; Reg3γ, Regenerating islet-Derived Protein 3 gamma; Cgtf, Connective tissue growth factor; Arg, Arginase; XOS; Timp1, Metallopeptidase Inhibitor 1; IS, Indoxyl Sulfate; pCS, pCresil Sulfate.

5.2. Clinical Observations

Thus, it is now clear that SCFAs may have a central and promising role in the treatment of renal failure. Indeed, several clinical trials have already been initiated. In the inflammation and oxidative stress observed in CKD, uremic toxins of intestinal origin also play a central role, promoting excess morbidity and mortality. This may be due to intestinal dysbiosis and the insufficient consumption of fermentable, complex carbohydrates, which consequently lead to reduced SCFA concentrations. Thus, a pilot study was conducted at the 'A Landolfi' Hospital (Solofra, Italy) in which 20 stable patients aged between 18 and 90 years were recruited, of which the most frequent causes of renal failure were diabetes mellitus and chronic glomerulonephritis. All of the subjects suffered from vascular and cardiac complications. Biochemical analyses were performed on the sera, and elevated levels of inflammatory and pro-oxidant markers were observed. However, when SCFAs, in particular sodium propionate, were administered, significant improvements were observed: no patient discontinued the treatment, and their body weight remained stable, there was a significant decrease in pro-inflammatory and pro-oxidant parameters such as high-sensitivity C-reactive protein (hs-CRP), IL-2, IL-6, IL-10, IL-17a, TNF-α, INF (Interferon)-γ, TGF-β, and endotoxins/lipopolysaccharides compared to the significant increase in the anti-inflammatory cytokine IL-10. In addition, the levels of MDA and uremic toxins, indoxyl sulphate and p-cresyl sulphate, were reduced. This study, therefore, from its conclusion, provided new information on the benefits of SCFAs for treating systemic inflammation, oxidative stress, and metabolic disorders [158]. Considering that elevated blood pressure and cardiovascular morbidity occur very often in patients with CKD. Some studies have shown that SCFAs can improve cardiovascular outcomes in CKD patients with kidney disease [159,160]. In fact, in 2019, the first clinical study was conducted to verify that SCFAs can bind to both the Olfr78 receptors expressed in the kidney on the afferent arteriole of the juxtaglomerular apparatus involved in the production of renin and the GPR41 receptor in the renal vascular system with contrasting effects on blood pressure [161–164]. Jadoon and colleagues examined the potential link between SCFAs and cardiovascular outcomes in patients with chronic renal failure. In a subcohort of 214 patients with CKD in the Clinical Phenotyping Resource and Biobank Core (CPROBE), including 81 patients with coronary artery disease (CAD) and self-reported cardiovascular disease (CVD), they measured the plasma levels of SCFAs by liquid chromatography-mass spectrometry and high-performance liquid chromatography. The results showed improved cardiovascular function in CKD patients, which was linked to significantly higher levels of SCFAs [165]. Furthermore, SCFAs have also been shown to significantly decrease systolic blood pressure in hemodialysis patients [166]. SCFA levels improved by diet also seems to have a positive effect on CKD. In fact, diet can improve the course of CKD by reducing urea levels [167], metabolic acidosis [168], and insulin resistance [169], as well as positively modulating the intestinal microbiome and, consequently, increasing SCFA concentrations [170,171]. Type 2-resistant starch-enriched biscuits (RS2) were administered to hemodialysis patients with chronic renal failure for 4 weeks. The results showed an increase in SCFA-producing bacteria *Roseburia* and *Ruminococcus gauvreauii* and a downregulation of the pro-inflammatory parameters [172]. While, in the course of another prospective, randomised, crossover study (Medika Study), for the first time, the effect of different diets on the modulation of the intestinal microbiota and, consequently, on the modification of the serum levels of IS and pCS were evaluated in patients with chronic renal failure. Sixty patients with grade 3B-4 chronic renal failure were recruited and given a free diet (FD), a very-low protein diet (VLPD) and a Mediterranean diet (MD). The stool and serum samples were collected at the end of each dietary regimen for the evaluation of IS and pCS levels or serum D-lactate levels. The results indicated that MD and VLPD increased bacterial species with anti-inflammatory potential and butyrate producers, circulating levels of IS and pCS were reduced, and an improvement in structural integrity and intestinal permeability was observed. Furthermore, VLPD reduced serum D-lactate and improved systolic blood pressure [173]. Wu and colleagues, on the other hand, evaluated changes in the composition of the gut microbiota in patients with chronic renal failure who followed a low-protein diet (LPD). In this study, 43 patients with chronic renal failure were involved, and changes in bacterial population, SCFAs production and uremic toxins were evaluated. These results also confirmed that nutritional therapy based on low protein intake improved renal function, reduced IS and pCS levels, and increased butyrate-producing bacterial populations [174].

The study sections and results are summarised in Table 3.

Table 3. Clinical studies report a related improvement in SCFA levels both in in vitro and animal models.

Clinical Studies	Treatment	Parameters Evaluated	Effect	References
20 patients with CKD and related complications	Sodium Propionate	Biochemical analyse on sera for hs-CRP, IL-2, IL-6, IL-10, IL-17a, TNF-α, INFγ, TGF-β, IL-10, MDA, and endotoxins/lipopolysaccharides	Sodium Propionate reduced inflammatory markers and improved anti-inflammatory parameters	Marzocco et al., 2018 [147]
43 patients with CKD	LPD	Analysis of bacterial populations and IS and pCS levels	LPD modulates gut dysbiosis and positively impacts the outcome of patients with CKD	Wu et al., 2020 [158]
Patients in HD with CKD	RS2	Evaluation of biochemical and clinical parameters, analysis of serum and plasma samples, genomic sequencing analysis	Mitigate inflammation and oxidative stress in hemodialysis patients by positively altering SCFA-producing bacteria	Kemp et al., 2021 [156]
214 patients with CKD and CVD	Addition of valerate	Evaluation of anthropometric, biochemical and clinical parameters, measurement of plasma levels of SCFAs	The addition of valerate to a model of hypertension, diabetes mellitus, and other complications significantly improved there conditions of patients	Jadoon et al., 2019 [154]
60 patients with grade 3B-4 CKD	FD, MD, VLPD	Anthropometri, clinical, and biochemical parameters obtained from stool and serum samples	Increased Lachnospiraceae, Ruminococcaceae, Prevotellaceae, Bifidobacteriaceae, Coprococcus, and Roseburia forming butyrate, increased anti-inflammatory potential, improved intestinal permeability and systolic blood pressure, reduced Enterobacteriaceae pathogens and circulating levels of IS, pCS, and D-Lactate	Di Iorio et al., 2018 [157]

Abbreviations: hs-CRP, high-sensitivity C-reactive protein; IL, Interleukin; INF-γ, Interferon gamma; MDA, Malondialdehyde; *TGF-β*, Transforming Growth Factor beta; TNF-α, Tumor Necrosis Factor alpha; IS, Indoxyl Sulfate; pCS, pCresil Sulfate; CVD, Cardiovascular disease; HD, Hemodialysis; CKD, Chronic Kidney Disease; LPD, Low-Protein Diet; SCFA, Short-chain Fatty Acids; FD, Free Diet; MD, Mediterranean Diet; VLPD, Very-Low Protein Diet.

6. Conclusions

SCFAs produced by microbial fermentation have been widely shown to reduce inflammation and oxidative stress, which are characteristic of several chronic diseases. CKD is a serious health problem, not least because of the systemic complications associated with it, and it is also a chronic condition that is very difficult to manage because of the underlying disease mechanisms. Therefore, the supplementation of short-chain fatty acids (e.g., acetate, propionate, or butyrate), either directly or by modulating the gut microbiota in favour of SCFA-producing bacterial species, including through dietary fibre or nutritional therapies, could have a positive impact on the management of chronic renal failure (Figure 3). However, further studies are still needed.

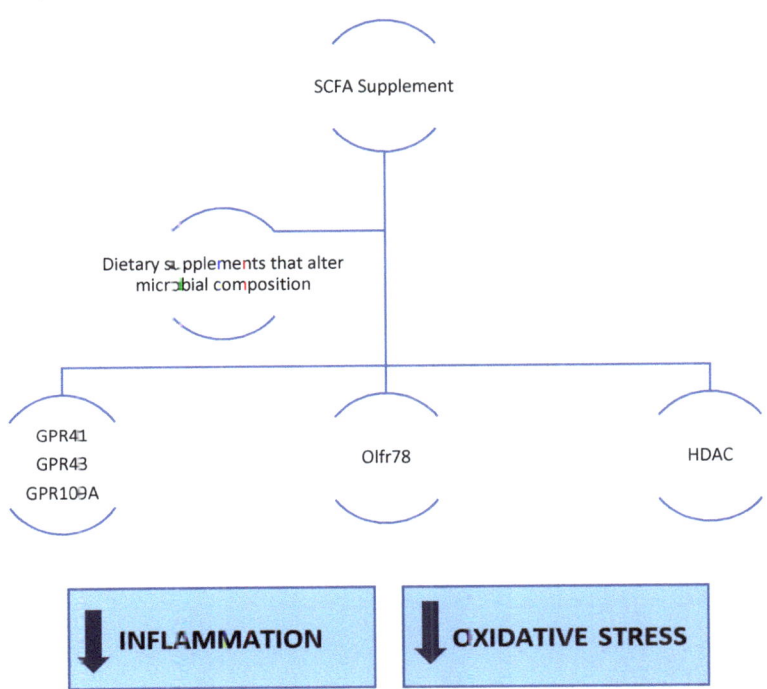

Figure 3. SCFAs result in increased activity on G-protein-coupled receptors and enhanced epigenetic regulatory activity through HDAC. SCFAs could be able to act positively on pro-inflammatory pathways (e.g., by negatively modulating the NF-κB signalling pathway) and pro-oxidant pathways (e.g., by positively modulating the Nrf2 pathway).

Author Contributions: S.M., B.R.D.I. and A.H. conceived the work; G.M. and S.M. wrote the manuscript; P.M., B.R.D.I. and A.H. edited the manuscript. All authors have read and agreed to the published version of the manuscript.

Funding: This research was founded by University of Salerno (FARB 2021- ORSA210342) granted to S.M.

Conflicts of Interest: The authors declare no conflict of interest.

References

1. Miele, L.; Giorgio, V.; Alberelli, M.A.; De Candia, E.; Gasbarrini, A.; Grieco, A. Impact of Gut Microbiota on Obesity, Diabetes, and Cardiovascular Disease Risk. *Curr. Cardiol. Rep.* **2015**, *12*, 120. [CrossRef] [PubMed]
2. Haghikia, A.; Jörg, S.; Duscha, A.; Berg, J.; Manzel, A.; Waschbisch, A.; Hammer, A.; Lee, D.H.; May, C.; Wilck, N.; et al. Dietary Fatty Acids Directly Impact Central Nervous System Autoimmunity via the Small Intestine. *Immunity* **2015**, *43*, 817–829. [CrossRef] [PubMed]
3. Lun, H.; Yang, W.; Zhao, S.; Jiang, M.; Xu, M.; Liu, F.; Wang, Y. Altered gut microbiota and microbial biomarkers associated with chronic kidney disease. *Microbiologyopen* **2019**, *4*, e00678. [CrossRef]
4. Vaziri, N.D.; Wong, J.; Pahl, M.; Piceno, Y.M.; Yuan, J.; De Santis, T.Z.; Ni, Z.; Nguyen, T.H.; Andersen, G.L. Chronic kidney disease alters intestinal microbial flora. *Kidney Int* **2013**, *83*, 308–315. [CrossRef] [PubMed]
5. Lau, W.L.; Savoj, J.; Nakata, M.B.; Vaziri, N.D. Altered microbiome in chronic kidney disease: Systemic effects of gut-derived uremic toxins. *Clin. Sci.* **2018**, *132*, 509–522. [CrossRef] [PubMed]
6. Vaziri, N.D.; Zhao, Y.Y.; Pahl, M.V. Altered intestinal microbial flora and impaired epithelial barrier structure and function in CKD: The nature, mechanisms, consequences and potential treatment. *Nephrol. Dial. Transplant.* **2016**, *31*, 737–746. [CrossRef]

7. Vaziri, N.D.; Yuan, J.; Norris, K. Role of urea in intestinal barrier dysfunction and disruption of epithelial tight junction in chronic kidney disease. *Am. J. Nephrol.* **2013**, *37*, 1–6. [CrossRef]
8. Moraes, C.; Fouque, D.; Amaral, A.C.; Mafra, D. Trimethylamine N-oxide from gut microbiota in chronic kidney disease patients: Focus on diet. *J. Ren. Nutr.* **2015**, *25*, 459–465. [CrossRef]
9. Ramezani, A.; Massy, Z.A.; Meijers, B.; Evenepoel, P.; Vanholder, R.; Raj, D.S. Role of the gut microbiome in uremia: A potential therapeutic target. *Am. J. Kidney Dis.* **2016**, *67*, 483–498. [CrossRef]
10. Yang, T.; Richards, E.M.; Pepine, C.J.; Raizada, M.K. The gut microbiota and the brain-gut-kidney axis in hypertension and chronic kidney disease. *Nat. Rev. Nephrol.* **2018**, *14*, 442–456. [CrossRef]
11. Barreto, F.C.; Barreto, D.V.; Liabeuf, S.; Meert, N.; Glorieux, G.; Temmar, M.; Choukroun, G.; Vanholder, R.; Massy, Z.A. European Uremic Toxin Work Group (EUTox). Serum indoxyl sulfate is associated with vascular disease and mortality in chronic kidney disease patients. *Clin. J. Am. Soc. Nephrol.* **2009**, *4*, 1551–1558. [CrossRef] [PubMed]
12. Di Iorio, B.R.; Marzocco, S.; Nardone, L.; Sirico, M.; De Simone, E.; Di Natale, G.; Di Micco, L. Urea and impairment of the Gut-Kidney axis in Chronic Kidney Disease. *G Ital. Nefrol.* **2017**, *34*, 1–12.
13. Cosola, C.; Rocchetti, M.T.; Sabatino, A.; Fiaccadori, E.; Di Iorio, B.R.; Gesualdo, L. Microbiota issue in CKD: How promising are gut-targeted approaches? *J. Nephrol.* **2019**, *32*, 27–37. [CrossRef]
14. Lau, W.L.; Kalantar-Zadeh, K.; Vaziri, N.D. The Gut as a Source of Inflammation in Chronic Kidney Disease. *Nephron* **2015**, *130*, 92–98. [CrossRef] [PubMed]
15. Diamanti, A.P.; Rosado, M.; Laganà, B.; D'Amelio, R. Microbiota and chronic inflammatory arthritis: An interwoven link. *J. Transl. Med.* **2016**, *14*, 233. [CrossRef] [PubMed]
16. Puddu, A.; Sanguineti, R.; Montecucco, F.; Viviani, G.L. Evidence for the gut microbiota short-chain fatty acids as key pathophysiological molecules improving diabetes. *Mediat. Inflamm.* **2014**, *2014*, 162021. [CrossRef]
17. Pisano, A.; D'Arrigo, G.; Coppolino, G.; Bolignano, D. Biotic Supplements for Renal Patients: A Systematic Review and Meta-Analysis. *Nutrients* **2018**, *10*, 1224. [CrossRef]
18. Pei, M.; Wei, L.; Hu, S.; Yang, B.; Si, J.; Yang, H.; Zhai, J. Probiotics, prebiotics and synbiotics for chronic kidney disease: Protocol for a systematic review and meta-analysis. *BMJ Open* **2018**, *8*, e020863. [CrossRef]
19. Harig, J.M.; Soergel, K.H.; Komorowski, R.A.; Wood, C.M. Treatment of diversion colitis with short-chain-fatty acid irrigation. *N. Engl. J. Med.* **1989**, *320*, 23–28. [CrossRef]
20. Khanna, S. Microbiota Replacement Therapies: Innovation in Gastrointestinal Care. *Clin. Pharm. Ther.* **2018**, *103*, 102–111. [CrossRef]
21. Ochoa-Repáraz, J.; Kirby, T.O.; Kasper, L.H. The Gut Microbiome and Multiple Sclerosis. *Cold Spring Harb. Perspect. Med.* **2018**, *8*, a029017. [CrossRef]
22. Iraporda, C.; Errea, A.; Romanin, D.E.; Cayet, D.; Pereyra, E.; Pignataro, O.; Sirard, J.C.; Garrote, G.L.; Abraham, A.G.; Rumbo, M. Lactate and short chain fatty acids produced by microbial fermentation downregulate proinflammatory responses in intestinal epithelial cells and myeloid cells. *Immunobiology* **2015**, *220*, 1161–1169. [CrossRef]
23. Vinolo, M.A.; Rodrigues, H.G.; Nachbar, R.T.; Curi, R. Regulation of inflammation by short chain fatty acids. *Nutrients* **2011**, *3*, 858–876. [CrossRef]
24. Maslowski, K.M.; Vieira, A.T.; Ng, A.; Kranich, J.; Sierro, F.; Yu, D.; Schilter, H.C.; Rolph, M.S.; Mackay, F.; Artis, D.; et al. Regulation of inflammatory responses by gut microbiota and chemoattractant receptor GPR43. *Nature* **2009**, *461*, 1282–1286. [CrossRef]
25. Richards, J.L.; Yap, Y.A.; McLeod, K.H.; Mackay, C.R.; Mariño, E. Dietary metabolites and the gut microbiota: An alternative approach to control inflammatory and autoimmune diseases. *Clin. Transl. Immunol.* **2016**, *5*, e82. [CrossRef]
26. Smith, P.M.; Howitt, M.R.; Panikov, N.; Michaud, M.; Gallini, C.A.; Bohlooly, Y.M.; Glickman, J.N.; Garrett, W.S. The microbial metabolites, short-chain fatty acids, regulate colonic Treg cell homeostasis. *Science* **2013**, *341*, 569–573. [CrossRef]
27. Park, J.; Kim, M.; Kang, S.G.; Jannasch, A.H.; Cooper, B.; Patterson, J.; Kim, C.H. Short-chain fatty acids induce both effector and regulatory T cells by suppression of histone deacetylases and regulation of the mTOR-S6K pathway. *Mucosal Immunol.* **2015**, *8*, 80–93. [CrossRef]
28. Macfarlane, G.T.; Macfarlane, S. Bacteria, colonic fermentation, and gastrointestinal health. *J. AOAC Int.* **2012**, *95*, 50–60. [CrossRef]
29. Bourriaud, C.; Robins, R.J.; Martin, L.; Kozlowski, F.; Tenailleau, E.; Cherbut, C.; Michel, C. Lactate is mainly fermented to butyrate by human intestinal microfloras but inter-individual variation is evident. *J. Appl. Microbiol.* **2005**, *99*, 201–212. [CrossRef]
30. Scott, K.P.; Martin, J.C.; Campbell, G.; Mayer, C.D.; Flint, H.J. Whole-genome transcription profiling reveals genes up-regulated by growth on fucose in the human gut bacterium "Roseburia inulinivorans". *J. Bacteriol.* **2006**, *188*, 4340–4349. [CrossRef]
31. Duncan, S.H.; Barcenilla, A.; Stewart, C.S.; Pryde, S.E.; Flint, H.J. Acetate utilization and butyryl coenzyme A (CoA): Acetate-CoA transferase in butyrate-producing bacteria from the human large intestine. *Appl. Environ. Microbiol.* **2002**, *68*, 5186–5190. [CrossRef] [PubMed]
32. Russell, W.R.; Gratz, S.W.; Duncan, S.H.; Holtrop, G.; Ince, J.; Scobbie, L.; Duncan, G.; Johnstone, A.M.; Lobley, G.E.; Wallace, R.J.; et al. High-protein, reduced-carbohydrate weight-loss diets promote metabolite profiles likely to be detrimental to colonic health. *Am. J. Clin. Nutr.* **2011**, *93*, 1062–1072. [CrossRef] [PubMed]

33. Wall, R.; Ross, R.P.; Shanahan, F.; O'Mahony, L.; O'Mahony, C.; Coakley, M.; Hart, O.; Lawlor, P.; Quigley, E.M.; Kiely, B.; et al. Metabolic activity of the enteric microbiota influences the fatty acid composition of murine and porcine liver and adipose tissues. *Am. J. Clin. Nutr.* **2009**, *89*, 1393–1401. [CrossRef] [PubMed]
34. Cummings, J.H.; Pomare, E.W.; Branch, W.J.; Naylor, C.P.; Macfarlane, G.T. Short chain fatty acids in human large intestine, portal, hepatic and venous blood. *Gut* **1987**, *28*, 1221–1227. [CrossRef]
35. Canani, R.B.; Costanzo, M.D.; Leone, L.; Pedata, M.; Meli, R.; Calignano, A. Potential beneficial effects of butyrate in intestinal and extraintestinal diseases. *World J. Gastroenterol.* **2011**, *17*, 1519–1528. [CrossRef]
36. Weitkunat, K.; Schumann, S.; Nickel, D.; Kappo, K.A.; Petzke, K.J.; Kipp, A.P.; Blaut, M.; Klaus, S. Importance of propionate for the repression of hepatic lipogenesis and improvement of insulin sensitivity in high-fat diet-induced obesity. *Mol. Nutr. Food Res.* **2016**, *60*, 2611–2621. [CrossRef]
37. Morrison, D.J.; Preston, T. Formation of short chain fatty acids by the gut microbiota and their impact on human metabolism. *Gut Microbes* **2016**, *7*, 189–200. [CrossRef]
38. Miyamoto, J.; Hasegawa, S.; Kasubuchi, M.; Ichimura, A.; Nakajima, A.; Kimura, I. Nutritional Signaling via Free Fatty Acid Receptors. *Int. J. Mol. Sci.* **2016**, *17*, 450. [CrossRef]
39. Kimura, I.; Ichimura, A.; Ohue-Kitano, R.; Igarashi, M. Free Fatty Acid Receptors in Health and Disease. *Physiol. Rev.* **2020**, *100*, 171–210. [CrossRef]
40. Haase, S.; Haghikia, A.; Wilck, N.; Müller, D.N.; Linker, R.A. Impacts of microbiome metabolites on immune regulation and autoimmunity. *Immunology* **2018**, *154*, 230–238. [CrossRef]
41. Schönfeld, P.; Wojtczak, L. Short-and medium-chain fatty acids in energy metabolism: The cellular perspective. *J. Lipid Res.* **2016**, *57*, 943–954. [CrossRef] [PubMed]
42. Li, L.; Ma, L.; Fu, P. Gut microbiota-derived short-chain fatty acids and kidney diseases. *Drug Des. Dev. Ther.* **2017**, *11*, 3531–3542. [CrossRef] [PubMed]
43. Marinissen, M.J.; Gutkind, J.S. G-protein-coupled receptors and signaling networks: Emerging paradigms. *Trends Pharmaco. Sci.* **2001**, *22*, 368–376. [CrossRef]
44. Brown, A.J.; Goldsworthy, S.M.; Barnes, A.A.; Eilert, M.M.; Tcheang, L.; Daniels, D.; Muir, A.I.; Wigglesworth, M.J.; Kinghorn, I.; Fraser, N.J.; et al. The Orphan G protein-coupled receptors GPR41 and GPR43 are activated by propionate and other short chain carboxylic acids. *J. Biol. Chem.* **2003**, *278*, 11312–11319. [CrossRef]
45. Hong, Y.H.; Nishimura, Y.; Hishikawa, D.; Tsuzuki, H.; Miyahara, H.; Gotoh, C.; Choi, K.C.; Feng, D.D.; Chen, C.; Lee, H.G.; et al. Acetate and propionate short chain fatty acids stimulate adipogenesis via GPCR43. *Endocrinology* **2005**, *146*, 5092–5099. [CrossRef]
46. Thangaraju, M.; Cresci, G.A.; Liu, K.; Ananth, S.; Gnanaprakasam, J.P.; Browning, D.D.; Mellinger, J.D.; Smith, S.B.; Digby, G.J.; Lambert, N.A.; et al. GPR109A is a G-protein-coupled receptor for the bacterial fermentation product butyrate and functions as a tumor suppressor in colon. *Cancer Res.* **2009**, *69*, 2826–2832. [CrossRef]
47. Tolhurst, G.; Heffron, H.; Lam, Y.S.; Parker, H.E.; Habib, A.M.; Diakogiannaki, E.; Cameron, J.; Grosse, J.; Reimann, F.; Gribble, F.M. Short-chain fatty acids stimulate glucagon-like peptide-1 secretion via the G-protein-coupled receptor FFAR2. *Diabetes* **2012**, *61*, 364–371. [CrossRef]
48. Koh, A.; De Vadder, F.; Kovatcheva-Datchary, P.; Bäckhed, F. From Dietary Fiber to Host Physiology: Short-Chain Fatty Acids as Key Bacterial Metabolites. *Cell* **2016**, *165*, 1332–1345. [CrossRef]
49. Arpaia, N.; Campbell, C.; Fan, X.; Dikiy, S.; van der Veeken, J.; de Roos, P.; Liu, H.; Cross, J.R.; Pfeffer, K.; Coffer, P.J.; et al. Metabolites produced by commensal bacteria promote peripheral regulatory T-cell generation. *Nature* **2013**, *504*, 451–455. [CrossRef]
50. Singh, N.; Gurav, A.; Sivaprakasam, S.; Brady, E.; Padia, R.; Shi, H.; Thangaraju, M.; Prasad, P.D.; Manicassamy, S.; Munn, D.H.; et al. Activation of Gpr109a, receptor for niacin and the commensal metabolite butyrate, suppresses colonic inflammation and carcinogenesis. *Immunity* **2014**, *40*, 128–139. [CrossRef]
51. Adom, D.; Nie, D. Regulation of autophagy by short chain fatty acids in colon cancer cells. In *Autophagy—A Double-Edged Sword—Cell Survival or Death?* Bailly, Y., Ed.; InTech: London, UK, 2013.
52. Nøhr, M.K.; Egerod, K.L.; Christiansen, S.H.; Gille, A.; Offermanns, S.; Schwartz, T.W.; Møller, M. Expression of the short chain fatty acid receptor GPR41/FFAR3 in autonomic and somatic sensory ganglia. *Neuroscience* **2015**, *290*, 126–137. [CrossRef] [PubMed]
53. Kimura, I.; Inoue, D.; Maeda, T.; Hara, T.; Ichimura, A.; Miyauchi, S.; Kobayashi, M.; Hirasawa, A.; Tsujimoto, G. Short-chain fatty acids and ketones directly regulate sympathetic nervous system via G protein-coupled receptor 41 (GPR41). *Proc. Natl. Acad. Sci. USA* **2011**, *108*, 8030–8035. [CrossRef] [PubMed]
54. Thorburn, A.N.; McKenzie, C.I.; Sher, S.; Stanley, D.; Macia, L.; Mason, L.J.; Roberts, L.K.; Wong, C.H.; Shim, R.; Robert, R.; et al. Evidence that asthma is a developmental origin disease influenced by maternal diet and bacterial metabolites. *Nat. Commun.* **2015**, *6*, 7320. [CrossRef] [PubMed]
55. Bultman, S.J. Interplay between diet, gut microbiota, epigenetic events, and colorectal cancer. *Mol. Nutr. Food Res.* **2017**, *61*, 10–1002. [CrossRef]
56. Go, A.S.; Chertow, G.M.; Fan, D.; McCulloch, C.E.; Hsu, C.Y. Chronic kidney disease and the risks of death, cardiovascular events, and hospitalizations. *N. Engl. Med.* **2004**, *351*, 1296–1305. [CrossRef]
57. Ammirati, A.L. Chronic Kidney Disease. *Rev. Assoc. Med. Bras.* **2020**, *66*, s03–s09. [CrossRef]

58. Ferenbach, D.A.; Bonventre, J.V. Acute kidney injury and chronic kidney disease: From the laboratory to the clinic. *Nephrol. Ther.* **2016**, *12*, S41–S48. [CrossRef]
59. Schrimpf, C.; Duffield, J.S. Mechanisms of fibrosis: The role of the pericyte. *Curr. Opin. Nephrol. Hypertens.* **2011**, *20*, 297–305. [CrossRef]
60. Yang, L.; Besschetnova, T.Y.; Brooks, C.R.; Shah, J.V.; Bonventre, J.V. Epithelial cell cycle arrest in G2/M mediates kidney fibrosis after injury. *Nat. Med.* **2010**, *16*, 535–543. [CrossRef]
61. Zafrani, L.; Ince, C. Microcirculation in Acute and Chronic Kidney Diseases. *Am. J. Kidney Dis.* **2015**, *66*, 1083–1094. [CrossRef]
62. Körner, A.; Eklöf, A.C.; Celsi, G.; Aperia, A. Increased renal metabolism in diabetes. Mechanism and functional implications. *Diabetes* **1994**, *43*, 629–633. [CrossRef] [PubMed]
63. Schofield, Z.V.; Woodruff, T.M.; Halai, R.; Wu, M.C.; Cooper, M.A. Neutrophils–a key component of ischemia-reperfusion injury. *Shock* **2013**, *40*, 463–470. [CrossRef] [PubMed]
64. Castoldi, A.; Braga, T.T.; Correa-Costa, M.; Aguiar, C.F.; Bassi, Ê.J.; Correa-Silva, R.; Elias, R.M.; Salvador, F.; Moraes-Vieira, P.M.; Cenedeze, M.A.; et al. TLR2, TLR4 and the MYD88 signaling pathway are crucial for neutrophil migration in acute kidney injury induced by sepsis. *PLoS ONE* **2012**, *7*, e37584. [CrossRef] [PubMed]
65. Dendooven, A.; Ishola DAJr Nguyen, T.Q.; Van der Giezen, D.M.; Kok, R.J.; Goldschmeding, R.; Joles, J.A. Oxidative stress in obstructive nephropathy. *Int. J. Exp. Pathol.* **2011**, *92*, 202–210. [CrossRef]
66. Drożdż, D.; Kwinta, P.; Sztefko, K.; Kordon, Z.; Drożdż, T.; Łątka, M.; Miklaszewska, M.; Zachwieja, K.; Rudziński, A.; Pietrzyk, J.A. Oxidative Stress Biomarkers and Left Ventricular Hypertrophy in Children with Chronic Kidney Disease. *Oxidative Med. Cell. Longev.* **2016**, *2016*, 7520231. [CrossRef] [PubMed]
67. Rosner, M.H.; Reis, T.; Husain-Syed, F.; Vanholder, R.; Hutchison, C.; Stenvinkel, P.; Blankestijn, P.J.; Cozzolino, M.; Juillard, L.; Kashani, K.; et al. Classification of Uremic Toxins and Their Role in Kidney Failure. *Clin. J. Am. Soc. Nephrol.* **2021**, *16*, 1918–1928. [CrossRef]
68. Basile, C.; Libutti, P.; Teutonico, A.; Lomonte, C. Tossine uremiche: Il caso dei "protein-bound compounds" [Uremic toxins: The case of protein-bound compounds]. *G Ital. Nefrol.* **2010**, *27*, 498–507.
69. El Chamieh, C.; Liabeuf, S.; Massy, Z. Uremic Toxins and Cardiovascular Risk in Chronic Kidney Disease: What Have We Learned Recently beyond the Past Findings? *Toxins* **2022**, *14*, 280. [CrossRef]
70. Adesso, S.; Magnus, T.; Cuzzocrea, S.; Campolo, M.; Rissiek, B.; Paciello, O.; Autore, G.; Pinto, A.; Marzocco, S. Indoxyl Sulfate Affects Glial Function Increasing Oxidative Stress and Neuroinflammation in Chronic Kidney Disease: Interaction between Astrocytes and Microglia. *Front. Pharmacol.* **2017**, *8*, 370. [CrossRef]
71. Adesso, S.; Ruocco, M.; Rapa, S.F.; Piaz, F.D.; Raffaele Di Iorio, B.; Popolo, A.; Autore, G.; Nishijima, F.; Pinto, A.; Marzocco, S. Effect of Indoxyl Sulfate on the Repair and Intactness of Intestinal Epithelial Cells: Role of Reactive Oxygen Species' Release. *Int. J. Mol. Sci.* **2019**, *20*, 2280. [CrossRef]
72. Marzocco, S.; Di Paola, R.; Ribecco, M.T.; Sorrentino, R.; Domenico, B.; Genesio, M.; Pinto, A.; Autore, G.; Cuzzocrea, S. Effect of methylguanidine in a model of septic shock induced by LPS. *Free Radic. Res.* **2004**, *38*, 1143–1153. [CrossRef] [PubMed]
73. Lisowska-Myjak, B. Uremic toxins and their effects on multiple organ systems. *Nephron Clin. Pract.* **2014**, *128*, 303–311. [CrossRef] [PubMed]
74. Marzocco, S.; Popolo, A.; Bianco, G.; Pinto, A.; Autore, G. Pro-apoptotic effect of methylguanidine on hydrogen peroxide-treated rat glioma cell line. *Neurochem. Int.* **2010**, *57*, 518–524. [CrossRef] [PubMed]
75. Borges, N.A.; Barros, A.F.; Nakao, L.S.; Dolenga, C.J.; Fouque, D.; Mafra, D. Protein-Bound Uremic Toxins from Gut Microbiota and Inflammatory Markers in Chronic Kidney Disease. *J. Ren. Nutr.* **2016**, *26*, 396–400. [CrossRef]
76. Rapa, S.F.; Prisco, F.; Popolo, A.; Iovane, V.; Autore, G.; Di Iorio, B.R.; Dal Piaz, F.; Paciello, O.; Nishijima, F.; Marzocco, S. Pro-Inflammatory Effects of Indoxyl Sulfate in Mice: Impairment of Intestinal Homeostasis and Immune Response. *Int. J. Mol. Sci.* **2021**, *22*, 1135. [CrossRef]
77. Marzocco, S.; Di Paola, R.; Genovese, T.; Sorrentino, R.; Britti, D.; Scollo, G.; Pinto, A.; Cuzzocrea, S.; Autore, G. Methylguanidine reduces the development of non septic shock induced by zymosan in mice. *Life Sci.* **2004**, *75*, 1417–1433. [CrossRef]
78. Marzocco, S.; Di Paola, R.; Serraino, I.; Sorrentino, R.; Meli, R.; Mattaceraso, G.; Cuzzocrea, S.; Pinto, A.; Autore, G. Effect of methylguanidine in carrageenan-induced acute inflammation in the rats. *Eur. J. Pharmacol.* **2004**, *484*, 341–350. [CrossRef]
79. Ahlawat, S.; Asha Sharma, K.K. Gut-organ axis: A microbial outreach and networking. *Lett. Appl. Microbiol.* **2021**, *72*, 636–668. [CrossRef]
80. Evenepoel, P.; Poesen, R.; Meijers, B. The gut-kidney axis. *Pediatr. Nephrol.* **2017**, *32*, 2005–2014. [CrossRef]
81. Meštrović, T.; Matijašić, M.; Perić, M.; Čipčić Paljetak, H.; Barešić, A.; Verbanac, D. The Role of Gut, Vaginal, and Urinary Microbiome in Urinary Tract Infections: From Bench to Bedside. *Diagnostics* **2020**, *11*, 7. [CrossRef]
82. Bien, J.; Sokolova, O.; Bozko, P. Role of Uropathogenic Escherichia coli Virulence Factors in Development of Urinary Tract Infection and Kidney Damage. *Int. J. Nephrol.* **2012**, *2012*, 681473. [CrossRef] [PubMed]
83. Magruder, M.; Sholi, A.N.; Gong, C.; Zhang, L.; Edusei, E.; Huang, J.; Albakry, S.; Satlin, M.J.; Westblade, L.F.; Crawford, C.; et al. Gut uropathogen abundance is a risk factor for development of bacteriuria and urinary tract infection. *Nat. Commun.* **2019**, *10*, 5521. [CrossRef] [PubMed]
84. Belyayeva, M.; Jeong, J.M. Acute pyelonephritis. In *StatPearls*; Stat Pearls Publishing: Treasure Island, FL, USA, 2020; pp. 2–3.

85. Nallu, A.; Sharma, S.; Ramezani, A.; Muralidharan, J.; Raj, D. Gut microbiome in chronic kidney disease: Challenges and opportunities. *Transl. Res.* **2017**, *179*, 24–37. [CrossRef] [PubMed]
86. Barrows, I.R.; Ramezani, A.; Raj, D.S. Gut Feeling in AKI: The Long Arm of Short–Chain Fatty Acids. *J. Am. Soc. Nephrol.* **2015**, *26*, 1755–1757. [CrossRef] [PubMed]
87. Al Khodor, S.; Shatat, I.F. Gut microbiome and kidney disease: A bidirectional relationship. *Pediatr. Nephrol.* **2017**, *32*, 921–931. [CrossRef] [PubMed]
88. Steenbeke, M.; Valkenburg, S.; Gryp, T.; Van Biesen, W.; Delanghe, J.R.; Speeckaert, M.M.; Glorieux, G. Gut Microbiota and Their Derived Metabolites, a Search for Potential Targets to Limit Accumulation of Protein-Bound Uremic Toxins in Chronic Kidney Disease. *Toxins* **2021**, *13*, 809. [CrossRef]
89. Hobby, G.P.; Karaduta, O.; Dusio, G.F.; Singh, M.; Zybailov, B.L.; Arthur, J.M. Chronic kidney disease and the gut microbiome. *Am. J. Physiol.-Ren. Physiol.* **2019**, *316*, F1211–F1217. [CrossRef]
90. Vaziri, N.D. Effect of synbiotic therapy on gut–derived uremic toxins and the intestinal microbiome in patients with CKD. *J. Am. Soc. Nephrol.* **2016**, *11*, 199–201. [CrossRef]
91. Pluznick, J.L. Gut microbiota in renal physiology: Focus on short-chain fatty acids and their receptors. *Kidney Int.* **2015**, *90*, 1191–1198. [CrossRef]
92. Mahmoodpoor, F.; Rahbar Saadat, Y.; Barzegari, A.; Ardalan, M.; Zununi Vahed, S. The impact of gut microbiota on kidney function and pathogenesis. *Biomed. Pharmacother.* **2017**, *93*, 412–419. [CrossRef]
93. Vijay, A.; Valdes, A.M. Role of the gut microbiome in chronic diseases: A narrative review. *Eur. J. Clin. Nutr.* **2021**, *28*, 1–13. [CrossRef] [PubMed]
94. Irazabal, M.; Torres, V.E. Reactive Oxygen Species and Redox Signaling in Chronic Kidney Disease. *Cells* **2020**, *9*, 1342. [CrossRef] [PubMed]
95. Akchurin, O.M.; Kaskel, F. Update on inflammation in chronic kidney disease. *Blood Purif.* **2015**, *39*, 84–92. [CrossRef] [PubMed]
96. Neagu, M.; Zipeto, D.; Popescu, I.D. Inflammation in Cancer: Part of the Problem or Part of the Solution? *J. Immunol. Res.* **2019**, *2019*, 5403910. [CrossRef]
97. Rapa, S.F.; Di Iorio, B.R.; Campiglia, P.; Heidland, A.; Marzocco, S. Inflammation and Oxidative Stress in Chronic Kidney Disease-Potential Therapeutic Role of Minerals, Vitamins and Plant-Derived Metabolites. *Int. J. Mol. Sci.* **2019**, *21*, 263. [CrossRef]
98. Roubicek, T.; Bartlova, M.; Krajickova, J.; Haluzikova, D.; Mraz, M.; Lacinova, Z.; Kudla, M.; Teplan, V.; Haluzik, M. Increased production of proinflammatory cytokines in adipose tissue of patients with end-stage renal disease. *Nutrition* **2009**, *25*, 762–768. [CrossRef]
99. Adesso, S.; Paterniti, I.; Cuzzocrea, S.; Fujioka, M.; Autore, G.; Magnus, T.; Pinto, A.; Marzocco, S. AST-120 Reduces Neuroinflammation Induced by Indoxyl Sulfate in Glial Cells. *J. Clin. Med.* **2018**, *7*, 365. [CrossRef]
100. Liu, T.; Zhang, L.; Joo, D.; Sun, S.C. NF-κB signaling in inflammation. *Signal Transduct. Target. Ther.* **2017**, *2*, 17023. [CrossRef]
101. Stockler-Pinto, M.B.; Saldanha, J.F.; Yi, D.; Mafra, D.; Fouque, D.; Soulage, C.O. The uremic toxin indoxyl sulfate exacerbates reactive oxygen species production and inflammation in 3T3-L1 adipose cells. *Free Radic. Res.* **2016**, *50*, 337–344. [CrossRef]
102. Duni, A.; Liakopoulos, V.; Roumeliotis, S.; Peschos, D.; Dounousi, E. Oxidative Stress in the Pathogenesis and Evolution of Chronic Kidney Disease: Untangling Ariadne's Thread. *Int. J. Mol. Sci.* **2019**, *20*, 3711. [CrossRef]
103. Kao, M.P.; Ang, D.S.; Pall, A.; Struthers, A.D. Oxidative stress in renal dysfunction: Mechanisms, clinical sequelae and therapeutic options. *J. Hum. Hypertens.* **2010**, *24*, 1–8. [CrossRef] [PubMed]
104. Descamps-Latscha, B.; Drüeke, T.; Witko-Sarsat, V. Dialysis-induced oxidative stress: Biological aspects, clinical consequences, and therapy. *Semin. Dial.* **2001**, *14*, 193–199. [CrossRef] [PubMed]
105. Modlinger, P.S.; Wilcox, C.S.; Aslam, S. Nitric oxide, oxidative stress, and progression of chronic renal failure. *Semin. Nephrol.* **2004**, *24*, 354–365. [CrossRef] [PubMed]
106. Di Meo, S.; Tanea, T.; Venditti, P.; Manuel, V. Role of ROS and RNS Sources in Physiological and Pathological Conditions. *Oxidative Med. Cell. Longev.* **2016**, *2016*, 1245049. [CrossRef]
107. Birben, E.; Murat, U.; Md, S.; Sackesen, C.; Erzurum, S.; Kalayci, O. Oxidative stress and antioxidant defense. *WAO J.* **2012**, *5*, 9–19. [CrossRef]
108. Krata, N.; Zagożdżon, R.; Foroncewicz, B.; Mucha, K. Oxidative Stress in Kidney Diseases: The Cause or the Consequence? *Arch. Immunol. Et. Ther. Exp.* **2018**, *66*, 211–220. [CrossRef]
109. Ratliff, B.B.; Abdulmahdi, W.; Pawar, R.; Wolin, M.S. Oxidant Mechanisms in Renal Injury and Disease. *Antioxid. Redox Signal.* **2016**, *25*, 119–146. [CrossRef]
110. Guijarro, C.; Egido, J. Transcription factor-κB (NF-κB) and renal disease. *Kidney Int.* **2001**, *59*, 415–424. [CrossRef]
111. Sanz, A.B.; Sanchez-Niño, M.D.; Ramos, A.M.; Moreno, J.A.; Santamaria, B.; Ruiz-Ortega, M.; Egido, J.; Ortiz, A. NF-κB in Renal Inflammation. *JASN* **2010**, *21*, 1254–1262. [CrossRef]
112. Yiu, W.H.; Wong, D.W.L.; Chan, L.Y.Y.; Leung, J.C.K.; Chan, K.W.; Lan, H.Y.; Lai, K.N.; Tang, S.C.W. Tissue Kallikrein Mediates Pro-Inflammatory Pathways and Activation of Protease-Activated Receptor-4 in Proximal Tubular Epithelial Cells. *PLoS ONE* **2014**, *9*, e88894. [CrossRef]
113. Kinugasa, E. Markers and possible uremic toxins: Japanese experiences. *Contrib. Nephrol.* **2011**, *168*, 134–138. [PubMed]
114. Boulanger, E.; Wautier, M.P.; Wautier, J.L.; Boval, B.; Panis, Y.; Wernert, N.; Danze, P.M.; Dequiedt, P. AGEs bind to mesothelial cells via RAGE and stimulate VCAM-1 expression. *Kidney Int.* **2002**, *61*, 148–156. [CrossRef] [PubMed]

115. Ruiz, S.; Pergola, P.E.; Zager, R.A.; Vaziri, N.D. Targeting the transcription factor Nrf2 to ameliorate oxidative stress and inflammation in chronic kidney disease. *Kidney Int.* **2013**, *83*, 1029–1041. [CrossRef] [PubMed]
116. Yamamoto, M.; Kensler, T.W.; Motohashi, H. The KEAP1-NRF2 System: A Thiol-Based Sensor-Effector Apparatus for Maintaining Redox Homeostasis. *Physiol. Rev.* **2018**, *98*, 1169–1203. [CrossRef] [PubMed]
117. Mann, G.E.; Forman, H.J. Introduction to Special Issue on Nrf2 Regulated Redox Signaling and Metabolism in Physiology and Medicine. *Free Radic. Biol. Med.* **2015**, *88*, 91–92. [CrossRef]
118. Cuadrado, A.; Rojo, A.I.; Wells, G.; Hayes, J.D.; Cousin, S.P.; Rumsey, W.L.; Attucks, O.C.; Franklin, S.; Levonen, A.L.; Kensler, T.W.; et al. Therapeutic targeting of the NRF2 and KEAP1 partnership in chronic diseases. *Nat. Rev. Drug Discov.* **2019**, *18*, 295–317. [CrossRef]
119. Wang, X.; He, G.; Peng, Y.; Zhong, W.; Wang, Y.; Zhang, B. Sodium butyrate alleviates adipocyte inflammation by inhibiting NLRP3 pathway. *Sci. Rep.* **2015**, *5*, 12676. [CrossRef]
120. Kobayashi, E.H.; Suzuki, T.; Funayama, R.; Nagashima, T.; Hayashi, M.; Sekine, H.; Tanaka, N.; Moriguchi, T.; Motohashi, H.; Nakayama, K.; et al. Nrf2 suppresses macrophage inflammatory response by blocking proinflammatory cytokine transcription. *Nat. Commun.* **2016**, *7*, 11624. [CrossRef]
121. Stenvinkel, P.; Chertow, G.M.; Devarajan, P.; Levin, A.; Andreoli, S.P.; Bangalore, S.; Warady, B.A. Chronic Inflammation in Chronic Kidney Disease Progression: Role of Nrf2. *Kidney Int. Rep.* **2021**, *6*, 1775–1787. [CrossRef]
122. Yuan, X.; Wang, L.; Bhat, O.M.; Lohner, H.; Li, P.L. Differential effects of short chain fatty acids on endothelial Nlrp3 inflammasome activation and neointima formation: Antioxidant action of butyrate. *Redox Biol.* **2018**, *16*, 21–31. [CrossRef]
123. Stempelj, M.; Kedinger, M.; Augenlicht, L.; Klampfer, L. Essential role of the JAK/STAT1 signaling pathway in the expression of inducible nitric-oxide synthase in intestinal epithelial cells and its regulation by butyrate. *J. Biol. Chem.* **2007**, *282*, 9797–9804. [CrossRef] [PubMed]
124. Chang, P.V.; Hao, L.; Offermanns, S.; Medzhitov, R. The microbial metabolite butyrate regulates intestinal macrophage function via histone deacetylase inhibition. *Proc. Natl. Acad. Sci. USA* **2014**, *111*, 2247–2252. [CrossRef] [PubMed]
125. Song, Y.; Li, X.; Li, Y.; Li, N.; Shi, X.; Ding, H.; Zhang, Y.; Li, X.; Liu, G.; Wang, Z. Non-esterified fatty acids activate the ROS-p38-p53/Nrf2 signaling pathway to induce bovine hepatocyte apoptosis in vitro. *Apoptosis* **2014**, *19*, 984–997. [CrossRef]
126. Wang, Y.; Li, C.; Li, J.; Wang, G.; Li, L. Non-Esterified Fatty Acid-Induced Reactive Oxygen Species Mediated Granulosa Cells Apoptosis Is Regulated by Nrf2/p53 Signaling Pathway. *Antioxidants* **2020**, *9*, 523. [CrossRef] [PubMed]
127. Zhang, M.; Wang, S.; Mao, L.; Leak, R.K.; Shi, Y.; Zhang, W.; Hu, X.; Sun, B.; Cao, G.; Gao, Y.; et al. Omega-3 fatty acids protect the brain against ischemic injury by activating Nrf2 and upregulating heme oxygenase 1. *J. Neurosci.* **2014**, *34*, 1903–1915. [CrossRef] [PubMed]
128. Wu, J.; Jiang, Z.; Zhang, H.; Liang, W.; Huang, W.; Zhang, H.; Li, Y.; Wang, Z.; Wang, J.; Jia, Y.; et al. Sodium butyrate attenuates diabetes-induced aortic endothelial dysfunction via P300-mediated transcriptional activation of Nrf2. *Free Radic. Biol. Med.* **2018**, *124*, 454–465. [CrossRef]
129. Yaku, K.; Enami, Y.; Kurajyo, C.; Matsui-Yuasa, I.; Konishi, Y.; Kojima-Yuasa, A. The enhancement of phase 2 enzyme activities by sodium butyrate in normal intestinal epithelial cells is associated with Nrf2 and p53. *Mol. Cell. Biochem.* **2012**, *370*, 7–14. [CrossRef]
130. Mihaylova, M.M.; Shaw, R.J. The AMPK signalling pathway coordinates cell growth, autophagy and metabolism. *Nat. Cell Biol.* **2011**, *13*, 1016–1023. [CrossRef]
131. Guo, W.; Liu, J.; Sun, J.; Gong, Q.; Ma, H.; Kan, X.; Cao, Y.; Wang, J.; Fu, S. Butyrate alleviates oxidative stress by regulating NRF2 nuclear accumulation and H3K9/14 acetylation via GPR109A in bovine mammary epithelial cells and mammary glands. *Free Radic. Biol. Med.* **2020**, *152*, 728–742. [CrossRef]
132. Srivastava, S.; Alfieri, A.; Siow, R.C.; Mann, G.E.; Fraser, P.A. Temporal and spatial distribution of Nrf2 in rat brain following stroke: Quantification of nuclear to cytoplasmic Nrf2 content using a novel immunohistochemical technique. *J. Physiol.* **2013**, *591*, 3525–3538. [CrossRef]
133. Faraonio, R.; Vergara, P.; Di Marzo, D.; Pierantoni, M.G.; Napolitano, M.; Russo, T.; Cimino, F. p53 suppresses the Nrf2-dependent transcription of antioxidant response genes. *J. Biol. Chem.* **2006**, *281*, 39776–39784. [CrossRef] [PubMed]
134. Logsdon, A.F.; Erickson, M.A.; Rhea, E.M.; Salameh, T.S.; Banks, W.A. Gut reactions: How the blood-brain barrier connects the microbiome and the brain. *Exp. Biol. Med.* **2018**, *243*, 159–165. [CrossRef] [PubMed]
135. Hoyles, L.; Snelling, T.; Umlai, U.K.; Nicholson, J.K.; Carding, S.R.; Glen, R.C.; McArthur, S. Microbiome-host systems interactions: Protective effects of propionate upon the blood-brain barrier. *Microbiome* **2018**, *6*, 55. [CrossRef] [PubMed]
136. Yin, Y.; Li, E.; Sun, G.; Yan, H.Q.; Foley, L.M.; Andrzejczuk, L.A.; Attarwala, I.Y.; Hitchens, T.K.; Kiselyov, K.; Dixon, C.E.; et al. Effects of DHA on Hippocampal Autophagy and Lysosome Function After Traumatic Brain Injury. *Mol. Neurobiol.* **2018**, *55*, 2454–2470. [CrossRef] [PubMed]
137. Duranton, F.; Cohen, G.; De Smet, R.; Rodriguez, M.; Jankowski, J.; Vanholder, R.; Argiles, A. European Uremic Toxin Work Group. Normal and pathologic concentrations of uremic toxins. *J. Am. Soc. Nephrol.* **2012**, *23*, 1258–1270. [CrossRef]
138. Chen, J.H.; Chiang, C.K. Uremic Toxins and Protein-Bound Therapeutics in AKI and CKD: Up-to-Date Evidence. *Toxins* **2021**, *14*, 8. [CrossRef]
139. Adesso, S.; Popolo, A.; Bianco, G.; Sorrentino, R.; Pinto, A.; Autore, G.; Marzocco, S. The uremic toxin indoxyl sulphate enhances macrophage response to LPS. *PLoS ONE* **2013**, *8*, e76778. [CrossRef]

140. Cheng, T.H.; Ma, M.C.; Liao, M.T.; Zheng, C.M.; Lu, K.C.; Liao, C.H.; Hou, Y.C.; Liu, W.C.; Lu, C.L. Indoxyl Sulfate, a Tubular Toxin, Contributes to the Development of Chronic Kidney Disease. *Toxins* **2020**, *12*, 684. [CrossRef]
141. Walther, C.P.; Nambi, V.; Hanania, N.A.; Navaneethan, S.D. Diagnosis and Management of Pulmonary Hypertension in Patients With CKD. *Am. J. Kidney Dis.* **2020**, *75*, 935–945. [CrossRef]
142. Stockler-Pinto, M.B.; Fouque, D.; Soulage, C.C.; Croze, M.; Mafra, D. Indoxyl sulfate and p-cresyl sulfate in chronic kidney disease. Could these toxins modulate the antioxidant Nrf2-Keap1 pathway? *J. Ren. Nutr.* **2014**, *24*, 286–291. [CrossRef]
143. Huang, W.; Guo, H.L.; Deng, X.; Zhu, T.T.; Xiong, J.F.; Xu, Y.H.; Xu, Y. Short-Chain Fatty Acids Inhibit Oxidative Stress and Inflammation in Mesangial Cells Induced by High Glucose and Lipopolysaccharide. *Exp. Clin. Endocrinol. Diabetes* **2017**, *125*, 98–105. [CrossRef] [PubMed]
144. Andrade-Oliveira, V.; Amano, M.T.; Correa-Costa, M.; Castoldi, A.; Felizardo, R.J.; de Almeida, D.C.; Bassi, E.J.; Moraes-Vieira, P.M.; Hiyane, M.I.; Rodas, A.C.; et al. Gut Bacteria Products Prevent AKI Induced by Ischemia-Reperfusion. *J. Am. Soc. Nephrol.* **2015**, *26*, 1877–1888. [CrossRef] [PubMed]
145. Huang, S.Y.; Chen, Y.A.; Chen, S.A.; Chen, Y.J.; Lin, Y.K. Uremic Toxins—Novel Arrhythmogenic Factor in Chronic Kidney Disease—Related Atrial Fibrillation. *Acta Cardiol. Sin.* **2016**, *32*, 259–264. [PubMed]
146. Marques, F.Z.; Nelson, E.; Chu, P.Y.; Horlock, D.; Fiedler, A.; Ziemann, M.; Tan, J.K.; Kuruppu, S.; Rajapakse, N.W.; El-Osta, A. et al. High-Fiber Diet and Acetate Supplementation Change the Gut Microbiota and Prevent the Development of Hypertension and Heart Failure in Hypertensive Mice. *Circulation* **2017**, *135*, 964–977. [CrossRef] [PubMed]
147. Zhang, Y.; Gao, F.; Tang, Y.; Xiao, J.; Li, C.; Ouyang, Y.; Hou, Y. Valproic acid regulates Ang II-induced pericyte-myofibroblast trans-differentiation via MAPK/ERK pathway. *Am. J. Transl. Res.* **2018**, *10*, 1976–1989.
148. Matsumoto, N.; Riley, S.; Fraser, D.; Al-Assaf, S.; Ishimura, E.; Wolever, T.; Phillips, G.O.; Phillips, A.O. Butyrate modulates TGF-beta1 generation and function: Potential renal benefit for Acacia(sen) SUPERGUM (gum arabic)? *Kidney Int.* **2006**, *69*, 257–265. [CrossRef]
149. Al-Harbi, N.O.; Nadeem, A.; Ahmad, S.F.; Alotaibi, M.R.; Al-Asmari, A.F.; Alanazi, W.A.; Al-Harbi, M.M.; El-Sherbeeny, A.M.; Ibrahim, K.E. Short chain fatty acid, acetate ameliorates sepsis-induced acute kidney injury by inhibition of NADPH oxidase signaling in T cells. *Int. Immunopharmacol.* **2018**, *58*, 24–31. [CrossRef]
150. Machado, R.A.; Constantino Lde, S.; Tomasi, C.D.; Rojas, H.A.; Vuolo, F.S.; Vitto, M.F.; Cesconetto, P.A.; de Souza, C.T.; Ritter, C.; Dal-Pizzol, F. Sodium butyrate decreases the activation of NF-κB reducing inflammation and oxidative damage in the kidney of rats subjected to contrast-induced nephropathy. *Nephrol. Dial. Transplant.* **2012**, *27*, 3136–3140. [CrossRef]
151. Liu, Y.; Li, Y.J.; Loh, Y.W.; Singer, J.; Zhu, W.; Macia, L.; Mackay, C.R.; Wang, W.; Chadban, S.J.; Wu, H. Fiber Derived Microbial Metabolites Prevent Acute Kidney Injury Through G-Protein Coupled Receptors and HDAC Inhibition. *Front. Cell Dev. Biol.* **2021**, *9*, 648639. [CrossRef]
152. Huang, W.; Man, Y.; Gao, C.; Zhou, L.; Gu, J.; Xu, H.; Wan, Q.; Long, Y.; Chai, L.; Xu, Y.; et al. Short-Chain Fatty Acids Ameliorate Diabetic Nephropathy via GPR43-Mediated Inhibition of Oxidative Stress and NF-κB Signaling. *Oxidative Med. Cell. Longev.* **2020**, *2020*, 4074832. [CrossRef]
153. Li, Y.J.; Chen, X.; Kwan, T.K.; Loh, Y.W.; Singer, J.; Liu, Y.; Ma, J.; Tan, J.; Macia, L.; Mackay, C.R.; et al. Dietary Fiber Protects against Diabetic Nephropathy through Short-Chain Fatty Acid-Mediated Activation of G Protein-Coupled Receptors GPR43 and GPR109A. *J. Am. Soc. Nephrol.* **2020**, *31*, 1267–1281. [CrossRef] [PubMed]
154. Felizardo, R.J.F.; de Almeida, D.C.; Pereira, R.L.; Watanabe, I.K.M.; Doimo, N.T.S.; Ribeiro, W.R.; Cenedeze, M.A.; Hiyane, M.I.; Amano, M.T.; Braga, T.T.; et al. Gut microbial metabolite butyrate protects against proteinuric kidney disease through epigenetic- and GPR109a-mediated mechanisms. *FASEB J.* **2019**, *33*, 11894–11908. [CrossRef] [PubMed]
155. Yang, H.; Zhang, Z.; Peng, R.; Zhang, L.; Liu, H.; Wang, X.; Tian, Y.; Sun, Y. RNA-Seq analysis reveals critical transcriptome changes caused by sodium butyrate in DN mouse models. *Biosci. Rep.* **2021**, *41*, BSR20203005. [CrossRef] [PubMed]
156. Hung, T.V.; Suzuki, T. Dietary Fermentable Fibers Attenuate Chronic Kidney Disease in Mice by Protecting the Intestinal Barrier. *J. Nutr.* **2018**, *148*, 552–561. [CrossRef]
157. Yang, J.; Li, Q.; Henning, S.M.; Zhong, J.; Hsu, M.; Lee, R.; Long, J.; Chan, B.; Nagami, G.T.; Heber, D.; et al. Effects of Prebiotic Fiber Xylooligosaccharide in Adenine-Induced Nephropathy in Mice. *Mol. Nutr. Food Res.* **2018**, *62*, e1800014. [CrossRef]
158. Marzocco, S.; Fazeli, G.; Di Micco, L.; Autore, G.; Adesso, S.; Dal Piaz, F.; Heidland, A.; Di Iorio, B. Supplementation of Short-Chain Fatty Acid, Sodium Propionate, in Patients on Maintenance Hemodialysis: Beneficial Effects on Inflammatory Parameters and Gut-Derived Uremic Toxins, A Pilot Study (PLAN Study). *J. Clin. Med.* **2018**, *7*, 315. [CrossRef]
159. Gansevoort, R.T.; Correa-Rotter, R.; Hemmelgarn, B.R.; Jafar, T.H.; Heerspink, H.J.; Mann, J.F.; Matsushita, K.; Wen, C.P. Chronic kidney disease and cardiovascular risk: Epidemiology, mechanisms, and prevention. *Lancet* **2013**, *382*, 339–352. [CrossRef]
160. Esgalhado, M.; Kemp, J.A.; Damasceno, N.R.; Fouque, D.; Mafra, D. Short-chain fatty acids: A link between prebiotics and microbiota in chronic kidney disease. *Future Microbiol.* **2017**, *12*, 1413–1425. [CrossRef]
161. Natarajan, N.; Hori, D.; Flavahan, S.; Steppan, J.; Flavahan, N.A.; Berkowitz, D.E.; Pluznick, J.L. Microbial short chain fatty acid metabolites lower blood pressure via endothelial G protein-coupled receptor 41. *Physiol. Genom.* **2016**, *48*, 826–834. [CrossRef]
162. Pluznick, J. A novel SCFA receptor, the microbiota, and blood pressure regulation. *Gut Microbes* **2014**, *5*, 202–207. [CrossRef]
163. Weber, G.J.; Foster, J.; Pushpakumar, S.B.; Sen, U. Altered microRNA regulation of short chain fatty acid receptors in the hypertensive kidney is normalized with hydrogen sulfide supplementation. *Pharmacol. Res.* **2018**, *134*, 157–165. [CrossRef] [PubMed]

164. Pevsner-Fischer, M.; Blacher, E.; Tatirovsky, E.; Ben-Dov, I.Z.; Elinav, E. The gut microbiome and hypertension. *Curr. Opin. Nephrol. Hypertens.* **2017**, *26*, 1–8. [CrossRef] [PubMed]
165. Jadoon, A.; Mathew, A.V.; Byun, J.; Gadegbeku, C.A.; Gipson, D.S.; Afshinnia, F.; Pennathur, S. For the Michigan Kidney Translational Core CPROBE Investigator Group. Gut Microbial Product Predicts Cardiovascular Risk in Chronic Kidney Disease Patients. *Am. J. Nephrol.* **2018**, *48*, 269–277. [CrossRef] [PubMed]
166. Karbach, S.H.; Schönfelder, T.; Brandão, I.; Wilms, E.; Hörmann, N.; Jäckel, S.; Schüler, R.; Finger, S.; Knorr, M.; Lagrange, J.; et al. Gut Microbiota Promote Angiotensin II-Induced Arterial Hypertension and Vascular Dysfunction. *J. Am. Heart Assoc.* **2016**, *5*, e003698. [CrossRef] [PubMed]
167. Di Iorio, B.R.; Marzocco, S.; Bellasi, A.; De Simone, E.; Dal Piaz, F.; Rocchetti, M.T.; Cosola, C.; Di Micco, L.; Gesualdo, L. Nutritional therapy reduces protein carbamylation through urea lowering in chronic kidney disease. *Nephrol. Dial. Transplant.* **2018**, *33*, 804–813. [CrossRef] [PubMed]
168. Di Iorio, B.R.; Di Micco, L.; Marzocco, S.; De Simone, E.; De Blasio, A.; Sirico, M.L.; Nardone, L. UBI Study Group. Very Low-Protein Diet (VLPD) Reduces Metabolic Acidosis in Subjects with Chronic Kidney Disease: The "Nutritional Light Signal" of the Renal Acid Load. *Nutrients* **2017**, *9*, 69. [CrossRef]
169. Bellasi, A.; Di Micco, L.; Santoro, D.; Marzocco, S.; De Simone, E.; Cozzolino, M.; Di Lullo, L.; Guastaferro, P.; Di Iorio, B. UBI study investigators. Correction of metabolic acidosis improves insulin resistance in chronic kidney disease. *BMC Nephrol.* **2016**, *17*, 158. [CrossRef]
170. Rocchetti, M.T.; Di Iorio, B.R.; Vacca, M.; Cosola, C.; Marzocco, S.; di Bari, I.; Calabrese, F.M.; Ciarcia, R.; De Angelis, M.; Gesualdo, L. Ketoanalogs' Effects on Intestinal Microbiota Modulation and Uremic Toxins Serum Levels in Chronic Kidney Disease (Medika2 Study). *J. Clin. Med.* **2021**, *10*, 840. [CrossRef]
171. Marzocco, S.; Dal Piaz, F.; Di Micco, L.; Torraca, S.; Sirico, M.L.; Tartaglia, D.; Autore, G.; Di Iorio, B. Very low protein diet reduces indoxyl sulfate levels in chronic kidney disease. *Blood Purif.* **2013**, *35*, 196–201. [CrossRef]
172. Kemp, J.A.; Regis de Paiva, B.; Fragoso Dos Santos, H.; Emiliano de Jesus, H.; Craven, H.; ZIjaz, U.; Alvarenga Borges, N.; GShiels, P.; Mafra, D. The Impact of Enriched Resistant Starch Type-2 Cookies on the Gut Microbiome in Hemodialysis Patients: A Randomized Controlled Trial. *Mol. Nutr. Food Res.* **2021**, *65*, e2100374. [CrossRef]
173. Di Iorio, B.R.; Rocchetti, M.T.; De Angelis, M.; Cosola, C.; Marzocco, S.; Di Micco, L.; di Bari, I.; Accetturo, M.; Vacca, M.; Gobbetti, M.; et al. Nutritional Therapy Modulates Intestinal Microbiota and Reduces Serum Levels of Total and Free Indoxyl Sulfate and P-Cresyl Sulfate in Chronic Kidney Disease (Medika Study). *J. Clin. Med.* **2019**, *8*, 1424. [CrossRef] [PubMed]
174. Wu, I.W.; Lee, C.C.; Hsu, H.J.; Sun, C.Y.; Chen, Y.C.; Yang, K.J.; Yang, C.W.; Chung, W.H.; Lai, H.C.; Chang, L.C.; et al. Compositional and Functional Adaptations of Intestinal Microbiota and Related Metabolites in CKD Patients Receiving Dietary Protein Restriction. *Nutrients* **2020**, *12*, 2799. [CrossRef] [PubMed]

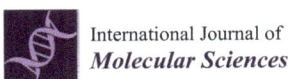

Review

Chronic Kidney Disease and Gut Microbiota: What Is Their Connection in Early Life?

Chien-Ning Hsu [1,2] and You-Lin Tain [3,4,*]

1. Department of Pharmacy, Kaohsiung Chang Gung Memorial Hospital, Kaohsiung 833, Taiwan; cnhsu@cgmh.org.tw
2. School of Pharmacy, Kaohsiung Medical University, Kaohsiung 807, Taiwan
3. Department of Pediatrics, Kaohsiung Chang Gung Memorial Hospital and Chang Gung University College of Medicine, Kaohsiung 833, Taiwan
4. Institute for Translational Research in Biomedicine, Kaohsiung Chang Gung Memorial Hospital and Chang Gung University College of Medicine, Kaohsiung 833, Taiwan
* Correspondence: tainyl@cgmh.org.tw; Tel.: +886-975-056-995; Fax: +886-7733-8009

Abstract: The gut–kidney interaction implicating chronic kidney disease (CKD) has been the focus of increasing interest in recent years. Gut microbiota-targeted therapies could prevent CKD and its comorbidities. Considering that CKD can originate in early life, its treatment and prevention should start in childhood or even earlier in fetal life. Therefore, a better understanding of how the early-life gut microbiome impacts CKD in later life and how to develop ideal early interventions are unmet needs to reduce CKD. The purpose of the current review is to summarize (1) the current evidence on the gut microbiota dysbiosis implicated in pediatric CKD; (2) current knowledge supporting the impact of the gut–kidney axis in CKD, including inflammation, immune response, alterations of microbiota compositions, short-chain fatty acids, and uremic toxins; and (3) an overview of the studies documenting early gut microbiota-targeted interventions in animal models of CKD of developmental origins. Treatment options include prebiotics, probiotics, postbiotics, etc. To accelerate the transition of gut microbiota-based therapies for early prevention of CKD, an extended comprehension of gut microbiota dysbiosis implicated in renal programming is needed, as well as a greater focus on pediatric CKD for further clinical translation.

Keywords: chronic kidney disease; hypertension; children; short-chain fatty acids; developmental origins of health and disease (DOHaD); gut microbiota; probiotics; prebiotics; trimethylamine-N-oxide

1. Introduction

Up to 10% of the population worldwide is affected by chronic kidney disease (CKD) [1]. CKD can be attributed to different negative conditions in early life [2–4], and therefore, World Kidney Day 2016 made efforts to keep the public informed of the need to focus on kidney disease in childhood and the antecedents of adult kidney disease [5]. During development, the fetal kidney is susceptible to a suboptimal in utero environment, resulting in alterations in function and structure by so-called renal programming [6]. The phenomenon of adverse conditions during organ development resulting in adult disease in later life is now termed "developmental origins of health and disease" (DOHaD) [7]. Conversely, adverse fetal programming could be reprogramming before clinical onset of the disease by early therapeutic intervention [8]. Accordingly, a shift of focus from treatment of established CKD towards the prevention of kidney disease in the earliest stage is highly needed.

Although various organ systems can be programmed in response to in utero suboptimal conditions, renal programming is considered key in the development of CKD and its comorbidities [6,9]. Renal programming is likely to constitute a first hit to the kidney, which makes the kidney more vulnerable to postnatal insults (i.e., second hit) to develop CKD in later life. Up to now, researchers have proposed some mechanisms associated with renal programming. These mechanisms, such as dysregulated nutrient-sensing signals [9], oxidative stress [10], nitric oxide (NO) signaling [11], aberrant activation of the renin–angiotensin system (RAS) [12], and gut microbiota dysbiosis [13,14], have been contributing to CKD in later life [2–4,6,8,9].

Due to the low antioxidant capacity of embryos [15], the developing kidney is extremely vulnerable to oxidant stress injury. As reviewed elsewhere [16], a number of animal models support that NO/reactive oxygen species imbalance-induced oxidative stress is involved in renal programming. On the other hand, increasing evidence suggests antioxidants can be used as reprogramming strategies to prevent kidney disease and hypertension of developmental origins [17]. In the developing kidney, the RAS components are highly expressed and play a key role in mediating proper physiological function and renal morphology [18]. A transient biphasic response with downregulation of the classical RAS axis in the neonatal stage becomes normalized with age [19,20]. Data from renal programming models reported that various early-life insults can disturb this normalization in adults, and consequently, the classical RAS axis is inappropriately activated, leading to the development of kidney disease in adulthood [6,19,20]. Conversely, emerging evidence supports that early RAS-based interventions could reverse programming processes to prevent kidney disease of developmental origins [12]. Additionally, nutrient-sensing signals play an essential role in normal renal physiology and the pathogenesis of kidney disease [21]. Early-life nutritional insults can impair nutrient-sensing signals that affect fetal development and, consequently, program chronic disease in later life [22]. Dysregulated nutrient-sensing signals, such as AMP-activated protein kinase (AMPK) and peroxisome proliferator-activated receptors (PPARs), have been linked to renal programming and the risks for developing kidney disease in later life [23,24]. Despite the fact that the complete mechanisms are still inconclusive, there seem to be interrelated aspects among them. Since detailed reviews of each mechanism are beyond the scope of this paper, readers are referred elsewhere [8–14].

Recent studies have focused on the impact of the gut microbiome in CKD and its associated complications [14]. Microbial metabolites can act as signaling compounds via systemic circulation [14]. Currently, there are some proposed mechanisms linking dysbiotic gut microbiota to CKD and related complications, such as alterations of the gut microbiome, dysregulation of short-chain fatty acids (SCFA) and their receptors, activation of aryl hydrocarbon receptor (AHR), increases of trimethylamine-N-oxide (TMAO), and microbiota-derived uremic toxins [14,25–29]. Maternal insults have been shown to change gut microbiome balance, leading to an increased risk of adult diseases [29]. Nevertheless, relatively little is known about whether and how diverse prenatal insults could influence gut microbiota, leading to CKD and its comorbidities in adult offspring.

This scoping review followed the Preferred Reporting Items for Systematic Reviews and Meta-Analyses extension for Scoping Reviews (PRISMA-ScR) to identify and examine the evidence around the impact of gut microbiota behind the programming of kidney disease evidence documenting prevention of CKD and its related complications by early-life gut microbiota-targeted therapy [30]. Our search strategy was designed to retrieve literature relating to DOHaD, gut microbiota, and pediatric kidney disease from PubMed/MEDLINE databases. We used the following search terms: "chronic kidney disease", "developmental programming", "DOHaD", "reprogramming", "gut microbiota", "probiotics", "prebiotics", "synbiotics", "postbiotics", "mother", "pregnancy", "gestation", "offspring", "progeny", "uremic toxin", "nephrogenesis", "nephron number", "kidney", "aryl hydrocarbon receptor", and "hypertension". Additional studies were then selected and assessed based on fitting references in eligible papers. The last search was conducted on 25 January 2022.

2. Human Evidence for Developmental Programming of CKD

The development of the human kidney starts at week 3 and ends at week 36 of gestation [31]. Hence, term neonates are born with a full complement of nephrons. In each kidney, the average number of nephrons, the basic unit of a kidney, is approximately 1 million with 10-fold interindividual differences [32]. Adverse in utero events could interfere with nephrogenesis, resulting in a reduction of nephron numbers and a wide range of congenital anomalies of the kidney and urinary tract (CAKUT) [33]. Reduced nephron number causes glomerular hyperfiltration and compensatory glomerular hypertrophy, consequently initiating a vicious cycle of further nephron loss [34]. Accordingly, reduced nephron number could act as a first trigger to increase the offspring's vulnerability to CKD throughout their later life.

Strong support for the developmental programming of CKD came from a number of epidemiological studies. Premature birth and low birth weight (LBW) are significant risk factors for CKD in later life [35–38]. A meta-analysis study recruiting more than 2 million babies revealed that LBW babies were 70% more likely to develop CKD in later life than those with normal birth weight [36]. In addition to premature birth and LBW, a case–control study of 1.6 million infants revealed that maternal gestational diabetes, maternal thalassemia/hemochromatosis, male gender, polyhydramnios or oligohydramnios, and first pregnancy are also risk factors for CAKUT [37]. Another case–control study recruiting 2000 CKD children acknowledged several early-life risk factors, such as LBW, prematurity, gestational diabetes, and maternal obesity, showed an increased risk of CKD in adult life [38]. As we reviewed elsewhere, a number of environmental risk factors are related to the developmental programming of CKD, such as maternal illness, nutritional imbalance, environmental chemicals, medication use, substance abuse, infection, and exogenous stress [4]. For example, maternal obesity and diabetes are correlated with an increased risk of kidney disease in adulthood [39,40]. Additionally, deficiencies in maternal total energy [41], folate [42], and vitamin A [43] during pregnancy were associated with detrimental influence on kidney structure and function. Epidemiological studies also showed that maternal exposure to polycyclic aromatic hydrocarbon, per- and polyfluoroalkyl substances, and polycyclic aromatic hydrocarbon, as well as air pollution associated with premature birth and LBW [44–47], are both risk factors for low nephron number. Moreover, a number of drugs administered to pregnant women have been known to affect kidney development, resulting in CAKUT [48]. These medications include angiotensin converting enzyme inhibitor, angiotensin receptor blockers, aminoglycosides, cyclosporine A, dexamethasone, furosemide, anti-epileptic drugs, cyclophosphamide, etc. [48].

Although the risk of CKD has been evaluated in plenty of human studies, interventions required to prove causation and to elucidate underlying molecular mechanisms remain unknown. Most of our knowledge regarding the critical window of vulnerability for insults, the types of insults driving renal programming, potential core mechanisms behind renal programming, and therapeutic strategy arise out of studies in animal models.

3. Gut Microbiota and Kidney Disease

Trillions of microbes living in the gut—the gut microbiota—have coexisted with humans in a state of mutually beneficial cohabitation. A diversity of environmental factors can induce gut microbial imbalance (i.e., dysbiosis), which in turn can affect human health and disease [49]. Although the role of gut microbiota in adulthood advanced CKD has been extensively reviewed elsewhere [14,25,50,51], less attention has been given to investigate its impact in early stages of kidney disease. Therefore, this section mainly discusses evidence supporting the role of early-life gut microbiota in humans, with an emphasis on pediatric CKD.

3.1. Early-Life Gut Microbiome

Although microbes colonize the neonatal gut immediately following birth [52], microbial colonization continues to develop and vary in species abundance until a typical adult-like gut microbiota is established at the age of 2–3 years [53]. A variety of maternal factors and early-life events determine the establishment of the gut microbiome, such as gestational age, type of delivery, maternal conditions, formula feeding, antibiotic exposure, and ecological factors [52–55].

During pregnancy and lactation, the mother gut microbiota can influence offspring gut microbial structure and composition, which highlights the importance of maternal factors in the establishment of early-life gut microbiome [55]. Several risk factors related to CKD of developmental origins have also been linked to alterations of gut microbiota, such as gestational diabetes [56], maternal obesity [57], prematurity [58], LBW [59], and maternal malnutrition [60]. Additionally, the establishment of the microbiome is highly interconnected with development of the immune system, and CKD has strong immune and inflammatory etiologies [61].

Moreover, several environmental chemicals that pregnant mothers are likely to be exposed to are associated with developmental origins of kidney disease [62]. Among them, exposure to heavy metals, polycyclic aromatic hydrocarbons, and dioxins also affect the gut microbiome, accompanied with the development of adult diseases [63]. All of these studies suggest that the early-life microbial alterations after the CKD-related adverse insults may be involved in the development of kidney disease in later life.

3.2. The Gut–Kidney Axis

The pathogenic interconnection between the gut microbiome and kidney diseases is termed the gut–kidney axis [14], which is implicated in CKD and its comorbidities. A paucity of data exists regarding how the gut–kidney axis functions in the pediatric population with CKD and what the impact of the gut microbiota is in this process. However, a great deal of work on the impact of the gut–kidney axis in established CKD has been conducted, including gut barrier dysfunction, inflammation, immune response, alterations of microbiota compositions, dysregulated SCFAs and their receptors, uremic toxins, etc. (Figure 1). Each of them are discussed.

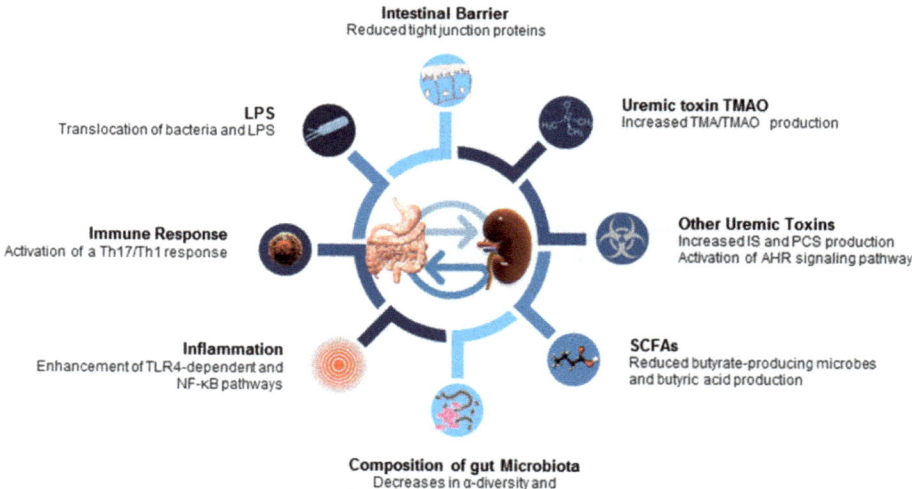

Figure 1. Schematic diagram summarizing the proposed mechanisms related to the gut–kidney axis involved in the pathogenesis of chronic kidney disease and its comorbidities. LPS = lipopolysaccharide; Th17 = T-helper 17 cell; Th1 = T-helper 1 cell; TLR4 = toll-like receptor 4; NF-κB = nuclear factor kappa B; SCFA = short-chain fatty acid; IS = indoxyl sulfate; PCS = p-cresyl sulfate; AHR = aryl hydrocarbon receptor; TMA = trimethylamine; TMAO = trimethylamine-N-oxide.

First, CKD can impair the intestinal barrier by disrupting the epithelial tight junction in a 5/6 nephrectomy rat model [64]. An apparent reduction of the tight junction proteins was reported in the gut mucosa of CKD animals, possibly attributed to uremic toxins [44]. As a result, an increased intestinal permeability and translocation of lipopolysaccharide (LPS) and bacteria across the intestinal barrier were reported. In CKD rats, gut bacteria could activate a T-helper 17 (Th17)/Th1 T-cell response and increase the production of inflammatory cytokines, and LPS could initiate innate immune cells through nuclear factor kappa B (NF-κB) and toll-like receptor 4 (TLR4) pathways, all triggering inflammation and immune response [65].

Second, changes in the composition of the gut microbiota are relevant to CKD. Uremia profoundly alters 190 and 175 bacterial operational taxonomic units (OTUs) of the gut microbiome in CKD humans [66] and rats [67], respectively. Specifically, the presence of aerobic bacteria such as those belonging to the phyla *Firmicutes*, *Actinobacteria*, and *Proteobacteria* in higher numbers, but fewer anaerobic bacteria, such as *Sutterellaceae*, *Bacteroidaceae*, and *Lactobacillaceae*, were observed in end stage kidney disease (ESKD) [45–47]. Notably, most research has consistently reported that animals and adult patients with CKD had low abundance of genus *Lactobacillus*, whereas the proportion of family *Enterobacteriaceae* were increased [14,66–69]. A systemic review recruiting 25 studies with 1436 CKD patients revealed that the α-diversity was decreased, and β-diversity of gut microbiota was significantly more distinct in ESKD patients than in healthy controls [69].

Third, the gut microbiota produces diverse metabolites, which are involved in multiple physiological processes, such as immunity and host energy metabolism [14]. Following dietary exposures to certain nutrients, particular microbiota-derived metabolites could be altered in ESKD patients [70]. Carbohydrates are fermented to generate SCFAs which signal the host to increase energy expenditure, enhance G protein-coupled receptor (GPCR) signaling, and act as an inhibitor for histone deacetylase (HDAC) [70–72]. SCFAs are made up of one to six carbon atoms (C1–C6), mainly consisting of acetic acid (C2), propionic acid (C3), and butyric acid (C4) [71]. In adult CKD patients, butyrate-producing microbes and butyric acid production reduced with disease severity [73].

Indoxyl sulfate (IS) and p-cresyl sulfate (PCS), both end-products of protein fermentation, and TMAO, an end-product of microbial carnitine/choline metabolism, are well-known microbiota-derived uremic toxins. Urinary excretion of several microbial tryptophan metabolites such as IS and PCS is decreased in patients with CKD. These tryptophan metabolites mainly from the indole metabolic pathway are accumulated as uremic toxins, which are ligands for AHR [74]. Activation of AHR is able to trigger inflammation, induce oxidative stress, and modulate the Th17 axis, contributing to CKD progression in vivo and in vitro [75,76]. The level of another uremic toxin, TMAO, is high in patients with ESKD and associated with increased risk of cardiovascular disease [77,78]. TMAO generation results from the fermentation by the gut microbiota of dietary carnitine/choline, which is converted to trimethylamine (TMA) and transformed into TMAO by flavin-containing monooxygenase (FMO) in the liver. Conversely, selective targeting of gut-microbiota-dependent TMAO generation has been reported to protect CKD progression in a murine model of CKD [79]. Although the uses of prebiotics, probiotics, postbiotics, and synbiotics have shown potential positive effects against uremic toxin generation, their evidence is still limited for the treatment and prevention of human CKD [80–82].

Together, the interaction between gut microbiota and CKD is bidirectional: CKD may affect the structure of the gut microbiota and contribute to gut dysbiosis, while dysbiosis in CKD patients may increase uremic toxin levels that in turn contribute to CKD progression. Considering the gut is a potential cause of CKD-related complications gut microbiota-targeted therapeutic strategies in CKD will have a considerable impact on CKD management.

3.3. Gut Microbiota in Pediatric CKD

Table 1 summarizes the alterations of gut microbiota and its related metabolites in pediatric kidney disease, as reported in the literature [83–89]. The study of the gut microbiome in children with kidney disease mainly focused on three types of dysbiosis: loss of diversity, shifts in keystone taxa, and alterations of microbial metabolites.

Table 1. Summary of studies investigated links between gut microbiota and pediatric chronic kidney disease.

Study	Study Population	Age (Years)	Alterations in Gut Microbiota and Metabolites
Crespo-Salgado et al., 2016 [83]	8 HD, 8 PD, 10 transplant, 13 controls	Control: 9.5 (3–16), HD: 13.6 (8–17), PD: 11.9 (3–17), transplant: 13.2 (2–18)	↓ Alpha diversity in PD and transplant ↓ Phyla *Firmicutes* and *Actinobacteria* but ↑ family *Enterobacteriaceae* in PD ↑ Phylum *Bacteroidetes* in HD ↑ Plasma levels of p-cresyl sulfate and indoxyl sulfate in HD and PD
Tsuji et al., 2018 [84]	12 INS, 11 controls	Controls: 5.1, relapsing INS: 3, non-relapsing INS: 4.3	↓ Butyrate-producing bacteria belonging to *Clostridium* clusters IV and XIVa ↓ Fecal butyric acid level
Hsu et al., 2018 [85]	60 CKD stage 1 26 CKD stage 2–3	11.3 (7.2–15.5) 11.3 (7.2–15.5)	↓ Urinary levels of DMA and TMAO in CKD stage 2–3 vs. CKD stage 1 ↓ Genus *Prevotella* in CKD children with an abnormal ABPM profile
Hsu et al., 2019 [86]	78 CKD stage 1–4	11.2 (7.4–15.2)	↑ Plasma levels of propionic acid and butyric acid in CKD children with an abnormal ABPM profile ↑ Phylum *Verrucomicrobia*, genus *Akkermansia*, and species ↓ *Bifidobacterium bifidum* in CKD children with CAKUT
Kang et al., 2019 [87]	20 INS	3.5 ± 2.1	↑ Genera *Romboutsia*, *Stomatobaculum* and *Cloacibacillus* after 4-week initial therapy
Hsu et al., 2020 [88]	115 CKD stage 1–4	11.3 (7.2–15.5)	↑ Plasma levels of DMA, TMA, and TMAO in children with CKD stage 2–4 vs. CKD stage 1 ↓ Phylum *Cyanobacteria*, genera *Subdoligranulum*, *Ruminococcus*, *Faecalibacterium*, and *Akkermansia* in CKD children with an abnormal ABPM profile
Yamaguchi et al., 2021 [89]	20 INS	INS with probiotics: 6.4 (3.7–10.6), INS without probiotics: 4.7 (3.5–7.8)	↓ Butyrate-producing bacteria

Data on age are presented as mean ± standard deviation or median (interquartile range); PD = peritoneal dialysis; HD = hemodialysis; CKD = chronic kidney disease; INS = idiopathic nephrotic syndrome; CAKUT = congenital anomalies of the kidney and urinary tract; DMA = dimethylamine; TMA = trimethylamine; TMAO = trimethylamine-N-oxide; ABPM = 24 h ambulatory blood pressure monitoring.

The pediatric gut microbiome in a uremic milieu has been evaluated in a small group of ESKD children who underwent hemodialysis (HD, $n = 8$), peritoneal dialysis (PD, $n = 8$), or kidney transplant ($n = 10$) [83]. Alpha diversity was decreased in children undergoing PD or transplant. ESKD children undergoing HD had increased abundance of phylum *Bacteroidetes*. Children on PD had an increase in the abundance of phyla *Firmicutes* and *Actinobacteria* but a decrease in abundance of family *Enterobacteriaceae*. Additionally, children on HD or PD had increased plasma levels of microbiota-derived uremic toxins, IS, and PCS [83]. A similar pattern of gut dysbiosis was reported in adult patients with ESKD [69,70].

In another small group of children ($n = 12$) with idiopathic nephrotic syndrome (INS), butyric acid level in the feces was decreased in relapsing INS children coinciding with decreased abundance of butyrate-producing bacteria belonging to *Clostridium* clusters IV and XIVa [84]. These microbes included *Clostridium orbiscindens*, *Faecalibacterium prausnitzii*,

Eubacterium hallii, *E. ramulus*, *E. rectale*, *E. ventriosum*, *Roseburia intestinalis*, *Eubacterium* spp., and *Butyrivibrio* spp.

One study recruiting 60 children diagnosed with CKD stage 1 and 26 stage 2–3 children showed that urinary levels of TMAO and dimethylamine (DMA, a metabolite of TMAO) were lower in children with CKD stages 2–3 than CKD stage 1 [85]. Additionally, the proportion of genus *Prevotella* was decreased in CKD children with blood pressure (BP) abnormalities.

In 78 children and adolescents with CKD stage 1–4 and a median age of 11.2 years, BP determined using 24 h ambulatory blood pressure monitoring (ABPM) was defined out of range, and BP was related to increased plasma levels of propionic acid and butyric acid [86]. Additionally, the abundance of phylum *Verrucomicrobia*, genus *Akkermansia*, and species *Bifidobacterium bifidum* were higher in CKD children with CAKUT compared to those with non-CAKUT.

In another study from our group, we recruited 115 children and adolescents with CKD stages 1–4 [88]. We found plasma levels of DMA, trimethylamine (TMA), and TMAO higher in children with CKD stage 2–4 vs. CKD stage 1. These data are consistent with previous studies in CKD adults [90,91], showing that TMAO is increased in CKD and that there is a negative association between circulating TMAO level and renal function. We also observed that phylum *Cyanobacteria*, genera *Subdoligranulum*, *Faecalibacterium*, *Ruminococcus*, and *Akkermansia* were decreased in CKD children stools with an abnormal ABPM profile.

CKD children with abnormal ABPM had a decreased proportion of genera *Gemella*, *Providencia*, and *Peptosreptoccocus*. Of note is that these genera of bacteria are involved in TMA production [92]. Accordingly, whether these microbes play a key role on the development of hypertension via the TMA–TMAO metabolic pathway in CKD children deserves further clarification.

In 20 children with INS who received oral prednisone therapy, abundance of genera *Romboutsia*, *Stomatobaculum*, and *Cloacibacillus* was increased after a 4-week initial therapy [87]. Another study recruited 20 children with INS and showed that probiotic treatment protected against relapse and coincided with increases in butyrate-producing bacteria and blood regulatory T cell (Treg) counts [89]. Considering gut microbiota shapes, the Th17/Treg balance, and Th17 involved in renal inflammation, probiotic treatment may have beneficial effects impacting the gut–kidney axis via immune regulation.

4. Gut Microbiota-Targeted Therapy

Recently, researchers have increasingly turned their attention on gut microbiota and its derived metabolites as a potential target for therapeutics [81,82,93,94]. In clinical practice, the most generally used gut microbiota-targeted therapies are probiotics and prebiotics. Probiotics are live bacteria that have health benefits when administered [93]. Prebiotics can promote the growth and activity of beneficial bacteria [93]. Synbiotics refer to a mixture comprising probiotic and prebiotics that also confers a health benefit. Additionally, the use of substances leased or produced through metabolism of the gut microbes, namely postbiotics, have shown a positive effect on the host [94]. Another gut microbiota-targeted therapy is fecal microbial transplantation (FMT). Although FMT is being broadly studied in microbiome-associated pathologies [95,96], its potential application for the treatment of CKD remains largely unknown. Moreover, treatment with oral intestinal absorbent AST-120 can reduce microbiota-derived uremic toxins [97]. Although AST-120 treatment has shown cardiovascular benefits in adult patients with CKD [98,99], its influence on gut microbiota compositions and other CKD-related complications remains limited. A summary of potential gut microbiota-targeted therapies in the treatment of developmental programming of CKD and its comorbidities is illustrated in Figure 2.

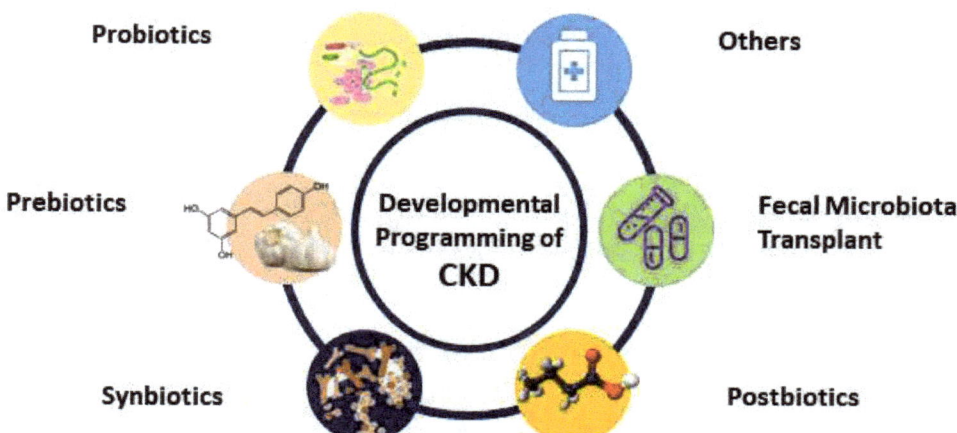

Figure 2. Schematic diagram of the potential gut microbiota-targeted therapy used for developmental programming of chronic kidney disease.

4.1. Human Evidence in Pediatric CKD

To date, limited data are available to examine whether alterations of gut microbiota by microbiota-targeted therapies can protect against CKD progression and its comorbidities in the pediatric population. For example, *Clostridium butyricum* is a butyrate-producing bacteria used as a probiotic [100]. Oral administration of *Clostridium butyricum* during remission was reported to reduce the frequency of relapse and the need for immunosuppressive agents in children with INS [89]. The protective effect of probiotic therapy was associated with increases in butyrate-producing bacteria and Treg cells. On the other hand, animal studies targeting gut microbiota to prevent the development of CKD and its associated complications have produced some compelling evidence.

4.2. Animal Models of Early-Life Gut Microbiota-Targeted Therapy

Here, we list in Table 2 a summary of studies documenting gut microbiota-targeted interventions in animal models of CKD of developmental origins and its comorbidities [101–110]. The therapeutic duration is during fetal and childhood stages. The literature review states that gut microbiota-targeted interventions used to prevent CKD and its comorbidities primarily include probiotics, prebiotics, and postbiotics.

As shown in Table 2, rats are the dominant species used by experiments, and hypertension is the most commonly studied CKD-related comorbidity. A variety of early-life insults can lead to structural and functional changes in the developing kidney by the so-called renal programming [6]. Unlike in humans, kidney development in rats continues up to postnatal week 1–2. According to DOHaD theory, adverse environmental insults during pregnancy and lactation period can interrupt kidney development, resulting in renal programming and adult kidney disease. Several models of renal programming have been used to examine gut microbiota-targeted interventions in CKD of developmental origins, such as maternal high-fructose diet [101,108], perinatal high-fat diet [102,107,109], perinatal 2,3,7,8-tetrachlorodibenzo-p-dioxin (TCDD) exposure [103], maternal adenine-induced CKD [104], maternal TMAO and ADMA exposure [105], and maternal high-fructose diet and TCDD exposure [110].

Table 2. Summary of early-life gut microbiota-targeted therapies for CKD and its comorbidities.

Gut Microbiota-Targeted Intervention	Animal Models	Species/Gender	Age at Evaluation	Effects on CKD and Its Comorbidities	Reference
Probiotics					
Daily oral gavage of *Lactobacillus casei rhamnosus* (2×10^8 CFU/day) to mother rats from pregnancy through lactation	Maternal high-fructose diet	SD rat/M	12 weeks	Prevented hypertension	Hsu et al., 2018 [101]
Daily oral gavage of *Lactobacillus casei rhamnosus* (2×10^8 CFU/day) to mother rats from pregnancy through lactation	Perinatal high-fat diet	SD rat/M	16 weeks	Prevented hypertension	Hsu et al., 2019 [102]
Prebiotics					
5% w/w long chain inulin to mother rats from pregnancy through lactation	Maternal high-fructose diet	SD rat/M	12 weeks	Prevented hypertension	Hsu et al., 2018 [101]
5% w/w long chain inulin to mother rats from pregnancy through lactation	Perinatal high-fat diet	SD rat/M	16 weeks	Prevented hypertension	Hsu et al., 2019 [102]
Resveratrol (50 mg/L) in drinking water to mother rats from pregnancy through lactation	Perinatal TCDD exposure model	SD rat/M	12 weeks	Prevented renal inflammation and hypertension	Hsu et al., 2021 [103]
Resveratrol (50 mg/L) in drinking water to mother rats from pregnancy through lactation	Maternal adenine-induced CKD	SD rat/M	12 weeks	Prevented hypertension	Hsu et al., 2020 [104]
Resveratrol (50 mg/L) in drinking water to mother rats from pregnancy through lactation	Maternal TMAO and ADMA exposure	SD rat/M	12 weeks	Prevented hypertension	Hsu et al., 2021 [105]
Resveratrol (50 mg/L) in drinking water to mother rats from week 6 to week 12	Pediatric adenine-induced CKD	SD rat/M	12 weeks	Prevented renal dysfunction and hypertension	Hsu et al., 2021 [106]
Resveratrol butyrate ester (25 mg/L or 50 mg/L) in drinking water to young rats from week 6 to week 12	Pediatric adenine-induced CKD	SD rat/M	12 weeks	Prevented renal dysfunction and hypertension	Hsu et al., 2021 [106]
Daily oral gavage of garlic oil (100 mg/kg/day) to mother rats from pregnancy through lactation	Perinatal high-fat diet	SD rat/M	16 weeks	Prevented hypertension	Hsu et al., 2021 [107]
Postbiotics					
Magnesium acetate (200 mmol/L) in drinking water to mother rats from pregnancy through lactation	Maternal high-fructose diet	SD rat/M	12 weeks	Prevented hypertension	Hsu et al., 2019 [108]
1% conjugated linoleic acid to mother rats from pregnancy through lactation	Maternal high-fat diet	SD rat/M	18 weeks	Prevented hypertension	Gray et al., 2015 [109]
Others					
1% DMB in drinking water to mother rats from pregnancy through lactation	Maternal high-fructose diet	SD rat/M	12 weeks	Prevented hypertension	Hsu et al., 2019 [108]
1% DMB in drinking water to mother rats from pregnancy through lactation	Maternal high-fructose diet and TCDD exposure	SD rat/M	12 weeks	Prevented hypertension	Hsu et al., 2020 [110]

Studies tabulated according to types of intervention, animal models, and age at evaluation. TCDD = 2,3,7,8-tetrachlorodibenzo-p-dioxin; CKD = chronic kidney disease; TMAO = trimethylamine-N-oxide; ADMA = asymmetric dimethylarginine; SD = Sprague-Dawley rat; DMB = 3,3-maternal dimethyl-1-butanol.

Taking the example of the maternal high-fructose diet model, high-fructose intake during pregnancy and lactation modified over 200 renal transcripts from nephrogenesis stage to adulthood [111]. Using whole-genome RNA next-generation sequencing (NGS), high-fructose-induced alterations of the renal transcriptome were reported in kidneys from 1-day-, 3-week-, and 3-month-old male offspring. NGS identified genes in arachidonic acid metabolism (*Cyp2c23*, *Hpgds*, *Ptgds* and *Ptges*) that contribute to renal programming and hypertension. Notably, this renal programming model has been used to examine the reprogramming effects of gut microbiota-targeted therapy on fructose-induced developmental programming [112]. Since the above-mentioned renal programming models have been established and linked to adverse renal outcomes in adult offspring, readers are referred to original references. There was only one study conducting an adenine-induced pediatric CKD model to determine the effects of probiotic resveratrol on CKD progression [106].

Review elsewhere showed that several probiotic microorganisms and prebiotics have benefits on adult CKD [81,82], while there was only very limited evidence regarding their role on CKD of developmental origins. Supplementation with *Lactobacillus casei rhamnosus* from pregnancy through lactation protected adult male rat progeny against hypertension programmed by a maternal high-fructose diet [101] or perinatal high-fat diet [102].

Additionally, inulin as a prebiotic has been examined for its protective effect in hypertension of developmental origins [101,102]. In a high-fat model [102], we previously demonstrated that inulin treatment protected against hypertension in adult rat offspring coinciding with alterations of the gut microbiota, particularly increasing the abundance of *Lactobacillus*, a well-known probiotic strain. Likewise, perinatal supplementing to rat dams with inulin protected adult offspring against maternal high-fructose diet-induced hypertension, which coincided with an increased plasma level of propionic acid [102].

Resveratrol can modulate gut microbiota composition, undergo biotransformation to activate metabolites via the intestinal microbiota, affect gut barrier function, modify the *Firmicutes* to *Bacteroidetes* (F/B) ratio, and reverse the gut microbial dysbiosis [113–116]. With a prebiotic effect for gut microbes, increasing evidence supports the beneficial effects of resveratrol on many diseases, including CKD [117,118]. One study revealed that perinatal resveratrol therapy could protect adult offspring against hypertension and CKD of developmental origins [119]. Studies using a maternal TCDD exposure rat model showed TCDD-induced renal hypertrophy and hypertension in adult progeny, and both are key features with early CKD. TCDD-induced hypertension is associated with activation of AHR signaling, induction of TH17-dependent renal inflammation, and alterations of gut microbiota compositions [103]. Conversely, the induction of AHR- and TH17-mediated renal inflammation could be counterbalanced by perinatal resveratrol supplementation. The beneficial effects of resveratrol are associated with reshaping the gut microbiome by augmenting microbes that can inhibit TH17 responses and reduce the F/B ratio, a microbial marker of hypertension [14]. In a maternal CKD model, adult offspring developed renal hypertrophy and hypertension [104]. Perinatal resveratrol therapy protected hypertension, coinciding with the restoration of microbial richness and diversity and an increase in *Lactobacillus* and *Bifidobacterium* [104]. Similar to TMAO, asymmetric dimethylarginine (ADMA) is a well-known uremic toxin [120]. Another study using a maternal TMAO plus ADMA exposure model demonstrated that adult offspring born to dams exposed to uremic toxins had renal dysfunction and hypertension [105]. Conversely, maternal treatment with resveratrol rescued hypertension induced by TMAO plus ADMA exposure, accompanied by increased butyrate-producing microbes and fecal butyric acid level.

Of note is that the low bioavailability of resveratrol diminishes its efficacy and clinical translation [121]. Accordingly, we produced resveratrol butyrate ester (RBE) via the esterification of resveratrol with the SCFA butyrate to improve the efficacy [122]. Using a pediatric CKD model [85], we recently found low-dose RBE (25 mg/L) is as effective as resveratrol (50 mg/L) in protecting against hypertension and renal dysfunction. The beneficial effects of RBE include regulation of SCFA receptors, decreased AHR signaling, and increased abundance of the beneficial microbes *Blautia* and *Enterococcus*.

Although there are many prebiotic foods, only garlic oil has shown beneficial effects against high-fat diet-induced hypertension in adult progeny [106]. These effects include increased α-diversity, increased plasma levels of acetic acid, butyric acid, and propionic acid, and increased beneficial bacteria *Lactobacillus* and *Bifidobacterium*.

In addition to probiotics and prebiotics, postbiotics is another gut microbiota-targeted therapy. Postbiotics include various components, such as microbial cell fractions, extracellular polysaccharides, functional proteins, cell lysates, extracellular vesicles, cell-wall-derived muropeptides, etc. [94]. Nevertheless, very limited information exists regarding the use of postbiotics in CKD. Acetate supplementation within gestation and lactation was reported to protect offspring against high-fructose-diet-induced hypertension, a major complication of CKD [108]. However, its protective effects on other complications of CKD are still waiting for clarification. Another example of postbiotic use in hypertension of developmental origins is conjugated linoleic acid [109]. Linoleic acid is a gut microbial metabolite derived from dietary polyunsaturated fatty acids (PUFA) [123]. Several gut microbes have been identified as producing PUFA-derived intermediate metabolites [124]. Administration of PUFA-derived bacterial metabolites such as linoleic acid has been shown to provoke anti-obesity and anti-inflammatory effects [125]. However, unlike probiotics and prebiotics [126,127], currently there is a lack of a clear definition for postbiotics. Considering the complex nature of postbiotics [94], a clear definition is important for future research from a regulatory perspective.

Moreover, there are other microbiota-related therapies applied for preventing CKD and its comorbidities. Microbe-dependent TMA and TMAO formation can be inhibited by 3,3-dimethyl-1-butanol (DMB), a structural analogue of choline [128]. Recently, two studies reported that maternal oral administration of DMB protected hypertension in adult rat progeny exposed to a maternal high-fructose diet [87] or high-fructose diet plus TCDD exposure [110]. This was accompanied by affecting the metabolic pathway of TMA-TMAO and reshaping gut microbiota [110].

As far as the multifaceted relationship between the gut and kidney, there might be other potential approaches by which the gut microbiota might prevent CKD and its associated complications. For example, RAS blockers are currently the most common therapies used for renoprotection and antihypertension [129]. Considering drug-mediated alterations in the gut microbiota compositions can have beneficial effects on the host [130], a greater understanding of mechanisms driving drug–gut microbiota interactions might aid in guiding the development of microbiota-targeted pharmacological interventions. Together, early microbiota-targeted therapies, in the long term, may enable the capacity to prevent the development of CKD and its comorbidities in a desired favorable direction. However, there is an urgent need to identify and fill the knowledge gaps on gut microbiota-targeted therapies between established CKD and CKD of developmental origins.

5. Conclusions and Perspectives

Mounting evidence in support of the link between gut microbiota and CKD starting in early life is intriguing but incomplete. One major unsolved problem is the gap in published child- and adult-focused clinical CKD research. Most pediatric CKD studies have limited power due to a small sample size. Although substantial evidence indicates an association between gut microbiota and CKD in adult patients with different stages of CKD and/or various comorbidities, we still lack such information in the pediatric population. Therefore, future work in large multicenter studies regarding CKD and its comorbidities is required to enable the establishment of more robust true relationships in the pediatric population.

Prior research has indicated that the early-life gut microbiome might influence renal programming and exert CKD in later life. Our review highlights the value of gut microbiota-targeted therapies, if applied early, to help prevent CKD and its related complications. Nevertheless, many probiotics and prebiotics used in adult CKD have not been examined in childhood CKD yet, especially in CKD of developmental origins.

In conclusion, gut microbiota dysbiosis is a highly pathogenetic link in the development of CKD and its comorbidities. After all of this significant growth in understanding of the gut microbiota in the pathophysiology of pediatric CKD and its targeted interventions, it may open new avenues for prevention of CKD in childhood or even earlier in fetal life.

Author Contributions: Conceptualization, C.-N.H. and Y.-L.T.; funding acquisition, C.-N.H. and Y.-L.T.; project administration, C.-N.H. and Y.-L.T.; data curation, C.-N.H. and Y.-L.T.; writing—original draft, C.-N.H. and Y.-L.T.; writing—review and editing, C.-N.H. and Y.-L.T. All authors have read and agreed to the published version of the manuscript.

Funding: This research was funded by grants MOST 110-2314-B-182-020-MY3 (Y.-L.T.) and MOST 110-2314-3-182A-029 (C.-N.H.) from the Ministry of Science and Technology, Taiwan, and the grants CORPG8M0081 and CORPG8M0151 from Chang Gung Memorial Hospital, Kaohsiung, Taiwan.

Institutional Review Board Statement: Not applicable.

Informed Consent Statement: Not applicable.

Data Availability Statement: All data are contained within the article.

Conflicts of Interest: The authors declare no conflict of interest.

References

1. Luyckx, V.A.; Tonelli, M.; Stanifer, J.W. The global burden of kidney disease and the sustainable development goals. *Bull. World Health Organ.* **2018**, *96*, 414–422. [CrossRef] [PubMed]
2. Chong, E.; Yosypiv, I.V. Developmental programming of hypertension and kidney disease. *Int. J. Nephrol.* **2012**, *2012*, 760580. [CrossRef] [PubMed]
3. Luyckx, V.A.; Bertram, J.F.; Brenner, B.M.; Fall, C.; Hoy, W.E.; Ozanne, S.E.; Vikse, B.E. Effect of fetal and child health on kidney development and long-term risk of hypertension and kidney disease. *Lancet* **2013**, *382*, 273–283. [CrossRef]
4. Tain, Y.L.; Hsu, C.N. The First Thousand Days: Kidney Health and Beyond. *Healthcare* **2021**, *9*, 1332. [CrossRef]
5. Ingelfinger, J.R.; Kalantar-Zadeh, K.; Schaefer, F.; World Kidney Day Steering Committee. World Kidney Day 2016: Averting the legacy of kidney disease-focus on childhood. *Pediatr. Nephrol.* **2016**, *31*, 343–348. [CrossRef] [PubMed]
6. Kett, M.M.; Denton, K.M. Renal programming: Cause for concern? *Am. J. Physiol. Regul. Integr. Comp. Physiol.* **2011**, *300*, R791–R803. [CrossRef] [PubMed]
7. Haugen, A.C.; Schug, T.T.; Collman, G.; Heindel, J.J. Evolution of DOHaD: The impact of environmental health sciences. *J. Dev. Orig. Health Dis.* **2014**, *6*, 55–64. [CrossRef]
8. Tain, Y.-L.; Joles, J.A. Reprogramming: A preventive strategy in hypertension focusing on the kidney. *Int. J. Mol. Sci.* **2016**, *17*, 23. [CrossRef] [PubMed]
9. Tain, Y.L.; Hsu, C.N. Developmental origins of chronic kidney disease: Should we focus on early life? *Int. J. Mol. Sci.* **2017**, *18*, 381. [CrossRef] [PubMed]
10. Hsu, C.N.; Tain, Y.L. Developmental origins of kidney disease: Why oxidative stress matters? *Antioxidants* **2021**, *10*, 33. [CrossRef]
11. Hsu, C.N.; Tain, Y.L. Regulation of nitric oxide production in the developmental programming of hypertension and kidney disease. *Int. J. Mol. Sci.* **2019**, *20*, 681. [CrossRef]
12. Hsu, C.N.; Tain, Y.L. Targeting the renin–angiotensin–aldosterone system to prevent hypertension and kidney disease of developmental origins. *Int. J. Mol. Sci.* **2021**, *22*, 2298. [CrossRef]
13. Hsu, C.N.; Hou, C.Y.; Hsu, W.H.; Tain, Y.L. Cardiovascular diseases of developmental origins: Preventive aspects of gut microbiota-targeted therapy. *Nutrients* **2021**, *13*, 2290. [CrossRef]
14. Yang, T.; Richards, E.M.; Pepine, C.J.; Raizada, M.K. The gut microbiota and the brain-gut-kidney axis in hypertension and chronic kidney disease. *Nat. Rev. Nephrol.* **2018**, *14*, 442–456. [CrossRef]
15. Dennery, P.A. Oxidative stress in development: Nature or nurture? *Free Radic. Biol. Med.* **2010**, *49*, 1147–1151. [CrossRef]
16. Tain, Y.L.; Hsu, C.N. Targeting on Asymmetric Dimethylarginine-Related Nitric Oxide-Reactive Oxygen Species Imbalance to Reprogram the Development of Hypertension. *Int. J. Mol. Sci.* **2016**, *17*, 2020. [CrossRef]
17. Hsu, C.N.; Tain, Y.L. Early Origins of Hypertension: Should Prevention Start Before Birth Using Natural Antioxidants? *Antioxidants* **2020**, *9*, 1034. [CrossRef]
18. Gubler, M.C.; Antignac, C. Renin-angiotensin system in kidney development: Renal tubular dysgenesis. *Kidney Int.* **2010**, *77*, 400–406. [CrossRef]
19. Vehaskari, V.M.; Stewart, T.; Lafont, D.; Soyez, C.; Seth, D.; Manning, J. Kidney angiotensin and angiotensin receptor expression in prenatally programmed hypertension. *Am. J. Physiol. Ren. Physiol.* **2004**, *287*, F262–F267. [CrossRef]
20. Grigore, D.; Ojeda, N.B.; Robertson, E.B.; Dawson, A.S.; Huffman, C.A.; Bourassa, E.A.; Speth, R.C.; Brosnihan, K.B.; Alexander, B.T. Placental insufficiency results in temporal alterations in the renin angiotensin system in male hypertensive growth restricted offspring. *Am. J. Physiol. Regul. Integr. Comp. Physiol.* **2007**, *293*, R804–R811. [CrossRef]
21. Efeyan, A.; Comb, W.C.; Sabatini, D.M. Nutrient-sensing mechanisms and pathways. *Nature* **2015**, *517*, 302–310. [CrossRef] [PubMed]
22. Tain, Y.L.; Hsu, C.N. Interplay between oxidative stress and nutrient sensing signaling in the developmental origins of cardiovascular disease. *Int. J. Mol. Sci.* **2017**, *18*, 841. [CrossRef] [PubMed]
23. Tain, Y.L.; Hsu, C.N. AMP-Activated Protein Kinase as a Reprogramming Strategy for Hypertension and Kidney Disease of Developmental Origin. *Int. J. Mol. Sci.* **2018**, *19*, 1744. [CrossRef] [PubMed]
24. Tain, Y.L.; Hsu, C.N.; Chan, J.Y. PPARs link early life nutritional insults to later programmed hypertension and metabolic syndrome. *Int. J. Mol. Sci.* **2015**, *17*, 20. [CrossRef]
25. Hobby, G.P.; Karaduta, O.; Dusio, G.F.; Singh, M.; Zybailov, B.L.; Arthur, J.M. Chronic kidney disease and the gut microbiome. *Am. J. Physiol. Renal Physiol.* **2019**, *316*, F1211–F1217. [CrossRef]
26. Al Khodor, S.; Shatat, I.F. Gut microbiome and kidney disease: A bidirectional relationship. *Pediatr. Nephrol.* **2017**, *32*, 921–931. [CrossRef]
27. Hsu, C.N.; Tain, Y.L. Developmental programming and reprogramming of hypertension and kidney disease: Impact of tryptophan metabolism. *Int. J. Mol. Sci.* **2020**, *21*, 8705. [CrossRef]

28. Sallée, M.; Dou, L.; Cerini, C.; Poitevin, S.; Brunet, P.; Burtey, S. The aryl hydrocarbon receptor-activating effect of uremic toxins from tryptophan metabolism: A new concept to understand cardiovascular complications of chronic kidney disease. *Toxins* 2014, 6, 934–949. [CrossRef]
29. Chu, D.M.; Meyer, K.M.; Prince, A.L.; Aagaard, K.M. Impact of maternal nutrition in pregnancy and lactation on offspring gut microbial composition and function. *Gut Microbes* 2016, 7, 459–470. [CrossRef]
30. Tricco, A.C.; Lillie, E.; Zarin, W.; O'Brien, K.K.; Colquhoun, H.; Levac, D.; Moher, D.; Peters, M.D.J.; Horsley, T.; Weeks, L.; et al. PRISMA Extension for Scoping Reviews (PRISMA-ScR): Checklist and Explanation. *Ann. Intern. Med.* 2018, 169, 467–473. [CrossRef]
31. Bertram, J.F.; Douglas-Denton, R.N.; Diouf, B.; Hughson, M.; Hoy, W. Human nephron number: Implications for health and disease. *Pediatr. Nephrol.* 2011, 26, 1529–1533. [CrossRef] [PubMed]
32. Luyckx, V.A.; Brenner, B.M. The clinical importance of nephron mass. *J. Am. Soc. Nephrol.* 2010, 21, 898–910. [CrossRef] [PubMed]
33. Murugapoopathy, V.; Gupta, I.R. A primer on congenital anomalies of the kidneys and urinary tracts (CAKUT). *Clin. J. Am. Soc. Nephrol.* 2020, 15, 723–731. [CrossRef] [PubMed]
34. Schnaper, H.W. Remnant nephron physiology and the progression of chronic kidney disease. *Pediatr. Nephrol.* 2014, 29, 193–202. [CrossRef]
35. Luyckx, V.A.; Brenner, B.M. Birth weight, malnutrition and kidney-associated outcomes—A global concern. *Nat. Rev. Nephrol.* 2015, 11, 135–149. [CrossRef]
36. White, S.L.; Perkovic, V.; Cass, A.; Chang, C.L.; Poulter, N.R.; Spector, T.; Haysom, L.; Craig, J.C.; Salmi, I.A.; Chadban, S.J.; et al. Is low birth weight an antecedent of CKD in later life? A systematic review of observational studies. *Am. J. Kidney Dis.* 2009, 54, 248–261. [CrossRef]
37. Tain, Y.L.; Luh, H.; Lin, C.Y.; Hsu, C.N. Incidence and risks of congenital anomalies of kidney and urinary tract in newborns: A population-based case-control study in Taiwan. *Medicine* 2016, 95, e2659. [CrossRef] [PubMed]
38. Hsu, C.W.; Yamamoto, K.T.; Henry, R.K.; de Roos, A.J.; Flynn, J.T. Prenatal risk factors for childhood CKD. *J. Am. Soc. Nephrol.* 2014, 25, 2105–2111. [CrossRef]
39. Lee, Y.Q.; Collins, C.E.; Gordon, A.; Rae, K.; Pringle, K.G. The relationship between maternal obesity and diabetes during pregnancy on offspring kidney structure and function in humans: A systematic review. *J. Dev. Orig. Health Dis.* 2018, 10, 406–419. [CrossRef]
40. Macumber, I.; Schwartz, S.; Leca, N. Maternal obesity is associated with congenital anomalies of the kidney and urinary tract in offspring. *Pediatr. Nephrol.* 2016, 32, 635–642. [CrossRef]
41. Painter, R.C.; Roseboom, T.J.; van Montfrans, G.A.; Bossuyt, P.M.; Krediet, R.T.; Osmond, C.; Barker, D.J.; Bleker, O.P. Microalbuminuria in adults after prenatal exposure to the Dutch famine. *J. Am. Soc. Nephrol.* 2005, 16, 189–194. [CrossRef] [PubMed]
42. Miliku, K.; Mesu, A.; Franco, O.; Hofman, A.; Steegers, E.A.; Jaddoe, V.W. Maternal and fetal folate, vitamin B 12, and homocysteine concentrations and childhood kidney outcomes. *Am. J. Kidney Dis.* 2017, 69, 521–530. [CrossRef] [PubMed]
43. Goodyer, P.; Kurpad, A.; Rekha, S.; Muthayya, S.; Dwarkanath, P.; Iyengar, A.; Philip, B.; Mhaskar, A.; Benjamin, A.; Maharaj, S.; et al. Effects of maternal vitamin A status on kidney development: A pilot study. *Pediatr. Nephrol.* 2007, 22, 209–214. [CrossRef] [PubMed]
44. Sol, C.M.; Santos, S.; Asimakopoulos, A.G.; Martinez-Moral, M.P.; Duijts, L.; Kannan, K.; Trasande, L.; Jaddoe, V.W. Associations of maternal phthalate and bisphenol urine concentrations during pregnancy with childhood blood pressure in a population-based prospective cohort study. *Environ. Int.* 2020, 138, 105677. [CrossRef] [PubMed]
45. Gao, X.; Ni, W.; Zhu, S.; Wu, Y.; Cui, Y.; Ma, J.; Liu, Y.; Qiao, J.; Ye, Y.; Yang, P.; et al. Per- and polyfluoroalkyl substances exposure during pregnancy and adverse pregnancy and birth outcomes: A systematic review and meta-analysis. *Environ. Res.* 2021, 201, 111632. [CrossRef]
46. Kumar, S.N.; Saxena, P.; Patel, R.; Sharma, A.; Pradhan, D.; Singh, H.; Deval, R.; Bhardwaj, S.K.; Borgohain, D.; Akhtar, N.; et al. Predicting risk of low birth weight offspring from maternal features and blood polycyclic aromatic hydrocarbon concentration. *Reprod. Toxicol.* 2020, 94, 92–100. [CrossRef]
47. Uwak, I.; Olson, N.; Fuentes, A.; Moriarty, M.; Pulczinski, J.; Lam, J.; Xu, X.; Taylor, B.D.; Taiwo, S.; Koehler, K.; et al. Application of the navigation guide systematic review methodology to evaluate prenatal exposure to particulate matter air pollution and infant birth weight. *Environ. Int.* 2021, 148, 106378. [CrossRef]
48. Schreuder, M.F.; Bueters, R.R.; Huigen, M.C.; Russel, F.G.; Masereeuw, R.; van den Heuvel, L.P. Effect of drugs on renal development. *Clin. J. Am. Soc. Nephrol.* 2011, 6, 212–217. [CrossRef]
49. Lynch, S.V.; Pedersen, O. The Human Intestinal Microbiome in Health and Disease. *N. Engl. J. Med.* 2016, 375, 2369–2379. [CrossRef] [PubMed]
50. Antza, C.; Stabouli, S.; Kotsis, V. Gut microbiota in kidney disease and hypertension. *Pharmacol. Res.* 2018, 130, 198–203. [CrossRef]
51. Armani, R.G.; Ramezani, A.; Yasir, A.; Sharama, S.; Canziani, M.E.F.; Raj, D.S. Gut Microbiome in Chronic Kidney Disease. *Curr. Hypertens. Rep.* 2017, 19, 29. [CrossRef] [PubMed]

52. Milani, C.; Duranti, S.; Bottacini, F.; Casey, E.; Turroni, F.; Mahony, J.; Belzer, C.; Delgado Palacio, S.; Arboleya Montes, S.; Mancabelli, L.; et al. The First Microbial Colonizers of the Human Gut: Composition, Activities, and Health Implications of the Infant Gut Microbiota. *Microbiol. Mol. Biol. Rev.* **2017**, *81*, e00036-17. [CrossRef] [PubMed]
53. Matamoros, S.; Gras-Leguen, C.; Le Vacon, F.; Potel, G.; De La Cochetiere, M.-F. Development of intestinal microbiota in infants and its impact on health. *Trends Microbiol.* **2013**, *21*, 167–173. [CrossRef] [PubMed]
54. Arrieta, M.C.; Stiemsma, L.T.; Amenyogbe, N.; Brown, E.M.; Finlay, B. The intestinal microbiome in early life: Health and disease. *Front. Immunol.* **2014**, *5*, 427. [CrossRef]
55. Sarkar, A.; Yoo, J.Y.; Valeria Ozorio Dutra, S.; Morgan, K.H.; Groer, M. The Association between Early-Life Gut Microbiota and Long-Term Health and Diseases. *J. Clin. Med.* **2021**, *10*, 459. [CrossRef]
56. Mehta, S.H.; Kruger, M.; Sokol, R.J. Is maternal diabetes a risk factor for childhood obesity? *J. Matern. Neonatal Med.* **2012**, *25*, 41–44. [CrossRef]
57. Zhou, L.; Xiao, X. The role of gut microbiota in the effects of maternal obesity during pregnancy on offspring metabolism. *Biosci. Rep.* **2018**, *38*, BSR20171234. [CrossRef]
58. Groer, M.; Luciano, A.A.; Dishaw, L.J.; Ashmeade, T.L.; Miller, E.M.; Gilbert, J.A. Development of the preterm infant gut microbiome: A research priority. *Microbiome* **2014**, *2*, 38. [CrossRef]
59. Unger, S.; Stintzi, A.; Shah, P.; Mack, D.; O'Connor, D.L. Gut microbiota of the very- low-birth-weight infant. *Pediatr. Res.* **2015**, *77*, 205–213. [CrossRef]
60. Mischke, M.; Plösch, T. More than just a gut instinct–the potential interplay between a baby's nutrition, its gut microbiome, and the epigenome. *Am. J. Physiol. Integr. Comp. Physiol.* **2013**, *304*, R1065–R1069. [CrossRef]
61. Sato, Y.; Yanagita, M. Immune cells and inflammation in AKI to CKD progression. *Am. J. Physiol. Renal Physiol.* **2018**, *315*, F1501–F1512. [CrossRef] [PubMed]
62. Hsu, C.N.; Tain, Y.L. Adverse Impact of Environmental Chemicals on Developmental Origins of Kidney Disease and Hypertension. *Front. Endocrinol.* **2021**, *12*, 745716. [CrossRef] [PubMed]
63. Tsiaoussis, J.; Antoniou, M.N.; Koliarakis, I.; Mesnage, R.; Vardavas, C.I.; Izotov, B.N.; Psaroulaki, A.; Tsatsakis, A. Effects of single and combined toxic exposures on the gut microbiome: Current knowledge and future directions. *Toxicol. Lett.* **2019**, *312*, 72–97. [CrossRef] [PubMed]
64. Vaziri, N.D.; Yuan, J.; Rahimi, A.; Ni, Z.; Said, H.; Subramanian, V.S. Disintegration of colonic epithelial tight junction in uremia: A likely cause of CKD-associated inflammation. *Nephrol. Dial. Transplant.* **2012**, *27*, 2686–2693. [CrossRef]
65. Andersen, K.; Kesper, M.S.; Marschner, J.A.; Konrad, L.; Ryu, M.; Kumar Vr, S.; Kulkarni, O.P.; Mulay, S.R.; Romoli, S.; Demleitner, J.; et al. Intestinal Dysbiosis, Barrier Dysfunction, and Bacterial Translocation Account for CKD-Related Systemic Inflammation. *J. Am. Soc. Nephrol.* **2017**, *28*, 76–83. [CrossRef]
66. Vaziri, N.D.; Wong, J.; Pahl, M.; Piceno, Y.M.; Yuan, J.; DeSantis, T.Z.; Ni, Z.; Nguyen, T.H.; Andersen, G.L. Chronic kidney disease alters intestinal microbial flora. *Kidney Int.* **2013**, *83*, 308–315. [CrossRef]
67. Yoshifuji, A.; Wakino, S.; Irie, J.; Tajima, T.; Hasegawa, K.; Kanda, T.; Tokuyama, H.; Hayashi, K.; Itoh, H. Gut Lactobacillus protects against the progression of renal damage by modulating the gut environment in rats. *Nephrol. Dial. Transplant.* **2016**, *31*, 401–412. [CrossRef]
68. Kikuchi, M.; Ueno, M.; Itoh, Y.; Suda, W.; Hattori, M. Uremic toxin-producing gut microbiota in rats with chronic kidney disease. *Nephron* **2017**, *135*, 51–60. [CrossRef]
69. Zhao, J.; Ning, X.; Liu, B.; Dong, R.; Bai, M.; Sun, S. Specific alterations in gut microbiota in patients with chronic kidney disease: An updated systematic review. *Ren Fail.* **2021**, *43*, 102–112. [CrossRef]
70. Wong, J.; Piceno, Y.M.; Desantis, T.Z.; Pahl, M.; Andersen, G.L.; Vaziri, N.D. Expansion of urease- and uricase-containing, indole and p-cresol-forming and contraction of short-chain fatty acid producing intestinal microbiota in ESRD. *Am. J. Nephrol.* **2014**, *39*, 230–237. [CrossRef]
71. Pluznick, J.L. Microbial short-chain fatty acids and blood pressure regulation. *Curr. Hypertens. Rep.* **2017**, *19*, 25. [CrossRef] [PubMed]
72. Ratajczak, W.; Ryl, A.; Mizerski, A.; Walczakiewicz, K.; Sipak, O.; Laszczyn'ska, M. Immunomodulatory potential of gut microbiome-derived short-chain fatty acids (SCFAs). *Acta Biochim. Pol.* **2019**, *66*, 1–12. [CrossRef] [PubMed]
73. Gao, B.; Jose, A.; Alonzo-Palma, N.; Malik, T.; Shankaranarayanan, D.; Regunathan-Shenk, R.; Raj, D.S. Butyrate producing microbiota are reduced in chronic kidney diseases. *Sci. Rep.* **2021**, *11*, 23530. [CrossRef] [PubMed]
74. Scott, S.A.; Fu, J.; Chang, P.V. Microbial tryptophan metabolites regulate gut barrier function via the aryl hydrocarbon receptor. *Proc. Natl. Acad. Sci. USA* **2020**, *117*, 19376–19387. [CrossRef] [PubMed]
75. Liu, J.R.; Miao, H.; Deng, D.Q.; Vaziri, N.D.; Li, P.; Zhao, Y.Y. Gut microbiota-derived tryptophan metabolism mediates renal fibrosis by aryl hydrocarbon receptor signaling activation. *Cell Mol. Life Sci.* **2021**, *78*, 909–922. [CrossRef] [PubMed]
76. Ichii, O.; Otsuka-Kanazawa, S.; Nakamura, T.; Ueno, M.; Kon, Y.; Chen, W.; Rosenberg, A.Z.; Kopp, J.B. Podocyte injury caused by indoxyl sulfate, a uremic toxin and aryl-hydrocarbon receptor ligand. *PLoS ONE* **2014**, *9*, e108448. [CrossRef] [PubMed]
77. Schiattarella, G.G.; Sannino, A.; Toscano, E.; Giugliano, G.; Gargiulo, G.; Franzone, A.; Trimarco, B.; Esposito, G.; Perrino, C. Gut microbe-generated metabolite trimethylamine-N-oxide as cardiovascular risk biomarker: A systematic review and dose-response meta-analysis. *Eur. Heart J.* **2017**, *38*, 2948–2956. [CrossRef]

78. Velasquez, M.T.; Ramezani, A.; Manal, A.; Raj, D.S. Trimethylamine N-Oxide: The good, the bad and the unknown. *Toxins* 2016, *8*, 326. [CrossRef]
79. Gupta, N.; Buffa, J.A.; Roberts, A.B.; Sangwan, N.; Skye, S.M.; Li, L.; Ho, K.J.; Varga, J.; DiDonato, J.A.; Tang, W.H.W.; et al. Targeted Inhibition of Gut Microbial Trimethylamine N-Oxide Production Reduces Renal Tubulointerstitial Fibrosis and Functional Impairment in a Murine Model of Chronic Kidney Disease. *Arterioscler. Thromb. Vasc. Biol.* 2020, *40*, 1239–1255. [CrossRef]
80. Sumida, K.; Lau, W.L.; Kovesdy, C.P.; Kalantar-Zadeh, K.; Kalantar-Zadeh, K. Microbiome modulation as a novel therapeutic approach in chronic kidney disease. *Curr. Opin. Nephrol. Hypertens.* 2021, *30*, 75–84. [CrossRef] [PubMed]
81. Pei, M.; Wei, L.; Hu, S.; Yang, B.; Si, J. Yang, H.; Zhai, J. Probiotics, prebiotics and synbiotics for chronic kidney disease: Protocol for a systematic review and meta-analysis. *BMJ Open* 2018, *8*, e020863. [CrossRef] [PubMed]
82. Zheng, H.J.; Guo, J.; Wang, Q.; Wang, L.; Wang, Y.; Zhang, F.; Huang, W.J.; Zhang, W.; Liu, W.J.; Wang, Y. Probiotics, prebiotics, and synbiotics for the improvement of metabolic profiles in patients with chronic kidney disease: A systematic review and meta-analysis of randomized controlled trials. *Crit. Rev. Food Sci. Nutr.* 2021, *61*, 577–598. [CrossRef] [PubMed]
83. Crespo-Salgado, J.; Vehaskari, V.M.; Stewart, T.; Ferris, M.; Zhang, Q.; Wang, G.; Blanchard, E.E.; Taylor, C.M.; Kallash, M.; Greenbaum, L.A.; et al. Intestinal microbiota in pediatric patients with end stage renal disease: A Midwest Pediatric Nephrology Consortium study. *Microbiome* 2016, *4*, 50. [CrossRef] [PubMed]
84. Tsuji, S.; Suruda, C.; Hashiyada, M.; Kimata, T.; Yamanouchi, S.; Kitao, T.; Kino, J.; Akane, A.; Kaneko, K. Gut microbiota dysbiosis in children with relapsing idiopathic nephrotic syndrome. *Am. J. Nephrol.* 2018, *47*, 164–170. [CrossRef]
85. Hsu, C.N.; Lu, P.C.; Lo, M.H.; Lin, I.C.; Chang-Chien, G.P.; Lin, S.; Tain, Y.L. Gut Microbiota-Dependent Trimethylamine N-Oxide Pathway Associated with Cardiovascular Risk in Children with Early-Stage Chronic Kidney Disease. *Int. J. Mol. Sci.* 2018, *19*, 3699. [CrossRef]
86. Hsu, C.N.; Lu, P.C.; Hou, C.Y.; Tain, Y.L. Blood Pressure Abnormalities Associated with Gut Microbiota-Derived Short Chain Fatty Acids in Children with Congenital Anomalies of the Kidney and Urinary Tract. *J. Clin. Med.* 2019, *8*, 1090. [CrossRef]
87. Kang, Y.; Feng, D.; Law, H.K.; Qu, W.; Wu, Y.; Zhu, G.H.; Huang, W.Y. Compositional alterations of gut microbiota in children with primary nephrotic syndrome after initial therapy. *BMC Nephrol.* 2019, *20*, 434. [CrossRef]
88. Hsu, C.N.; Chang-Chien, G.P.; Lin, S. Hou, C.Y.; Ku, P.C.; Tain, Y.L. Association of trimethylamine, trimethylamine N-oxide and dimethylamine with cardiovascular risk in children with chronic kidney disease. *J. Clin. Med.* 2020, *9*, 336. [CrossRef]
89. Yamaguchi, T.; Tsuji, S.; Akagawa, S.; Akagawa, Y.; Kino, J.; Yamanouchi, S.; Kimata, T.; Hashiyada, M.; Akane, A.; Kaneko, K. Clinical Significance of Probiotics for Children with Idiopathic Nephrotic Syndrome. *Nutrients* 2021, *13*, 365. [CrossRef]
90. Pelletier, C.C.; Croyal, M.; Ene, L.; Aguesse, A.; Billon-Crossouard, S.; Krempf, M.; Lemoine, S.; Guebre-Egziabher, F.; Juillard, L.; Soulage, C.O. Elevation of Trimethylamine-N-Oxide in Chronic Kidney Disease: Contribution of Decreased Glomerular Filtration Rate. *Toxins* 2019, *11*, 635. [CrossRef]
91. Zeng, Y.; Guo, M.; Fang, X.; Teng, F.; Tan, X.; Li, X.; Wang, M.; Long, Y.; Xu, Y. Gut Microbiota-Derived Trimethylamine N-Oxide and Kidney Function: A Systematic Review and Meta-Analysis. *Adv. Nutr.* 2021, *12*, 1286–1304. [CrossRef] [PubMed]
92. Nelson, T.M.; Borgogna, J.L.; Brotman, R.M.; Ravel, J.; Walk, S.T.; Yeoman, C.J. Vaginal biogenic amines: Biomarkers of bacterial vaginosis or precursors to vaginal dysbiosis? *Front. Physiol.* 2015, *6*, 253. [CrossRef]
93. Pandey, K.R.; Naik, S.R.; Vakil, B.V. Probiotics, prebiotics and synbiotics-A review. *J. Food Sci. Technol.* 2015, *52*, 7577–7587. [CrossRef]
94. Żółkiewicz, J.; Marzec, A.; Ruszczyński, M.; Feleszko, W. Postbiotics-A step beyond pre- and probiotics. *Nutrients* 2020, *12*, 2189. [CrossRef]
95. Leshem, A.; Horesh, N.; Elinav, E. Fecal microbial transplantation and its potential application in cardiometabolic syndrome. *Front. Immunol.* 2019, *10*, 1341. [CrossRef] [PubMed]
96. Zhou, Y.; Xu, H.; Huang, H.; Li, Y.; Chen, H.; He, J.; Du, Y.; Chen, Y.; Zhou, Y.; Nie, Y. Are There Potential Applications of Fecal Microbiota Transplantation beyond Intestinal Disorders? *Biomed. Res. Int.* 2019, *2019*, 3469754. [CrossRef]
97. Sanaka, T.; Sugino, N.; Teraoka, S.; Ota, K. Therapeutic effects of oral sorbent in undialyzed uremia. *Am. J. Kidney Dis.* 1988, *12*, 97–103. [CrossRef]
98. Toyoda, S.; Hashimoto, R.; Tezuka, T.; Sakuma, M.; Abe, S.; Ishikawa, T.; Taguchi, I.; Inoue, T. Antioxidative effect of an oral adsorbent, AST-120, and long-term outcomes in chronic kidney disease patients with cardiovascular disease. *Hypertens. Res.* 2020, *43*, 1128–1131. [CrossRef]
99. Lee, C.T.; Hsu, C.Y.; Tain, Y.L.; Ng, H.Y.; Cheng, B.C.; Yang, C.C.; Wu, C.H.; Chiou, T.T.; Lee, Y.T.; Liao, S.C. Effects of AST-120 on blood concentrations of protein-bound uremic toxins and biomarkers of cardiovascular risk in chronic dialysis patients. *Blood Purif.* 2014, *37*, 76–83. [CrossRef]
100. Takahashi, M.; Taguchi, H.; Yamaguchi, H.; Osaki, T.; Kamiya, S. Studies of the effect of Clostridium butyricum on Helicobacter pylori in several test models including gnotobiotic mice. *J. Med. Microbiol.* 2000, *49*, 635–642. [CrossRef]
101. Hsu, C.-N.; Lin, Y.-J.; Hou, C.-Y.; Tain, Y.-L. Maternal administration of probiotic or prebiotic prevents male adult rat offspring against developmental programming of hypertension induced by high fructose consumption in pregnancy and lactation. *Nutrients* 2018, *10*, 1229. [CrossRef] [PubMed]
102. Hsu, C.N.; Hou, C.; Chan, J.Y.H.; Lee, C.T.; Tain, Y.L. Hypertension programmed by perinatal high-fat diet: Effect of maternal gut microbiota-targeted therapy. *Nutrients* 2019, *11*, 2908. [CrossRef] [PubMed]

103. Hsu, C.N.; Hung, C.H.; Hou, C.Y.; Chang, C.I.; Tain, Y.L. Perinatal Resveratrol Therapy to Dioxin-Exposed Dams Prevents the Programming of Hypertension in Adult Rat Offspring. *Antioxidants* **2021**, *10*, 1393. [CrossRef] [PubMed]
104. Hsu, C.N.; Hou, C.Y.; Chang-Chien, G.P.; Lin, S.; Yang, H.W.; Tain, Y.L. Perinatal Resveratrol Therapy Prevents Hypertension Programmed by Maternal Chronic Kidney Disease in Adult Male Offspring: Implications of the Gut Microbiome and Their Metabolites. *Biomedicines* **2020**, *8*, 567. [CrossRef] [PubMed]
105. Hsu, C.N.; Hou, C.Y.; Chang-Chien, G.P.; Lin, S.; Chan, J.Y.H.; Lee, C.T.; Tain, Y.L. Maternal resveratrol therapy protected adult rat offspring against hypertension programmed by combined exposures to asymmetric dimethylarginine and trimethylamine-N-oxide. *J. Nutr. Biochem.* **2021**, *93*, 108630. [CrossRef] [PubMed]
106. Hsu, C.N.; Hou, C.Y.; Chang, C.I.; Tain, Y.L. Resveratrol Butyrate Ester Protects Adenine-Treated Rats against Hypertension and Kidney Disease by Regulating the Gut-Kidney Axis. *Antioxidants* **2021**, *11*, 83. [CrossRef] [PubMed]
107. Hsu, C.N.; Hou, C.Y.; Chang-Chien, G.P.; Lin, S.; Tain, Y.L. Maternal Garlic Oil Supplementation Prevents High-Fat Diet-Induced Hypertension in Adult Rat Offspring: Implications of H2S-Generating Pathway in the Gut and Kidneys. *Mol. Nutr. Food Res.* **2021**, *65*, e2001116. [CrossRef]
108. Hsu, C.N.; Chang-Chien, G.P.; Lin, S.; Hou, C.Y.; Tain, Y.L. Targeting on gut microbial metabolite trimethylamine-N-Oxide and short-chain fatty acid to prevent maternal high-fructose-diet-induced developmental programming of hypertension in adultmale offspring. *Mol. Nutr. Food Res.* **2019**, *63*, e1900073. [CrossRef]
109. Gray, C.; Vickers, M.H.; Segovia, S.A.; Zhang, X.D.; Reynolds, C.M. A maternal high fat diet programmes endothelial function and cardiovascular status in adult male offspring independent of body weight, which is reversed by maternal conjugated linoleic acid (CLA) supplementation. *PLoS ONE* **2015**, *10*, e0115994.
110. Hsu, C.N.; Chan, J.Y.H.; Yu, H.R.; Lee, W.C.; Wu, K.L.H.; Chang-Chien, G.P.; Lin, S.; Hou, C.Y.; Tain, Y.L. Targeting on gut microbiota-derived metabolite trimethylamine to protect adult male rat offspring against hypertension programmed by combined maternal high-fructose intake and dioxin exposure. *Int. J. Mol. Sci.* **2020**, *21*, 5488. [CrossRef]
111. Tain, Y.L.; Wu, K.L.; Lee, W.C.; Leu, S.; Chan, J.Y. Maternal fructose-intake-induced renal programming in adult male offspring. *J. Nutr. Biochem.* **2015**, *26*, 642–650. [CrossRef] [PubMed]
112. Hsu, C.N.; Yu, H.R.; Chan, J.Y.H.; Wu, K.L.H.; Lee, W.C.; Tain, Y.L. The Impact of Gut Microbiome on Maternal Fructose Intake-Induced Developmental Programming of Adult Disease. *Nutrients* **2022**, *14*, 1031. [CrossRef] [PubMed]
113. Chen, M.L.; Yi, L.; Zhang, Y.; Zhou, X.; Ran, L.; Yang, J.; Zhu, J.D.; Zhang, Q.Y.; Mi, M.T. Resveratrol Attenuates TrimethylamineN-Oxide (TMAO)-Induced Atherosclerosis by Regulating TMAO Synthesis and Bile Acid Metabolism via Remodeling of the Gut Microbiota. *mBio* **2016**, *7*, e02210–e02215. [CrossRef] [PubMed]
114. Qiao, Y.; Sun, J.; Xia, S.; Tang, X.; Shi, Y.; Le, G. Effects of resveratrol on gut microbiota and fat storage in a mouse model with high-fat-induced obesity. *Food Funct.* **2014**, *5*, 1241–1249. [CrossRef]
115. Etxeberria, U.; Arias, N.; Boqué, N.; Macarulla, M.T.; Portillo, M.P.; Martínez, J.A.; Milagro, F.I. Reshaping faecal gut microbiota composition by the intake of trans-resveratrol and quercetin in high-fat sucrose diet-fed rats. *J. Nutr. Biochem.* **2015**, *26*, 651–660. [CrossRef]
116. Bird, J.K.; Raederstorff, D.; Weber, P.; Steinert, R.E. Cardiovascular and Antiobesity Effects of Resveratrol Mediated through the Gut Microbiota. *Adv. Nutr.* **2017**, *8*, 839–849. [CrossRef]
117. Den Hartogh, D.J.; Tsiani, E. Health Benefits of Resveratrol in Kidney Disease: Evidence from In Vitro and In Vivo Studies. *Nutrients* **2019**, *11*, 1624. [CrossRef]
118. Song, J.Y.; Shen, T.C.; Hou, Y.C.; Chang, J.F.; Lu, C.L.; Liu, W.C.; Chen, P.J.; Chen, B.H.; Zheng, C.M.; Lu, K.C. Influence of Resveratrol on the Cardiovascular Health Effects of Chronic Kidney Disease. *Int. J. Mol. Sci.* **2020**, *21*, 6294. [CrossRef]
119. Hsu, C.N.; Hou, C.Y.; Tain, Y.L. Preventive Aspects of Early Resveratrol Supplementation in Cardiovascular and Kidney Disease of Developmental Origins. *Int. J. Mol. Sci.* **2021**, *22*, 4210. [CrossRef]
120. Tain, Y.L.; Hsu, C.N. Toxic Dimethylarginines: Asymmetric Dimethylarginine (ADMA) and Symmetric Dimethylarginine (SDMA). *Toxins* **2017**, *9*, 92. [CrossRef]
121. Walle, T.; Hsieh, F.; DeLegge, M.H.; Oatis, J.E., Jr.; Walle, U.K. High absorption but very low bioavailability of oral resveratrol in humans. *Drug Metab. Dispos.* **2004**, *32*, 1377–1382. [CrossRef]
122. Tain, Y.L.; Chang, S.K.C.; Liao, J.X.; Chen, Y.W.; Huang, H.T.; Li, Y.L.; Hou, C.Y. Synthesis of Short-Chain-Fatty-Acid Resveratrol Esters and Their Antioxidant Properties. *Antioxidants* **2021**, *10*, 420. [CrossRef]
123. Miyamoto, J.; Igarashi, M.; Watanabe, K.; Karaki, S.I.; Mukouyama, H.; Kishino, S.; Li, X.; Ichimura, A.; Irie, J.; Sugimoto, Y.; et al. Gut microbiota confers host resistance to obesity by metabolizing dietary polyunsaturated fatty acids. *Nat. Commun.* **2019**, *10*, 4007. [CrossRef]
124. Kishino, S.; Takeuchi, M.; Park, S.B.; Hirata, A.; Kitamura, N.; Kunisawa, J.; Kiyono, H.; Iwamoto, R.; Isobe, Y.; Arita, M.; et al. Polyunsaturated fatty acid saturation by gut lactic acid bacteria affecting host lipid composition. *Proc. Natl. Acad. Sci. USA* **2013**, *110*, 17808–17813. [CrossRef]
125. Miyamoto, J.; Mizukure, T.; Park, S.B.; Kishino, S.; Kimura, I.; Hirano, K.; Bergamo, P.; Rossi, M.; Suzuki, T.; Arita, M.; et al. A gut microbial metabolite of linoleic acid, 10-hydroxy-cis-12-octadecenoic acid, ameliorates intestinal epithelial barrier impairment partially via GPR40-MEK-ERK pathway. *J. Biol. Chem.* **2015**, *290*, 2902–2918. [CrossRef]

126. Gibson, G.R.; Hutkins, R.; Sanders, M.E.; Prescott, S.L.; Reimer, R.A.; Salminen, S.J.; Scott, K.; Stanton, C.; Swanson, K.S.; Cani, P.D.; et al. Expert consensus document: The international scientific association for probiotics and prebiotics (isapp) consensus statement on the definition and scope of prebiotics. *Nat. Rev. Gastroenterol. Amp. Hepatol.* **2017**, *14*, 491. [CrossRef]
127. Food and Agriculture Organization of the United Nations/World Health Organization (FAO/WHO). Guidelines for the Evaluation of Probiotics in Food. In *Joint Fao/Who Working Group on Drafting Guidelines for the Evaluation of Probiotics in Food*; WHO: London, UK; Ontario, ON, Canada, 2002.
128. Wang, Z.; Roberts, A.B.; Buffa, J.A.; Levison, B.S.; Zhu, W.; Org, E.; Gu, X.; Huang, Y.; Zamanian-Daryoush, M.; Culley, M.K.; et al. Non-lethal Inhibition of Gut Microbial Trimethylamine Production for the Treatment of Atherosclerosis. *Cell* **2015**, *163*, 1585–1595. [CrossRef]
129. Cravedi, P.; Ruggenenti, P.; Remuzzi, G. Which antihypertensive drugs are the most nephroprotective and why? *Expert Opin. Pharmacother.* **2010**, *11*, 2651–2663. [CrossRef]
130. Walsh, J.; Griffin, B.T.; Clarke, G.; Hyland, N.P. Drug-gut microbiota interactions: Implications for neuropharmacology. *Br. J. Pharmacol.* **2018**, *175*, 4415–4429. [CrossRef]

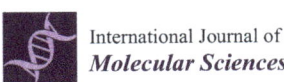

Article

In Vivo Inhibition of TRPC6 by SH045 Attenuates Renal Fibrosis in a New Zealand Obese (NZO) Mouse Model of Metabolic Syndrome

Zhihuang Zheng [1,2], Yao Xu [3], Ute Krügel [4], Michael Schaefer [4], Tilman Grune [5,6], Bernd Nürnberg [7], May-Britt Köhler [2], Maik Gollasch [1,5,*], Dmitry Tsvetkov [3,*] and Lajos Markó [2,6,8,9,*]

1. Department of Nephrology/Intensive Care, Charité—Universitätsmedizin Berlin, Corporate Member of Freie Universität Berlin and Humboldt-Universität zu Berlin, 10117 Berlin, Germany; zhihuang.zheng@charite.de
2. Experimental and Clinical Research Center, a Joint Cooperation of the Charité—University Medicine Berlin and Max Delbrück Center for Molecular Medicine in the Helmholtz Association, 13125 Berlin, Germany; may-britt.koehler@charite.de
3. Department of Internal Medicine and Geriatrics, University Medicine Greifswald, 17475 Greifswald, Germany; yao.xu@med.uni-greifswald.de
4. Rudolf Boehm Institute for Pharmacology and Toxicology, Leipzig University, 04107 Leipzig, Germany; ute.kruegel@medizin.uni-leipzig.de (U.K.); michael.schaefer@medizin.uni-leipzig.de (M.S.)
5. Department of Molecular Toxicology, German Institute of Human Nutrition Potsdam-Rehbruecke (DIfE), 14558 Nuthetal, Germany; tilman.grune@dife.de
6. DZHK (German Centre for Cardiovascular Research), Partner Site, 10785 Berlin, Germany
7. Department of Pharmacology, Experimental Therapy and Toxicology and Interfaculty Center of Pharmacogenomics and Drug Research, University of Tübingen, 72076 Tübingen, Germany; bernd.nuernberg@uni-tuebingen.de
8. Berlin Institute of Health at Charité-Universitätsmedizin Berlin, 10178 Berlin, Germany
9. Charité-Universitätsmedizin Berlin, Corporate Member of Freie Universität Berlin and Humboldt-Universität zu Berlin, 10117 Berlin, Germany
* Correspondence: maik.gollasch@med.uni-greifswald.de (M.G.); dmitry.tsvetkov@med.uni-greifswald.de (D.T.); lajos.marko@charite.de (L.M.)

Citation: Zheng, Z.; Xu, Y.; Krügel, U.; Schaefer, M.; Grune, T.; Nürnberg, B.; Köhler, M.-B.; Gollasch, M.; Tsvetkov, D.; Markó, L. In Vivo Inhibition of TRPC6 by SH045 Attenuates Renal Fibrosis in a New Zealand Obese (NZO) Mouse Model of Metabolic Syndrome. *Int. J. Mol. Sci.* **2022**, *23*, 6870. https://doi.org/10.3390/ijms23126870

Academic Editors: Luís Belo and Márcia Carvalho

Received: 18 March 2022
Accepted: 16 June 2022
Published: 20 June 2022

Publisher's Note: MDPI stays neutral with regard to jurisdictional claims in published maps and institutional affiliations.

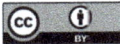

Copyright: © 2022 by the authors. Licensee MDPI, Basel, Switzerland. This article is an open access article distributed under the terms and conditions of the Creative Commons Attribution (CC BY) license (https://creativecommons.org/licenses/by/4.0/).

Abstract: Metabolic syndrome is a significant worldwide public health challenge and is inextricably linked to adverse renal and cardiovascular outcomes. The inhibition of the transient receptor potential cation channel subfamily C member 6 (TRPC6) has been found to ameliorate renal outcomes in the unilateral ureteral obstruction (UUO) of accelerated renal fibrosis. Therefore, the pharmacological inhibition of TPRC6 could be a promising therapeutic intervention in the progressive tubulo-interstitial fibrosis in hypertension and metabolic syndrome. In the present study, we hypothesized that the novel selective TRPC6 inhibitor SH045 (larixyl N-methylcarbamate) ameliorates UUO-accelerated renal fibrosis in a New Zealand obese (NZO) mouse model, which is a polygenic model of metabolic syndrome. The in vivo inhibition of TRPC6 by SH045 markedly decreased the mRNA expression of pro-fibrotic markers (*Col1α1*, *Col3α1*, *Col4α1*, *Acta2*, *Ccn2*, *Fn1*) and chemokines (*Cxcl1*, *Ccl5*, *Ccr2*) in UUO kidneys of NZO mice compared to kidneys of vehicle-treated animals. Renal expressions of intercellular adhesion molecule 1 (ICAM-1) and α-smooth muscle actin (α-SMA) were diminished in SH045- versus vehicle-treated UUO mice. Furthermore, renal inflammatory cell infiltration (F4/80+ and CD4−) and tubulointerstitial fibrosis (Sirius red and fibronectin staining) were ameliorated in SH045-treated NZO mice. We conclude that the pharmacological inhibition of TRPC6 might be a promising antifibrotic therapeutic method to treat progressive tubulo-interstitial fibrosis in hypertension and metabolic syndrome.

Keywords: TRPC6; UUO; NZO mice; inflammation; fibrosis; CKD; SH045

1. Introduction

Chronic kidney disease (CKD) is characterized by progressive loss of kidney function. The main risk factors of developing CKD are the combination of obesity, diabetes and hypertension, which is commonly referred to as metabolic syndrome. Other contributors are autoimmune diseases (e.g., glomerulonephritis), environmental exposures and genetic risk factors [1,2]. Morphologically, persistent low-grade renal inflammation and tubulointerstitial fibrosis are key hallmarks of CKD [3,4]. The complex interplay of fibroblasts, lymphocytes, tubular, and other cell types in the kidney lead to excessive extracellular matrix deposition and the further deterioration of renal function [5,6]. Although unspecific treatments strategies are available (e.g., medications lowering blood pressure), CKD progression is still poorly controlled.

In recent years, novel drug targets, such as transient receptor potential cation channel, subfamily C, and member 6 (TRPC6), emerged [7,8]. TRPC6 mutations lead to glomerular injury and proteinuria, presumably involving the Ca^{2+} signaling pathway and resulting in progressive kidney failure [9–12]. Both TRPC6 gain-of-function and loss-of-function cause familial forms of focal segmental glomerulosclerosis (FSGS) [11,13]. Interestingly, in a murine model of kidney injury (unilateral ureteral obstruction (UUO)), $Trpc6^{-/-}$ deficiency and pharmacological blockade with BI-749327 ameliorated renal fibrosis in C57BL/6J mice [7,8]. Remarkably, these beneficial effects were not observed in the acute stage of kidney injury (AKI) [14]. Thus, TRPC6 inhibition may have effects on renal fibrogenesis during AKI-to-CKD transition. Given this state of affairs, TRPC6 inhibition seems to represent a promising new therapeutic approach to combat progressive renal failure since it potentially affects CKD at later stages after kidney injury. However, it is unknown whether TRPC6 inhibition is effective for inhibiting progressive tubulo-interstitial fibrosis in hypertension and metabolic syndrome.

Recently, by the chemical diversification of (+)-larixol originating from *Larix decidua* resin traditionally used for inhalation, its methylcarbamate congener, named SH045, was developed as a novel, highly potent, subtype-selective inhibitor of TRPC6 [15]. In the present study, we hypothesized that this novel selective TRPC6 inhibitor (SH045) [15] could ameliorate renal fibrogenesis in the New Zealand obese (NZO) mouse model, which is a polygenic model of metabolic syndrome [16]. We studied the therapeutic effects of the in vivo inhibition of TRPC6 by the novel blocker SH045 in the UUO mouse model of accelerated renal fibrogenesis utilizing these mice.

2. Results

2.1. SH045 Treatment Does Not Affect Renal Function and Trpc Expression in UUO Model

To investigate the impact of in vivo TRPC6 inhibition on renal function, target molecules and fibrosis, we performed UUO in the NZO mice. During the one week period, we administrated SH045 (TRPC6 inhibitor) or vehicle once daily (Figure 1A). After 7 days, urinary tract obstruction led to hydronephrosis (Figure S1). Consistent with our previous findings, *Trpc6* expression significantly increased in UUO kidneys. SH045 affected neither *Trpc6* mRNA expression nor the expression of other TRPC channels, including *Trpc1*, *Trpc2*, *Trpc3* and *Trpc4* (Figure 1B and Figure S2A–D). SH045 had no impact on renal function. Serum creatinine ($p = 0.1098$; Figure 1B) and blood urea nitrogen (BUN) ($p = 0.928$; Figure 1C), serum cystatin C, urine albumin, and urine albumin-to-creatinine ratio in SH045-treated mice were unchanged (Figure 1D–F). In addition, we found no differences in serum levels of glucose, sodium, potassium, ionized calcium, total CO_2, hemoglobin, hematocrit, and anion gap in SH045-treated animals compared to the vehicle group (Table S1). SH045-treated mice exhibited a slightly higher serum chloride concentration ($p = 0.047$), albeit within the normal physiological range.

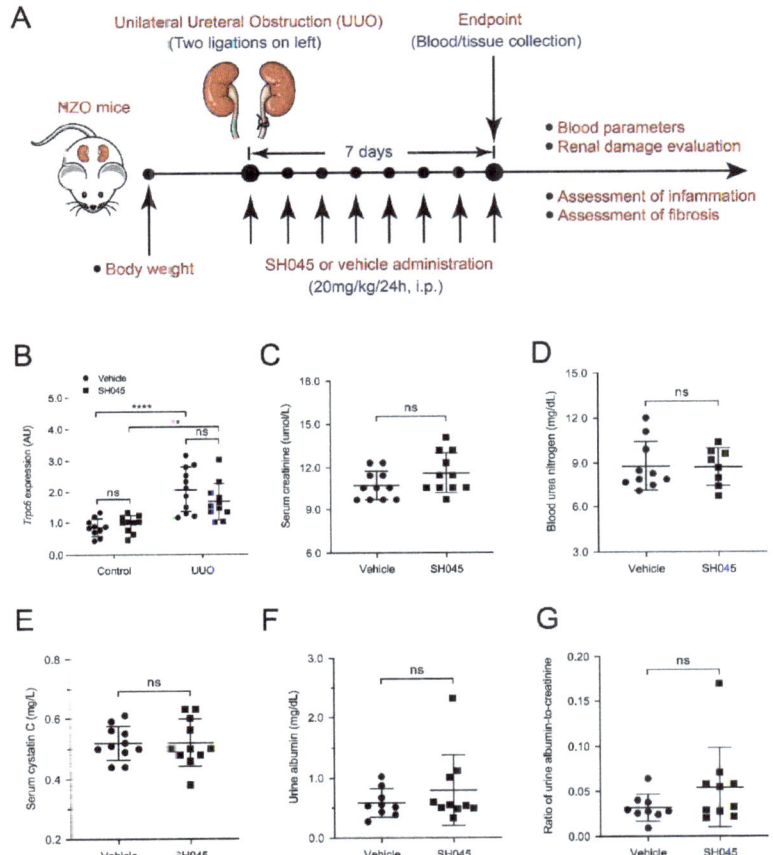

Figure 1. Impact of SH045 administration on renal function and Trpc6 expression in UUO model. (**A**) Experimental design of unilateral ureteral obstruction (UUO) model. NZO mice were subjected to UUO and then injected with SH045 ($n = 11$) or vehicle ($n = 11$) once every 24 h between day 0 and day 7. All mice were euthanized on day 7 after UUO surgery. (**B**) Renal mRNA levels of *Trpc6* (control $n = 10$, UUO $n = 11$). Control group includes kidneys that were not subjected to the UUO. (**C**) Serum levels of creatinine, (**D**) blood urea nitrogen, and (**E**) cystatin C in the experimental UUO groups. (**F**) Urine albumin and (**G**) ratio of albumin to creatinine in the experimental UUO groups (UUO vehicle $n = 10$–11, UUO SH045 $n = 8$–11). Data expressed as means ± SD. Two-way ANOVA followed by Sidak's multiple comparisons post hoc test. ** $p < 0.01$ and **** $p < 0.0001$ defined as significant. ns, not statistically significant. AU, arbitrary units.

2.2. SH045 Treatment Does Not Alter Kidney Parenchymal Damage

Morphologically, UUO increased mesangial matrix deposition, leading to glomerular hypertrophy, and tubular dilatation (Figure 2A–D). The expressions of renal damage markers, kidney injury molecule-1 (*Havcr1*) and Lipocalin-2 (*Lcn2*), were increased in UUO kidneys compared to control (Figure 2E,F). However, SH045 did not affect these parameters in both UUO and control kidneys (Figure 2A–F). These results indicate that TRPC6 inhibition per se has no impact on the damage to renal parenchyma (glomerular or tubular) caused by UUO.

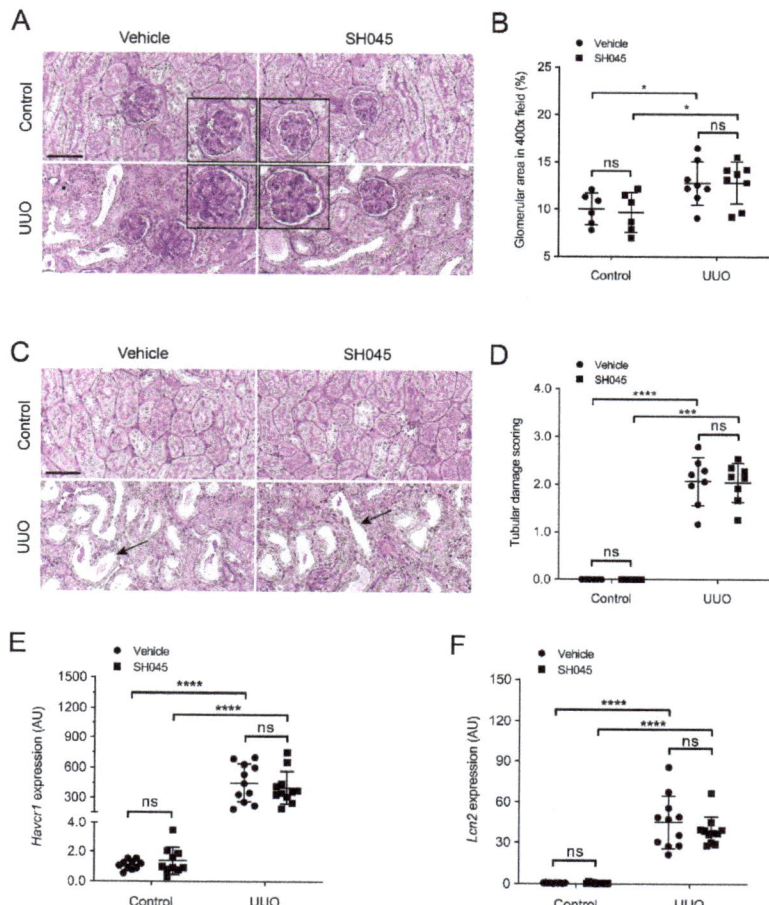

Figure 2. SH045 impact on kidney histopathology after UUO. (**A**) Representative images of UUO-injured glomerulus (magnification: 400×). Kidney sections were stained with periodic acid–Schiff staining (PAS). (**B**) Quantification of glomerular damage (control $n = 6$, UUO $n = 8$). (**C**) Representative images of UUO-injured tubules (magnification: 400×). Kidneys sections were stained with periodic acid–Schiff staining (PAS). Arrows indicate tubular injury. Scale bars are 50 μm. (**D**) Semi-quantification of tubular damage (control $n = 6$, UUO $n = 8$). (**E**) Renal mRNA levels of kidney injury molecule 1 (*Havcr1*) and (**F**) Lipocalin 2 (*Lcn2*) (control $n = 10$, UUO $n = 11$). Data expressed as means ± SD. Two-way ANOVA followed by Sidak's multiple comparisons post hoc test. * $p < 0.05$, *** $p < 0.001$ and **** $p < 0.0001$ defined as significant. ns, not statistically significant. AU, arbitrary units.

2.3. SH045 Treatment Ameliorates Renal Expression of Inflammatory Markers

Next, we measured the renal mRNA expression of inflammatory cytokines and chemokines using qRT-PCR. The expression of inflammatory molecules was markedly increased in kidneys subjected to UUO compared to control groups (Figure 3). The mRNA expression of chemokine (C-X-C motif) ligand 1 (*Cxcl1*), chemokine (C-C motif) ligand 5 (*Ccl5*), and chemokine (C-C motif) receptor 2 (*Ccr2*) was significantly lower in UUO kidneys of SH045-treated mice (SH045 UUO kidneys) compared to UUO kidneys of vehicle-treated mice (vehicle UUO kidneys) (Figure 3A–C). The expressions of chemokine (C-C motif) ligand 2 (*Ccl2*), chemokine (C-X-C motif) ligand 2 (*Cxcl2*), and intercellular adhesion molecule 1 (*Icam1*) were increased in both SH045 UUO and vehicle UUO kidneys compared to control kidneys, although there were no differences between SH045 UUO and vehicle UUO kidneys ($p = 0.056$, $p = 0.068$ and $p = 0.076$, respectively) (Figure 3D–F). Furthermore, immunofluorescence staining of ICAM-1 markedly increased in UUO kidneys in comparison to control kidneys (Figure S3A–C). Additionally, the pharmacological inhibition of TRPC6 by SH045 decreased ICAM-1 expression after UUO in comparison to vehicle-treated kidneys (Figure S3A–C). Whereas ICAM1 expression was similar in the vessels of UUO kidneys, vehicle-treated kidneys had a much higher expression in SH045-treated UUO kidneys due to more ICAM-1-positive immune cell infiltration (Figure S3A).

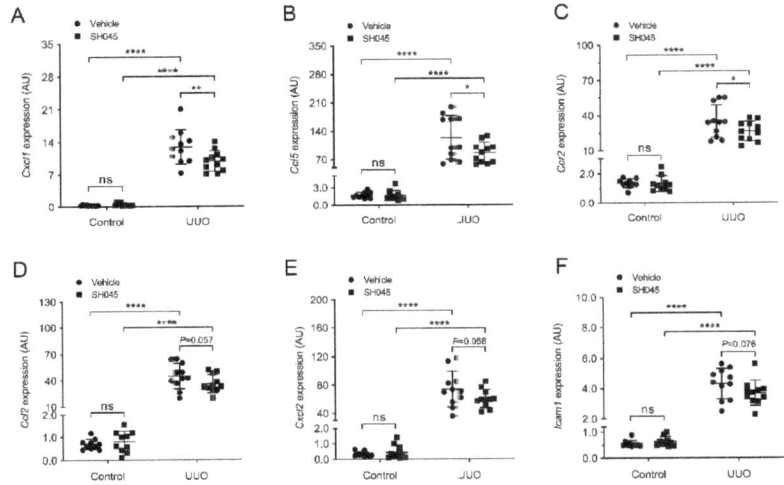

Figure 3. SH045 impact on renal expression of inflammatory markers. (**A**) Renal mRNA levels of chemokine (C-X-C motif) ligand 1 (*Cxcl1*), (**B**) chemokine (C-C motif) ligand 5 (*Ccl5*), (**C**) chemokine (C-C motif) receptor 2 (*Ccr2*), (**D**) chemokine (C-C motif) ligand 2 (*Ccl2*), (**E**) chemokine (C-X-C motif) ligand 2 (*Cxcl2*), and (**F**) intercellular adhesion molecule-1 (*Icam1*) (control $n = 10$, UUO $n = 11$). Data expressed as means ± SD. Two-way ANOVA followed by Sidak's multiple comparisons post hoc test. * $p < 0.05$, ** $p < 0.01$, and **** $p < 0.0001$ defined as significant. ns, not statistically significant. AU, arbitrary units.

2.4. SH045 Treatment Leads to Less Renal Immune Cell Infiltration

To evaluate inflammatory cell infiltration in UUO kidneys, we examined macrophages and T cell presence using immunofluorescence. Kidney cross sections were immunolabelled with the macrophage marker F4/80 and T cell marker CD4 as described previously [17]. As shown in Figure 4A,B, excessive CD4-positive cells infiltration was observed in renal interstitium of UUO kidneys in comparison to control kidneys (Figure 4A,B). Similarly the number of F4/80-positive cells in UUO kidneys was also markedly increased compared to control kidneys (Figure 4C,D). In accordance with ameliorated inflammatory cytokine and chemokine expression, SH045 treatment decreased UUO-induced macrophage and T cell infiltration (Figure 4A–D). Thus, these data suggest that TRPC6 inhibition reduces renal inflammation in the UUO model of NZO mice.

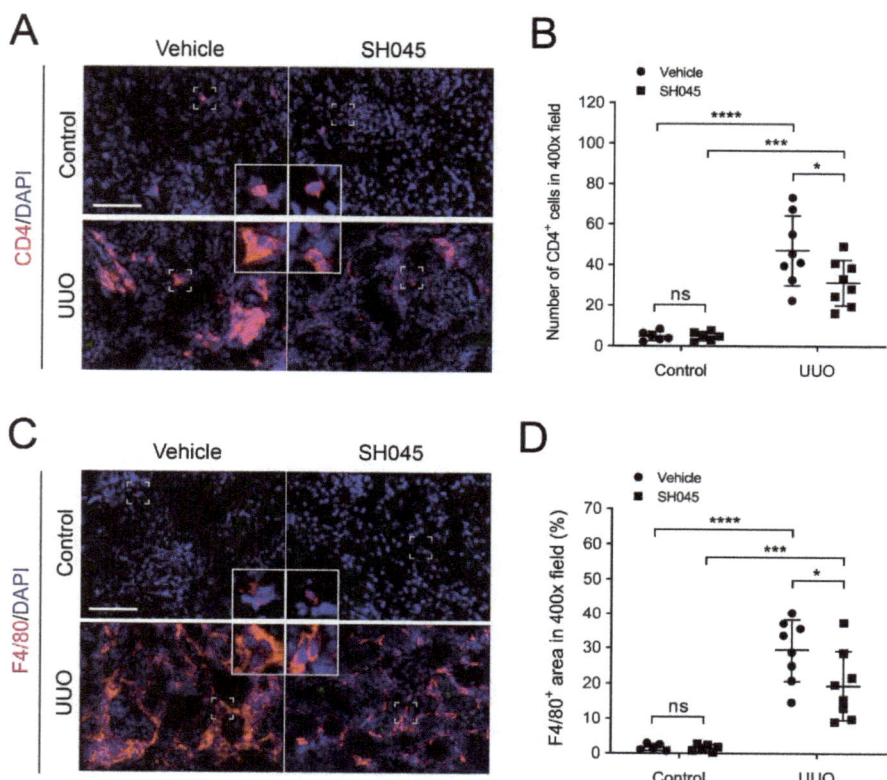

Figure 4. SH045 impact on renal inflammatory cell accumulation after UUO. (**A**) Representative images of control and UUO-injured kidneys stained with CD4+ T cells (magnification: 400×). Rectangles represent single-cell magnifications. Scale bars are 50 µm. (**B**) Quantification in renal infiltration of CD4+ T cells (control $n = 6$, UUO $n = 8$). (**C**) Representative images of control and UUO-injured kidneys stained with F4/80+ macrophages (magnification: 400×). Rectangles represent single-cell magnifications. Scale bars are 50 µm. (**D**) Quantification in renal infiltration of F4/80+ macrophages (control $n = 6$, UUO $n = 8$). Data expressed as means ± SD. Two-way ANOVA followed by Sidak's multiple comparisons post hoc test. * $p < 0.05$, *** $p < 0.001$, and **** $p < 0.0001$ defined as significant. ns, not statistically significant. AU, arbitrary units.

2.5. SH045 Treatment Reduces Renal Expression of Fibrotic Markers

Since progressive fibrosis is a typical lesion occurring after UUO [18], we examined the impact of SH045 administration on renal fibrosis. We measured the renal mRNA expression of pro-fibrotic markers, including collagen I (*Col1a2*), collagen III (*Col3a1*), collagen IV (*Col4a3*), α-smooth muscle actin (*Acta2*), connective tissue growth factor (*Ccn2*), and fibronectin (*Fn1*). All these fibrosis-associated genes were upregulated after UUO (Figure 5A–F). Notably, SH045 treatment significantly reduced *Col1a2*, *Col3a1*, *Col4a3*, *Acta2*, *Ccn2*, and *Fn1* expressions in the UUO kidney (Figure 5A–F).

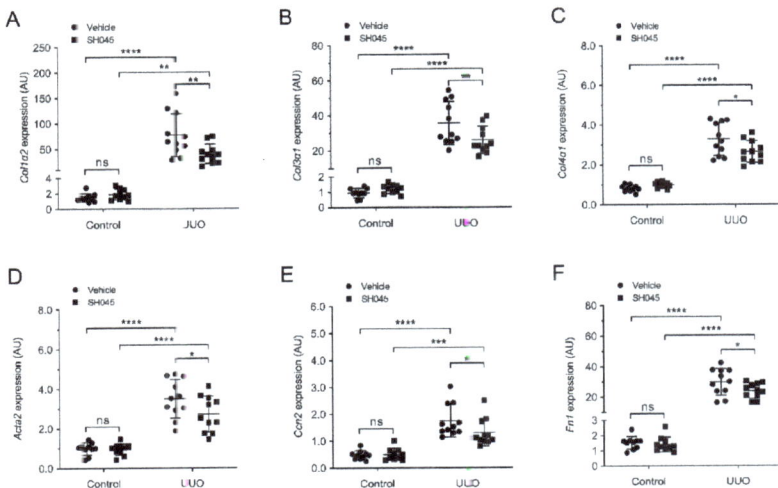

Figure 5. SH045 impact on expression of renal fibrotic markers UUO. (**A**) Renal mRNA levels of collagen type I α 1 (*Col1α2*), (**B**) Collagen type III α 1 (*Col3α1*), (**C**) Collagen type IV α 1 (*Col4α1*), (**D**) α-Smooth muscle actin (*Acta2*), (**E**) Connective tissue growth factor (*Ccn2*), and (**F**) Fibronectin (*Fn1*) (Control $n = 10$, UUO $n = 11$). Data expressed as means ± SD. Two-way ANOVA followed by Sidak's multiple comparisons post hoc test. * $p < 0.05$, ** $p < 0.01$, *** $p < 0.001$ and **** $p < 0.0001$ defined as significant. ns, not statistically significant. AU, arbitrary units.

To further confirm our qPCR data, Sirius red (SR) and fibronectin immunofluorescence staining was performed. Control kidneys exhibited small SR-positive (+) areas. In contrast, UUO kidneys displayed markedly increased SR$^+$ areas compared to control kidneys, indicating that UUO caused considerable collagen deposition (Figure 6A,B). SH045 effectively decreased this collagen deposition (Figure 6A,B). Similarly, immunofluorescence staining revealed increased fibronectin deposition and chromogenic immunohistochemistry increased α-smooth muscle actin (α-SMA) expression in UUO kidneys in comparison to control kidneys, which were reduced by SH045 treatment (Figure 6C–F). Taken together, these data suggest that renal fibrosis and inflammatory reactions are ameliorated in response to in vivo TRPC6 inhibition by SH045.

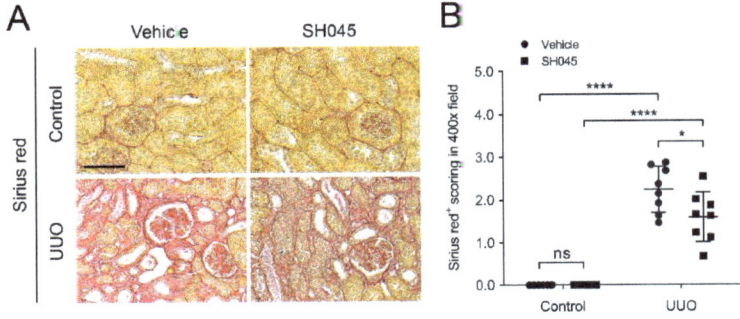

Figure 6. *Cont.*

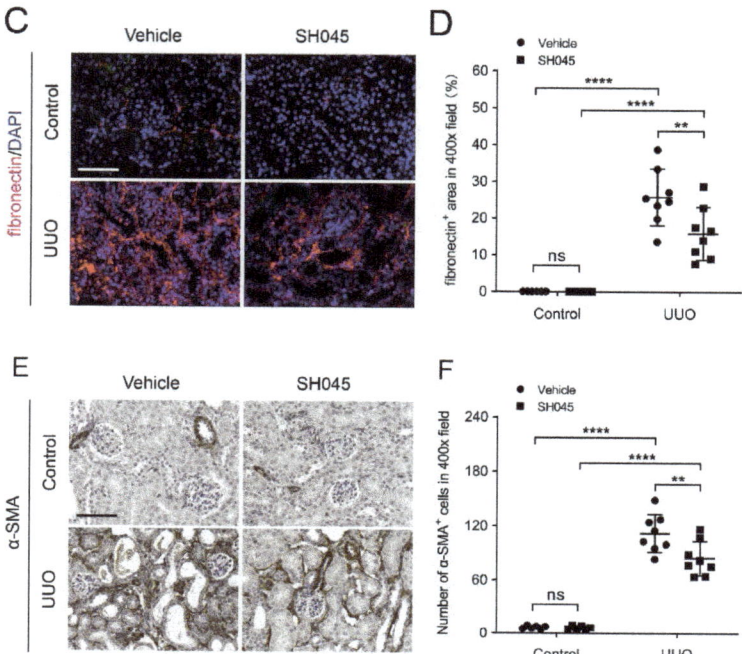

Figure 6. SH045 impact on renal fibrogenesis after UUO. (A) Representative images of control and UUO-injured kidneys stained with Sirius red (magnification: 400×). Scale bars are 50 μm. (B) Semi-quantification in renal Sirius red+ area proportion (control n = 6, UUO n = 8). (C) Representative images of control and UUO-injured kidneys stained with fibronectin (magnification: 400×). Scale bars are 50 μm. (D) Quantification in fibronectin+ area (control n = 6, UUO n = 8). (E) Representative images of control and UUO-injured kidneys stained with α-SMA (magnification: 400×). Scale bars are 50 μm. (F) Quantification of α-SMA+ staining (control n = 6, UUO n = 8). Data expressed as means ± SD. Two-way ANOVA followed by Sidak's multiple comparisons post hoc test. * $p < 0.05$, ** $p < 0.01$, and **** $p < 0.0001$ defined as significant. ns, not statistically significant.

3. Discussion

Renal fibrosis is the final common outcome of progressive CKD, which is often observed in metabolic syndrome [19]. To date, there are few clinical treatments that successfully target fibrosis in CKD. Thus, developing new drug treatments is the current focus. Increasing evidence indicates that TRPC6 could play a critical role in kidney fibrosis [20]. In our previous study using $Trpc6^{-/-}$ mice, we found that TRPC6 deficiency ameliorated renal fibrosis and immune cellular infiltration in the UUO model [7]. However, the results were difficult to interpret due to confounding genomic and non-genomic effects of other TRPC channels, e.g., TPRC1, TRPC3, TRPC4 and TRPC5. Previous studies identified SH045 (larixyl N-methylcarbamate) as a novel, highly potent, subtype-selective inhibitor of TRPC6 channels [15]. In our previous study, we found that the in vivo inhibition of TRPC6 by SH045 had no effects on acute kidney injury (AKI) [14]. However, there are no studies on the effects of SH045 in kidney fibrosis. In the present study, we tested the hypothesis that SH045 ameliorates UUO-accelerated renal fibrosis in NZO mice.

Our results show that SH045 ameliorates fibrotic processes in UUO kidneys. Expressions of all investigated fibrosis or fibrosis-related genes were ameliorated by SH045 treatment. The histological assessment of deposited collagen and extracellular matrix protein confirmed the expression data of the genes. Of note, renal fibrosis arises after an insult, whereas resident kidney fibroblasts and cells of hematopoietic origin differentiate into myofibroblasts [21–23]. Myofibroblasts acquire a contractile/proliferative phenotype upon activation by profibrotic factors and become principal kidney collagen-producing cells [24]. Considerable evidence indicates that renal inflammation plays a central role in the initiation and progression of fibrosis [19]. Myofibroblasts are regulated by a variety of means, including paracrine signals derived from lymphocytes and macrophages. Critical chemokines recruiting macrophages and lymphocytes are CCL2/CCR2, CCL5, and CXCL1/2. ICAM-1 is an endothelial- and leukocyte-associated transmembrane protein in facilitating leukocyte endothelial transmigration [25]. Interestingly, our results show that SH045 inhibits the overexpression of these chemokines and the infiltration of numerous immune cells, suggesting that TRPC6 inhibition may antagonize renal fibrosis by affecting inflammatory processes. TRPC6 is expressed in a wide range of cell types, including neutrophils, lymphocytes, platelets and the endothelium, which might be a modulator of tissue susceptibility to inflammatory injuries [26,27]. Some studies suggested that TRPC6 channels may enhance chemotactic responses by increasing Ca^{2+} concentration, which promotes actin-based cytoskeleton remodeling [28,29]. Furthermore, Ca^{2+} currents within T-lymphocytes are influenced by TRPC6, which can affect the function of T-lymphocytes [30]. Novel myeloid cell subsets could be targeted to ameliorate injury or enhance repair, including an *Arg1*+ monocyte subset present during injury and *Mmp12*+ macrophages present during repair [31]. It is intriguing to speculate that TRPC6 inhibition might ameliorate fibrotic processes in UUO kidneys by modulating the function(s) of theses cell types.

On the other hand, TRPC6 was also reported to contribute to fibroblast transdifferentiation and healing in vivo [32]. Thus, the beneficial effects of TRPC6 inhibition seen in the UUO model might also involve fibroblasts. A TPRC6 blockade may decrease Ca^{2+} dependent activation of MEK/ERK signaling pathway [33]. Of note, this pathway was implemented in the detrimental differentiation and expansion of kidney fibroblasts [34]. The inhibition of the ERK1/2 pathway by trametinib ameliorated UUO-induced fibrosis through the mammalian target of rapamycin complex 1 (mTORC1) and its downstream targets.

In the present study, SH045 did not affect renal function parameters in 7-day-UUO mice, which is not surprising. In this short-term UUO model, the kidney function of contralateral undamaged kidney remained preserved and compensated for the loss of the obstructed kidney at the early stage [35]. We used the NZO inbred obese mouse strain, which carries susceptibility genes for diabetes and hypertension, conditions similar to metabolic syndrome and CKD in humans [36]. Our data observed in UUO induced fibrosis in NZO mice, and thus might be of importance in mimicking human CKD pathophysiology.

Renal fibrosis involves complex interactions among multiple cells and cytokine signaling pathways. Further studies of the TRPC6 modulation of renal fibrosis using single-cell RNA sequencing could help to better understand the exact mechanism(s) of action in the different cell types. Single-cell RNA sequencing enables the precise discrimination of specific cell type(s) or cell state(s) enriched in certain conditions (e.g., UUO) [31]. Thus, selecting cellular labels based on gene expression markers could represent a novel approach to determine cell type(s) or cell state(s) predominantly influenced by the inhibition of TRPC6 (by SH045) in the UUO model. Understanding the mechanisms behind TRPC6-induced fibrogenesis is essential for developing novel therapies to slow the progression of CKD.

Our study demonstrates that the in vivo administration of SH045 ameliorates immune cell infiltration and fibrosis in NZO mice subjected to UUO, which makes SH045 a promising therapeutic drug strategy in CKD treatment for metabolic syndrome.

4. Materials and Methods

4.1. Animals

Male NZO mice (n = 22, NZO/BomHIDife genetic background) from Max-Rubner-Laboratory, German Institute of Human Nutrition Potsdam-Rehbrücke (Nuthetal, Germany) were used. These mice had increased weight (45.90 ± 4.11g b.w) and were previously characterized [7]. Mice were held in specific-pathogen-free (SPF) condition, in a 12:12 h light–dark cycle, with free access to food and drinking water. All experimental procedures were approved by the Berlin Animal Review Board, Berlin, Germany and followed the restrictions in the Berlin State Office for Health and Social Affairs (LaGeSo) [37]. All experiments were performed in accordance with ARRIVE guidelines [38].

4.2. UUO Model

UUO mouse model was performed as described earlier [7]. Briefly, NZO mice were anaesthetized by isoflurane (2.2%) supplied with air flow at approximately 350 mL/min. During the surgery mice were placed on a heating pad to prevent hypothermia. Preemptive analgesia with carprofen (5–10 mg/kg b.w) was subcutaneously used. Body temperature was maintained at 37.5 °C and monitored during surgery using a temperature controller with a heating pad (TCAT-2, Physitemp Instruments, Clifton, NJ, USA). In deep anesthesia, the anterior abdominal skin was shaved. Then, a midline laparotomy was conducted via an incision of the avascular linea alba, and the left ureter was exposed from left side. The ureter was then ligated twice close to the renal pelvis using a 5–0 polyglycolic acid (PGA) suture wire (Resorba®, Nürnberg, Germany). The linea alba and skin were closed separately. The wound was sanitized with a silver aluminium spray (Henry Schein®, Berlin, Germany), and 0.5 mL of warm (37 °C) isotonic sodium chloride solution was intraperitoneally injected. Subsequently, each mouse was placed in a cage in front of an infrared (IR) lamp and monitored until they recovered consciousness. For the following two days, mice received carprofen (2.5 mg/mL) in their drinking water (1:50) with a final concentration of 0.05 mg/mL. After surgery mice had free access to drinking water and chow. Seven days after UUO surgery, mice were sacrificed by overdose of isoflurane and cervical dislocation. The blood samples were collected for further analysis and left kidneys were removed immediately. The kidneys were divided into three portions. Upper part of the kidney tissue was frozen in isopthane. Middle part of kidney was immersed in 4% phosphate–buffered saline (PBS)-buffered formalin for histological assessment. The other left tissue was snap frozen in liquid nitrogen for RNA preparation.

4.3. TRPC6 Inhibitor

SH045 (Larixyl-6-N-methylcarbamate) was previously described [15]. SH045 was initially dissolved in DMSO (final concentration of DMSO is 0.5%) and then in 5% Cremophor EL® solution with 0.9% NaCl and used for intraperitoneal injection (i.p.). Mice subjected to UUO were treated with SH045 (20 mg/kg once per day, i.p.) or vehicle daily until day 7 after surgery.

4.4. Blood Measurements and Drugs

The blood measurements of sodium, potassium, chloride, ionized calcium, total carbon dioxide, glucose, urea nitrogen, creatinine, hematocrit, hemoglobin, and anion gap were performed at endpoint. Nighty-five microliters of blood were taken from the facial vein, and parameters were measured using i-STAT system with Chem8+ cartridges (Abbott GmbH, Wiesbaden, Germany).

4.5. Quantitative Real-Time (qRT)-PCR

The qRT-PCR was performed as previously described [7]. Briefly, total mRNA from mice was isolated from snap-frozen kidneys using RNeasy RNA isolation kit (Qiagen, Australia), according to the manufacturer's instructions. The concentration and quality of RNA were determined by NanoDrop-1000 spectrophotometer (Thermo Fisher Scientific, Waltham, MA, USA). Next, RNA was transcribed to cDNA using a reaction kit (Applied Biosystems, Waltham, MA, USA). Quantitative analysis of target marker was performed with qRT-PCR using the relative standard curve method. TaqMan or SYBR green analysis was conducted by using an Applied Biosystems 7500 Sequence Detector (Applied Biosystems, Waltham, MA, USA). The expression levels were normalized to 18S rRNA. All primer sequences are provided in Table S2.

4.6. Kidney Histopathology

Histological kidney assessment was performed as previously reported [39]. Formalin-fixed, paraffin-embedded sections (2 µm) of kidneys were subjected to periodic acid–Schiff (PAS) and Sirius red (SR) staining. The PAS reaction visualized the basement membranes of the capillary loops of the glomeruli, through which the glomerular damage can be evaluated [7]. In each group, 10 fields of view were randomly selected from each kidney sample section under a 400× magnification, and the average ratio of glomerular section area to total area within the view was calculated using the software ImageJ. SR staining allows for a quantification of interstitial fibrosis. The severity of tubule interstitial fibrosis was graded from 0 to 3 according to the distribution of lesions: 0, no lesion; 1, less than 20%; 2, 20–50%; 3, more than 50% [40]. Semi-quantitative glomerular damage and renal fibrotic scoring were performed in a blinded manner at 400× magnification per sample. All measurements were repeated three times.

4.7. Immunofluorescence and Immunohistochemistry

We performed immunostaining as previously described [7,41]. Immunofluorescence or immunohistochemistry was performed on 3-µm ice-cold acetone-fixed cryosections of kidneys using the following primary antibodies: anti-fibronectin, anti-CD4, anti-F4/80, anti-ICAM-1, anti-α-SMA (AbD Serotec, Oxford, UK). For indirect immunostaining, non-specific binding sites were blocked with 10% normal donkey serum for 30 min. Then, sections were incubated with the primary antibody for 1 h at room temperature or overnight at 4 °C. All incubations were performed in a humid chamber. For fluorescence visualization of bound primary antibodies, sections were further incubated with Cy3-conjugated secondary antibodies (Jackson Immuno Research, WG, USA) for 1 h in a humid chamber at room temperature. Slides were analyzed using a Zeiss Axioplan-2 imaging microscope with the computer program AxioVision 4.8 (Zeiss, Jena, Germany). For immunohistochemistry, after incubation with the primary antibody directed against α-SMA, biotinylated secondary antibody (Dako REAL™ EnVision™; Dako Denmark A/S, Glostrup, Denmark) was used. Immunohistochemical positive staining was consecutively revealed by the 3,3′-Diaminobenzidine Peroxidase Substrate Kit (Dako REAL™ EnVision™; Dako Denmark A/S, Glostrup, Denmark) in accordance with the manufacturer's instructions.

Quantitative analyses of infiltrating cells (CD4+ and F4/80+) and fibroblasts (α-SMA–) were counted in 15 non-overlapping, randomly chosen fields per kidney section under a 400× magnification. The average ratio of the fibronectin or ICAM-1-labeled area to the total area in the view (400×) was calculated using the software ImageJ (NIH, Bethesda, MD, USA). In addition, ICAM-1 expression was also analyzed using software ImageJ to calculate the mean gray value (integrated density to area).

4.8. Statistics

Statistical analysis was performed using GraphPad 5.04 software. Study groups were analyzed by two-way ANOVA using Sidak's multiple comparisons post hoc test. Data are presented as mean $\pm$ SD. p values < 0.05 were considered statistically significant.

Supplementary Materials: The following are available online at: https://www.mdpi.com/article/10.3390/ijms23126870/s1.

Author Contributions: Conceptualization, M.G., D.T. and L.M.; Data curation, Z.Z.; Formal analysis, Z.Z. and Y.X.; Funding acquisition, M.S., B.N. and M.G.; Investigation, Z.Z. and Y.X.; Methodology, Z.Z., U.K., M.S., B.N. and M.-B.K.; Project administration, M.G., D.T. and L.M.; Resources, U.K., T.C., M.G. and L.M.; Software, Z.Z., D.T. and L.M.; Supervision, M.G., D.T. and L.M.; Validation, D.T. and L.M.; Writing—original draft, Z.Z.; Writing—review and editing, M.G., D.T. and L.M. All authors agree to be accountable for all aspects of the work in ensuring that questions related to the accuracy or integrity of any part of the work are appropriately investigated and resolved. All authors made substantial contributions to conception, design, drafting and completion of the article. All authors have read and agreed to the published version of the manuscript.

Funding: This work was supported by the Deutsche Forschungsgemeinschaft (DFG) to M.G. (GO766/18-2, GO 766/12-3, SFB 1365), B.N. (NU 53/12-2) and M.S. (TRR 152) and Werner Jackstädt-Stiftung.

Institutional Review Board Statement: The animal study protocol was approved by the Berlin Animal Review Board, Berlin, Germany and followed the restrictions in the Berlin State Office for Health and Social Affairs (Landesamt für Gesundheit und Soziales, LaGeSo) (license No. G0175/18, 11 Sep. 2018). All experiments were performed in accordance with ARRIVE guidelines.

Informed Consent Statement: Not applicable.

Data Availability Statement: Represented data are publicly archived datasets. For further information, please contact the corresponding author.

Acknowledgments: We thank Mario Kaßmann for his administrative support. We thank Jana Czychi, Gabriele N'diaye, and Juliane Ulrich for their technical help. We acknowledge financial support from the Open Access Publication Fund of Charité—Universitätsmedizin Berlin and the German Research Foundation (DFG).

Conflicts of Interest: The authors declare no conflict of interest.

References

1. Jha, V.; Garcia-Garcia, G.; Iseki, K.; Li, Z.; Naicker, S.; Plattner, B.; Saran, R.; Wang, A.Y.; Yang, C.W. Chronic kidney disease: Global dimension and perspectives. *Lancet* **2013**, *382*, 260–272. [CrossRef]
2. Genovese, G.; Friedman, D.J.; Ross, M.D.; Lecordier, L.; Uzureau, P.; Freedman, B.I.; Bowden, D.W.; Langefeld, C.D.; Oleksyk, T.K.; Uscinski Knob, A.L.; et al. Association of trypanolytic ApoL1 variants with kidney disease in African Americans. *Science* **2010**, *329*, 841–845. [CrossRef]
3. Li, X.; Pan, J.; Li, H.; Li, G. DsbA-L mediated renal tubulointerstitial fibrosis in UUO mice. *Nat. Commun.* **2020**, *11*, 4467. [CrossRef]
4. Black, L.; Lever, J.M.; Traylor, A.M.; Chen, B.; Yang, Z.; Esman, S.; Jiang, Y.; Cutter, G.; Boddu, R.; George, J.; et al. Divergent effects of AKI to CKD models on inflammation and fibrosis. *Am. J. Physiol. Ren. Physiol.* **2018**, *315*, F1107–F1118. [CrossRef]
5. Schlondorff, J. TRPC6 and kidney disease: Sclerosing more than just glomeruli? *Kidney Int.* **2017**, *91*, 773–775. [CrossRef] [PubMed]
6. Eddy, A.A. Overview of the cellular and molecular basis of kidney fibrosis. *Kidney Int Suppl (2011).* **2014**, *4*, 2–8. [CrossRef] [PubMed]
7. Kong, W.; Haschler, T.N.; Nürnberg, B.; Krämer, S.; Gollasch, M.; Markó, L. Renal Fibrosis, Immune Cell Infiltration and Changes of TRPC Channel Expression after Unilateral Ureteral Obstruction in Trpc6-/- Mice. *Cell Physiol. Biochem.* **2019**, *52*, 1484–1502. [PubMed]
8. Lin, B.L.; Matera, D.; Doerner, J.F.; Zheng, N.; Del Camino, D.; Mishra, S.; Bian, H.; Zeveleva, S.; Zhen, X.; Blair, N.T.; et al. In vivo selective inhibition of TRPC6 by antagonist BI 749327 ameliorates fibrosis and dysfunction in cardiac and renal disease. *Proc. Natl. Acad. Sci. USA* **2019**, *116*, 10156–10161. [CrossRef]
9. Ilatovskaya, D.V.; Staruschenko, A. TRPC6 channel as an emerging determinant of the podocyte injury susceptibility in kidney diseases. *Am. J. Physiol. Ren. Physiol.* **2015**, *309*, F393–F397. [CrossRef]
10. Dryer, S.E.; Roshanravan, H.; Kim, E.Y. TRPC channels: Regulation, dysregulation and contributions to chronic kidney disease. *Biochim. Biophys. Acta Mol. Basis Dis.* **2019**, *1865*, 1041–1066. [CrossRef]
11. Winn, M.P.; Conlon, P.J.; Lynn, K.L.; Farrington, M.K.; Creazzo, T.; Hawkins, A.F.; Daskalakis, N.; Kwan, S.Y.; Ebersviller, S.; Burchette, J.L.; et al. A mutation in the TRPC6 cation channel causes familial focal segmental glomerulosclerosis. *Science* **2005**, *308*, 1801–1804. [CrossRef] [PubMed]
12. Reiser, J.; Polu, K.R.; Moller, C.C.; Kenlan, P.; Altintas, M.M.; Wei, C.; Faul, C.; Herbert, S.; Villegas, I.; Avila-Casado, C.; et al. TRPC6 is a glomerular slit diaphragm-associated channel required for normal renal function. *Nat. Genet.* **2005**, *37*, 739–744. [CrossRef] [PubMed]
13. Riehle, M.; Buscher, A.K.; Gohlke, B.O.; Kassmann, M.; Kolatsi-Joannou, M.; Brasen, J.H.; Nagel, M.; Becker, J.U.; Winyard, P.; Hoyer, P.F.; et al. TRPC6 G757D Loss-of-Function Mutation Associates with FSGS. *J. Am. Soc. Nephrol.* **2016**, *27*, 2771–2783. [CrossRef] [PubMed]
14. Zheng, Z.; Tsvetkov, D.; Bartolomaeus, T.U.P.; Erdogan, C.; Krügel, U.; Schleifenbaum, J.; Schaefer, M.; Nürnberg, B.; Chai, X.; Ludwig, F.A.; et al. Role of TRPC6 in kidney damage after acute ischemic kidney injury. *Sci. Rep.* **2022**, *12*, 3038. [CrossRef] [PubMed]
15. Häfner, S.; Burg, F.; Kannler, M.; Urban, N.; Mayer, P.; Dietrich, A.; Trauner, D.; Broichhagen, J.; Schaefer, M. A (+)-Larixol Congener with High Affinity and Subtype Selectivity toward TRPC6. *ChemMedChem* **2018**, *13*, 1028–1035. [CrossRef] [PubMed]
16. Breyer, M.D.; Böttinger, E.; Brosius, F.C., 3rd; Coffman, T.M.; Harris, R.C.; Heilig, C.W.; Sharma, K. Mouse models of diabetic nephropathy. *J. Am. Soc. Nephrol.* **2005**, *16*, 27–45. [CrossRef]
17. Markó, L.; Park, J.K.; Henke, N.; Rong, S.; Balogh, A.; Klamer, S.; Bartolomaeus, H.; Wilck, N.; Ruland, J.; Forslund, S.K.; et al. B-cell lymphoma/leukaemia 10 and angiotensin II-induced kidney injury. *Cardiovasc. Res.* **2020**, *116*, 1059–1070. [CrossRef]

18. Chevalier, R.L.; Forbes, M.S.; Thornhill, B.A. Ureteral obstruction as a model of renal interstitial fibrosis and obstructive nephropathy. *Kidney Int.* **2009**, *75*, 1145–1152. [CrossRef]
19. Lv, W.; Booz, G.W.; Wang, Y.; Fan, F.; Roman, R.J. Inflammation and renal fibrosis: Recent developments on key signaling molecules as potential therapeutic targets. *Eur. J. Pharmacol.* **2018**, *820*, 65–76. [CrossRef]
20. Wu, Y.L.; Xie, J.; An, S.W.; Oliver, N.; Barrezueta, N.X.; Lin, M.H.; Birnbaumer, L.; Huang, C.L. Inhibition of TRPC6 channels ameliorates renal fibrosis and contributes to renal protection by soluble klotho. *Kidney Int.* **2017**, *91*, 830–841. [CrossRef] [PubMed]
21. LeBleu, V.S.; Taduri, G.; O'Connell, J.; Teng, Y.; Cooke, V.G.; Woda, C.; Sugimoto, H.; Kalluri, R. Origin and function of myofibroblasts in kidney fibrosis. *Nat. Med.* **2013**, *19*, 1047–1053. [CrossRef]
22. Zeisberg, E.M.; Potenta, S.E.; Sugimoto, H.; Zeisberg, M.; Kalluri, R. Fibroblasts in kidney fibrosis emerge via endothelial-to-mesenchymal transition. *J. Am. Soc. Nephrol.* **2008**, *19*, 2282–2287. [CrossRef] [PubMed]
23. Lu, Y.A.; Liao, C.T.; Raybould, R. Single-Nucleus RNA Sequencing Identifies New Classes of Proximal Tubular Epithelial Cells in Kidney Fibrosis. *J. Am. Soc. Nephrol.* **2021**, *32*, 2501–2516. [CrossRef] [PubMed]
24. Tomasek, J.J.; Gabbiani, G.; Hinz, B.; Chaponnier, C.; Brown, R.A. Myofibroblasts and mechano-regulation of connective tissue remodelling. *Nat. Rev. Mol. Cell Biol.* **2002**, *3*, 349–363. [CrossRef]
25. Shlipak, M.G.; Fried, L.F.; Crump, C.; Bleyer, A.J.; Manolio, T.A.; Tracy, R.P.; Furberg, C.D.; Psaty, B.M. Elevations of inflammatory and procoagulant biomarkers in elderly persons with renal insufficiency. *Circulation* **2003**, *107*, 87–92. [CrossRef]
26. Chen, Q.; Zhou, Y.; Zhou, L.; Fu, Z.; Yang, C.; Zhao, L.; Li, S.; Chen, Y.; Wu, Y.; Ling, Z.; et al. TRPC6-dependent Ca(2+) signaling mediates airway inflammation in response to oxidative stress via ERK pathway. *Cell Death Dis.* **2020**, *11*, 170. [CrossRef] [PubMed]
27. European Bioinformatics Institute (EMBL-EBI); SIB Swiss Institute of Bioinformatics (PIR). P.I.R. Universal Protein Resource (Uniprot). Available online: http://www.uniprot.org/ (accessed on 17 March 2022).
28. Damann, N.; Owsianik, G.; Li, S.; Poll, C.; Nilius, B. The calcium-conducting ion channel transient receptor potential canonical 6 is involved in macrophage inflammatory protein-2-induced migration of mouse neutrophils. *Acta Physiol.* **2009**, *195*, 3–11. [CrossRef] [PubMed]
29. Lindemann, O.; Umlauf, D.; Frank, S.; Schimmelpfennig, S.; Bertrand, J.; Pap, T.; Hanley, P.J.; Fabian, A.; Dietrich, A.; Schwab, A. TRPC6 regulates CXCR2-mediated chemotaxis of murine neutrophils. *J. Immunol.* **2013**, *190*, 5496–5505. [CrossRef]
30. Carrillo, C.; Hichami, A.; Andreoletti, P.; Cherkaoui-Malki, M.; del Mar Cavia, M.; Abdoul-Azize, S.; Alonso-Torre, S.R.; Khan, N.A. Diacylglycerol-containing oleic acid induces increases in [Ca(2+)](i) via TRPC3/6 channels in human T-cells. *Biochim. Biophys. Acta* **2012**, *1821*, 618–626. [CrossRef]
31. Conway, B.R.; O'Sullivan, E.D. Kidney Single-Cell Atlas Reveals Myeloid Heterogeneity in Progression and Regression of Kidney Disease. *J. Am. Soc. Nephrol.* **2020**, *31*, 2833–2854. [CrossRef]
32. Davis, J.; Burr, A.R.; Davis, G.F.; Birnbaumer, L.; Molkentin, J.D. A TRPC6-dependent pathway for myofibroblast transdifferentiation and wound healing in vivo. *Dev. Cell* **2012**, *23*, 705–715. [CrossRef] [PubMed]
33. Agell, N.; Bachs, O.; Rocamora, N.; Villalonga, P. Modulation of the Ras/Raf/MEK/ERK pathway by Ca(2+), and calmodulin. *Cell Signal* **2002**, *14*, 649–654. [CrossRef]
34. Andrikopoulos, P.; Kieswich, J.; Pacheco, S.; Nadarajah, L.; Harwood, S.M.; O'Riordan, C.E.; Thiemermann, C.; Yaqoob, M.M. The MEK Inhibitor Trametinib Ameliorates Kidney Fibrosis by Suppressing ERK1/2 and mTORC1 Signaling. *J. Am. Soc. Nephrol.* **2019**, *30*, 33–49. [CrossRef] [PubMed]
35. Zeng, F.; Miyazawa, T.; Kloepfer, L.A.; Harris, R.C. ErbB4 deletion accelerates renal fibrosis following renal injury. *Am. J. Physiol. Ren Physiol.* **2018**, *314*, F773–F787. [CrossRef] [PubMed]
36. Mirhashemi, F.; Scherneck, S.; Kluth, O.; Kaiser, D.; Vogel, H.; Kluge, R.; Schürmann, A.; Neschen, S.; Joost, H.G. Diet dependence of diabetes in the New Zealand Obese (NZO) mouse: Total fat, but not fat quality or sucrose accelerates and aggravates diabetes. *Exp. Clin. Endocrinol. Diabetes* **2011**, *119*, 167–171. [CrossRef]
37. Restrictions in the State Office for Health and Social Affairs (LAGeSo). Animal Welfare. Available online: https://www.berlin.de/lageso/gesundheit/veterinaerwesen/tierschutz/ (accessed on 17 August 2021).
38. Kilkenny, C.; Browne, W.J.; Cuthill, I.C.; Emerson, M.; Altman, D.G. Improving bioscience research reporting: The ARRIVE guidelines for reporting animal research. *PLoS Biol.* **2010**, *8*, e1000412. [CrossRef]
39. Mannaa, M.; Markó, L.; Balogh, A.; Vigolo, E.; N'Diaye, G.; Kaßmann, M.; Michalick, L.; Weichelt, U.; Schmidt-Ott, K.M.; Liedtke, W.B.; et al. Transient Receptor Potential Vanilloid 4 Channel Deficiency Aggravates Tubular Damage after Acute Renal Ischaemia Reperfusion. *Sci. Rep.* **2018**, *8*, 4878. [CrossRef]
40. Zheng, Z.; Li, C.; Shao, G.; Li, J.; Xu, K.; Zhao, Z.; Zhang, Z.; Liu, J.; Wu, H. Hippo-YAP/MCP-1 mediated tubular maladaptive repair promote inflammation in renal failed recovery after ischemic AKI. *Cell Death Dis.* **2021**, *12*, 754. [CrossRef]
41. Zheng, Z.; Deng, G.; Qi, C.; Xu, Y.; Liu, X.; Zhao, Z.; Zhang, Z.; Chu, Y.; Wu, H.; Liu, J. Porous Se@SiO2 nanospheres attenuate ischemia/reperfusion (I/R)-induced acute kidney injury (AKI) and inflammation by antioxidative stress. *Int. J. Nanomed.* **2019**, *14*, 215–229. [CrossRef]

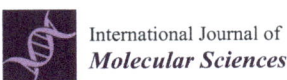

Review

New Insights on the Role of Marinobufagenin from Bench to Bedside in Cardiovascular and Kidney Diseases

Nazareno Carullo, Giuseppe Fabiano, Mario D'Agostino, Maria Teresa Zicarelli, Michela Musolino, Pierangela Presta, Ashour Michael, Michele Andreucci, Davide Bolignano and Giuseppe Coppolino *

Renal Unit "Magna Graecia" University of Catanzaro, 88100 Catanzaro, Italy
* Correspondence: gcoppolino@unicz.it; Tel.: +39-096-1369-7170

Abstract: Marinobufagenin (MBG) is a member of the bufadienolide family of compounds, which are natural cardiac glycosides found in a variety of animal species, including man, which have different physiological and biochemical functions but have a common action on the inhibition of the adenosine triphosphatase sodium-potassium pump (Na+/K+-ATPase). MBG acts as an endogenous cardiotonic steroid, and in the last decade, its role as a pathogenic factor in various human diseases has emerged. In this paper, we have collated major evidence regarding the biological characteristics and functions of MBG and its implications in human pathology. This review focused on MBG involvement in chronic kidney disease, including end-stage renal disease, cardiovascular diseases, sex and gender medicine, and its actions on the nervous and immune systems. The role of MBG in pathogenesis and the development of a wide range of pathological conditions indicate that this endogenous peptide could be used in the future as a diagnostic biomarker and/or therapeutic target, opening important avenues of scientific research.

Keywords: Marinobufagenin (MBG); chronic kidney disease; end-stage renal disease (ESRD); nervous and immune systems

1. Introduction

This review focuses on the recent discoveries on the role of Marinobufagenin (MBG) in CV and kidney diseases. MBG is one of the more interesting molecules belonging to the family of bufadienolides. They are part of the cardiac glycoside [1–3] group of molecules that have significant physiological and biochemical differences but share the ability to inhibit the adenosine triphosphatase sodium–potassium pump (Na^+/K^+-ATPase), an enzyme which is ubiquitous in cell membranes. They play a role in positive cardiac inotropism, as they have natriuretic and vasoconstrictive properties. Bufadienolides were initially found in several animal species, characterized by different phylogeny, suggesting their relevance in evolution (Table 1). We highlight, in particular, the role of MBG as a cardiotonic steroid in humans, as they have relevant roles in many different clinical conditions characterized by body fluid volume expansion, such as pre-eclampsia (PE), hypertension, heart failure and chronic kidney disease (CKD) (Table 2). In recent years, a growing interest has emerged in its role as a novel potential biomarker for cardiovascular (CV) disease.

Table 1. Principal known effects of MBG on several organs and systems in Pre-clinical conditions.

Organs and Systems	Pathological Conditions	Effects of MBG	Pre-Clinical Studies	
			Model	Results
Kidney and CV system	Volume-expanding conditions: essential hypertension, heart failure, PE, CKD complications: LVH, UC, myocardial fibrosis, diastolic dysfunction	Sodium and fluid retention, organ fibrosis and remodeling, vascular and microcirculation alterations, activation of oxidative stress pathways	Fedorova, O.V., et al. [4]; male Fisher 344XNB rats and anesthetized dogs	IV saline infusion to anesthetized rats induced a significant increase in MLF plasma levels and pituitary OLC. No changes in pituitary MLF levels. Two hours of plasma volume expansion in anesthetized dogs increased urinary release of MLF. No change in OLC immunoreactivity. Evidence for the presence of a bufadienolide EDLF in mammals. Volume expansion stimulates EDLF response with the stimulation of brain OLC and plasma bufadienolide.
			Bagrov, A.Y., et al. [5]; anesthetized dogs	Decreased urinary release of MLF after volume expansion, but no changes in OLC, suggesting a bufadienolide nature of mammalian EDLF.
			Kennedy, DJ., et al. [6]; male CD1 mice	Plasma MBG increased after PNx. PNx caused cardiac hypertrophy and fibrosis, inducing UC.
			Priyadarshi, S., et al. [7]; male Sprague Dawley rats, isolated cardiac myocytes	In rats subjected to remnant kidney surgery, the administration of green tea extract at the induced attenuation of LVH, hypertension and preserved cardiac Na-K-ATP-ase activity. In isolated cardiac myocytes, both MBG and ouabain increased ROS production, whereas the addition of green tea prevented the increase in ROS production.
			Kennedy, DJ., et al. [8]; male Sprague Dawley rats	Rats with PNx had a significant increase in MBG plasma levels and urinary excretion rates and developed UC.
			Elkareh, J., et al. [9]; male Sprague Dawley rats, isolated cardiac fibroblasts	PNx increased MBG levels. Heart tissue samples from rats subjected to MBG-infusion and PNx showed an important increase in collagen-1 and α smooth muscle actin, whereas immunization against MBG attenuated these effects. Cardiotonic steroids, such as MBG, play a substantial role in the pathogenesis of cardiac fibrosis.

Table 1. Cont.

Organs and Systems	Pathological Conditions	Effects of MBG	Pre-Clinical Studies	
			Model	Results
			Xie, Z., et al. [10]; neonatal ventricular myocytes cultures	Ouabain increases ROS production in cardiac myocytes, while preincubation with NAC and vitamin E reduced these effects. In cultured myocytes, the effects of ouabain on growth and growth-related genes can be dissociated from its effect on the resting intracellular Ca^{2+}, the latter being responsible for the positive inotropic effect of this drug. It remains to be clarified whether the redox state of the myocyte or the intact heart may alter the effects of cardiac glycosides on cardiac hypertrophy without affecting the positive inotropic effect of these drugs.
			Pamnani, M.B., et al. [11]; male Wistar rats	Bufalin infusion increased mean the arterial BP, HR and renal excretion of Na+ and water, while ouabain infusion in an equimolar dose produced a significantly smaller increase in these effects and had no effect on HR. Bufalin has a greater effect on CV contractility and renal excretion of Na+ and water in rats than ouabain.
			Vu, H.V., et al. [12]; pregnant female rats	MBG levels increased in pregnant female rats treated with deoxycorticosterone acetate and 0.9% saline compared with normal pregnant rats. The administration of MBG in normal pregnant female rats caused a significant increase in blood pressure and vasoconstrictive activity of uterine vessels, while no changes were observed with the infusion of ouabain or digoxin at the same concentration. There is a relationship between MBG and a PE-like syndrome in rats.
			Vu, H.V., et al. [13]; pregnant female rats	RBG administration reversed MBG effects on BP. Antagonism of MBG could be a future therapeutic strategy for PE.
			Agunanne, E., et al. [14]; pregnant female Sprague Dawley rats	RBG administration in early pregnancy prevented PE syndrome in a rat model. RBG also prevented IUGR and had no teratogenic effects. Treatment of PE can focus on drugs that do not compromise the fetus.
Feto-placental unit	Sex and gender medicine: pregnancy diseases, PE	Endothelial dysfunction, apoptosis, release of angiogenic factors, umbilical arteries fibrosis	Uddin, M.N., et al. [15]; human extra-villous CTB cell line SGHPL-4 derived from first trimester chronic villous tissue	MBG induces a negative effect on CTB cell function, including apoptosis. MBG has a role in abnormal placentation and altered vascular function typical of PE. Targeting the MBG signaling pathway may be a future therapeutic strategy in PE treatment.

Table 1. Cont.

Organs and Systems	Pathological Conditions	Effects of MBG	Pre-Clinical Studies	
			Model	Results
			La Marca, H.L., et al. [16]; human extra-villous CTB cell line SGHPL-4 derived from first trimester chorionic villous tissues	MBG has an anti-proliferative effect on CTB before CTB differentiation into an invasive pathway. MBG inhibits CTB cell migration and growth factor-induced invasion processes. MBG expression in the early phase of pregnancy has a role in abnormal placentation and altered vascular function.
Nervous system	Synaptic dysfunction, genesis of neurofibrillary tangles, neuronal death	Genesis of new isoforms of sodium Nax channels	Grigorova, Y.N., et al. [17]; young Dahl salt sensitive rats	HS diet prohypertensive and profibrotic effects can be at least partially attributed to MBG increase. MBG and HS diet had similar effects on CV system. MBG and HS diet upregulated the expression of fibrosis and Alzheimer's disease genes in LV of the rat model. Hippocampal neuronal density was not affected by MBG or HS diet. Brain plasticity in young rats probably helped the animals to sustain the MBG-induced central arterial stiffness, which is one of the underlying mechanisms of cognitive impairment.
Immune system	Inhibition of neutrophil migration, inhibition of pro-inflammatory cytokines	Anti-inflammatory activity in a dose-dependent manner	Carvalho, D.C.M., et al. [18]; Swiss mice peritoneal fluid	MBG inhibited polymorphonuclear leukocyte migration to the peritoneal cavity. MBG reduced the expression of different pro-inflammatory cytokines. MBG had no cytotoxicity effects on macrophages in peritoneum.

Legend: BP: blood pressure; CTB: cytotrophoblast; EDLF: endogenous digitalis-like factor; HR: heart rate; HS: high-salt; IUGR: intrauterine growth restriction; LV: left ventricle; LVH: left ventricular hypertrophy; MBG: marinobufagenin; MLF: marinobufagenin like-factor; NAC: N-acetylcysteine OLC: ouabain-like compound; PE: pre-eclampsia; PNx: partial nephrectomy; RBG: resinobufagenin; ROS: reactive oxygen species; UC: uremic cardiomyopathy.

Table 2. Principal known effects of MBG on several organs and systems in clinical conditions.

Organs and Systems	Pathological Processes	Effects of MBG	Clinical Studies	
			Population	Results
Kidney and CV system	Volume-expanding conditions: essential hypertension, heart failure, PE CKD complications: LVH, UC, myocardial fibrosis, diastolic dysfunction	Sodium and fluid retention, organ fibrosis and remodeling, vascular and microcirculation alterations, activation of oxidative stress pathways	Keppel, M.H., [19] et al.; in patients with arterial hypertension; plasma MBG levels were measured in 40 patients, of whom 11 patients had primary aldosteronism (PA) and 29 patients had essential hypertension after exclusion of PA.	MBG concentrations increased, but not significantly, and showed a direct correlation trend with albuminuria and proteinuria.
			Bolignano, D., [20] et al.; cohort of 29 patients on HD vs. healthy controls.	MBG levels in HD patients were significantly higher than in healthy controls and significantly reduced in HD patients experiencing IDH during follow-up. Inverse correlations were found between the absolute number of IDH episodes per person and, respectively pre-dialysis MBG, 2 h MBG and HD-end MBG. MBG levels remained basically unchanged in HD patients with no documented IDH episodes during follow-up.
			Piecha, G., et al. [21]; 68 HD patients vs. 68 age-, gender- and blood pressure-matched subjects without CKD.	Mean plasma MBG immunoreactivity was significantly higher in HD patients compared with subjects with normal kidney function. In HD patients, plasma MBG was higher in men than in women, while this difference was not observed in subjects with normal kidney function.
			Bolignano, D., et al. [22]; 46 HD patients vs. healthy controls.	MBG levels were significantly higher in HD patients than in healthy controls. A statistically significant trend in MBG levels was found across different patterns of LV geometry, with the highest values in eccentric LVH. MBG levels were higher in presence of diastolic dysfunction.
			Jablonski, K.L., et al. [23]; middle-aged/older adults with moderately elevated systolic BP, but otherwise free of CV disease, diabetes, kidney disease and other clinical disorders.	Urinary MBG excretion decreased after 5 weeks of low sodium diet compared with 5 weeks of high sodium, while plasma MBG levels were not different between sodium conditions. Urinary MBG excretion was related to urinary sodium excretion and blood pressure measurements

Table 2. *Cont.*

Organs and Systems	Pathological Processes	Effects of MBG	Clinical Studies	
			Population	Results
			Strauss, M., et al. [24]; young, apparently healthy Black and White adults (60).	A persistent positive association between carotid-femoral pulse wave velocity and MBG excretion was found in women but not in men. High endogenous MBG levels may contribute to large artery stiffness in women through pressure-independent mechanisms
			Strauss, M., et al. [25]; young, apparently healthy Black and White adults (63)	LV mass, end diastolic volume and stroke volume were positively related to MBG excretion. The relationship between LV mass and MBG excretion was evident in women but not in men. Women may be more sensitive to MBG effects on early structural cardiac changes
			Lopatin, D.A., et al. [26]; 6 non-pregnant women, 6 normotensive age-matched pregnant controls and 11 patients with PE.	MBG levels significantly increased in PE pregnant women. MBG induced a contractile response of isolated rings of human mesenteric arteries in a concentration-dependent manner. MBG has a pathogenic role in PE.
Feto-placental unit	Sex and gender medicine: pregnancy diseases, PE	Endothelial dysfunction, apoptosis, release of angiogenic factors, umbilical arteries fibrosis	Agunanne, E., et al. [14]; 17 pre-eclamptic women and 46 normotensive pregnant women in various gestational periods.	Serum and urinary levels of MBG were significantly greater in pre-eclamptic women than normotensive pregnant women. MBG can be used for prediction and diagnosis of PE.
			Nikitina, E.R., et al. [27]; 16 pre-eclamptic pregnant women and 14 gestational age-matched normal pregnant women.	Serum and urinary levels of MBG increased in pre-eclamptic women compared with normal pregnant women. MBG, through a Fli-1-dependent mechanism stimulates collagen synthesis in umbilical arteries, leading to the impairment of vasorelaxation. MBG may represent a potential target for PE therapy.

Legend: CKD: chronic kidney disease; CTB: cytotrophoblast; ESKD: end-stage kidney disease; Fli-1: friend leukemia integration 1 transcription factor; HD: hemodialysis; IDH: intradialytic hypotension; LV: left ventricle; LVH: left ventricular hypertrophy; MBG: marinobufagenin; PE: pre-eclampsia; UC: uremic cardiomyopathy. Specification: numbers in parentheses indicate the reference number in the text.

2. Biochemical Structure and Production

The cardiac glycosides include bufadienolides and cardenolides, which substantially differ from each other in both biochemical structure and the cellular [1,2] mechanism of action. Bufadienolides are steroid compounds with a δ-lactone ring at carbon C_{17}, primarily synthesized from cholesterol as a precursor via the mevalonate-independent pathway [28]. They have a double unsaturated six-membered lactone ring while cardenolides have an unsaturated five-membered lactone ring [29]. However, at present, the bufadienolide biosynthesis mechanism is still unknown [26].

Bufadienolides are found in both animals and plants [30,31] and those of mammalian origin are produced by the placenta [32] and adrenal cortex [33] under the control of the bile acid CYP27A1 enzyme, although other production sites cannot be excluded [34]. Bufadienolides are eliminated unchanged via renal excretion [13]. The bufadienolides are so named because they are extracted from the venom of a common toad, *bufo marinus* or *rhinella marina*, both members of the Bufonidae family [35]. Skin [36] and parotoid gland secretions [37] of *bufo marinus* are considered the main natural sources of MBG. This toad species is native to South and Central America and has remained almost unchanged since the late Miocene period. Later, the species was introduced to Australia and the Oceanian islands and is currently one of the worst invasive species in many countries. Both sexes of the *Bufo* species possess huge parotid glands, stretching through the retro-orbital level and releasing a venom composed of different types of molecules, such as alkaloids, peptides, biogenic amines, steroids (bufogenins and bufotoxins) and proteins [38–40], which have antimicrobial activity and a defense action against potential predators [41–43]. The chemical and pharmacological characteristics of the secretions from the parotid gland and skin of the family Bufonidae have been studied for some time [44], and as early as 1972, 50 compounds were recognized in 39 species collected from different locations around the world [45].

Mechanism of Action

The most studied of the bufadienolides is MBG, an endogenous mammalian natriuretic and cardiotonic compound with vasoconstrictive effects [1,46,47], which has a great affinity for the α1 isoform of Na^+/K^+-ATPase [48], the main form of the enzyme present in renal tubules [1]. In contrast, cardenolides act primarily on the α2 and α3 isoforms [48]. The Na^+/K^+-ATPase consists of an alpha subunit with catalytic action together with binding sites for ATP, cardiotonic steroids (CTS) and other ligands, as well as a beta subunit. Four α isoforms and three β isoforms are known for this enzyme. The α1β1 complex is largely present in various tissues, and the α2 isoform is mainly present in cardiac, smooth muscle and cerebral tissues. One of the peculiarities of the bufadienolides is represented by the fact that they exert a different action according to the receptor on which they act [49]. Currently, the Na^+/K^+-ATPase is recognized as having three major functions: as a pump, as an enzyme and as a receptor to cardiotonic steroids [50]. A "signalling" function has also been recognized, whereby the plasmalemmal Na^+/K^+-ATPases reside in the caveolae of cells with other key signaling proteins [51,52]. Indeed, two distinct pathways of MBG action have been described, by which MBG acts on the Na^+/K^+-ATPase [50]. According to the first (defined as the ionic pathway), MBG causes an altered transmembrane ion transport by inhibiting the Na^+/K^+ ATPase, and this, in the kidney, results in natriuresis as a physiological response to sodium load [4,46,53]. The inhibition of Na^+/K^+-ATPase in the vascular smooth muscle cells induces vasoconstriction [54,55] through an increase in intracellular sodium concentration and the concomitant reversal of the function of the vascular Na^+/Ca^{++}-exchanger. This results in an increased calcium influx within smooth muscle cells, consequently causing the further release of calcium from the sarcoplasmic reticulum. The result is vasoconstriction secondary to the actin–myosin interaction [50,56]. The second mode of action (the signaling function) can cause the activation of several intracellular signals, such as mitogen-activated protein kinases (MAPK) and reactive oxygen species (ROS) inducing fibrosis [50,57]. MBG has been suggested to cause cardiac [57,58] and vascular [57,59] fibrosis, simply through the activation of the above intracellular signaling cascades.

The inhibition of Na^+/K^+ ATPase, caused by MBG, has different effects, depending on the tissue in which it occurs. For example, in renal tubules, it stimulates natriuresis and, at the level of the proximal tubule, it promotes the internalization of the sodium pump with a reduction in the expression of the transport protein Na^+/H^+ (NHE3) in the apical membrane of the renal proximal tubule [60]. MBG, after binding to the enzyme Na^+/K^+-ATPase, slowly dissociates to induce the endocytosis of this enzyme. This reduces sodium absorption and increases sodium excretion in the proximal renal tubule. By decreasing the amount of Na^+/K^+-ATPase available, it also decreases the ability to respond to changes in Na^+ and water, leading to the promotion of water retention and volume expansion [61]. In mammals, sodium stimulates the synthesis and secretion of MBG via the angiotensin/sympathetic pathway [34]. Indeed, increased sodium intake promotes angiotensin II, aldosterone and sympathetic nervous system synthesis, resulting in the stimulation of adrenal MBG synthesis and secretion [62].

In healthy young adults, 24 h urinary MBG values were strongly linked with habitual salt intake. This is confirmed by data derived from studies in rats, whose stimulation of MBG through the intake of Na^+ or the infusion of MBG leads to cardiac hypertrophy and vascular fibrosis [24]. In one study, a four-week administration of MBG in rats caused a significant increase in plasma aldosterone and increased systolic blood pressure values. In another study on rats, MBG infusion caused renal fibrosis, subsequently attenuated by passive immunization and improving renal function [59,63]. The use of mineralocorticoid receptor antagonists (MRA) has also been shown to have a preventive effect on MBG-induced fibrosis by occupying the binding sites of the endogenous cardiotonic steroids [64].

With regard to profibrotic pathways, Drummond et al. [65] reported possible opposite relationships between MBG and the antifibrotic microRNA miR-29b-3p, which emerged from the regulation of cardiac fibrosis in a CKD murine model, because of the Na^+/K^+-ATPase signaling involvement in miR-29b-3p regulation. Similar results were observed in another study conducted in cardiac fibroblasts [66,67], in which cardiac tissue was obtained from rats treated with MBG or partial nephrectomy surgery, showing opposite trends between MBG and miR-29b-3p expression in relation to collagen expression and thereby the extent of fibrosis. All together, these data indicated that CTS mediate the Na^+/K^+-ATPase signaling-induced regulation of miR-29b-3p expression. The mechanistic phenomena underlying this crosstalk is still yet to be totally defined and are probably due to the convergent action on molecules and kinases common to several pathways.

3. Extraction Techniques

Several methods for assaying these compounds have been studied, mainly for the purpose of monitoring certain drugs used in traditional Chinese medicine. The main issue concerns the difficulty of obtaining access to standard material for the setup and validation of analytical methods required for MBG measurement [68–72]. Generally, bufadienolides are extracted through solvent treatment from the dry or fresh skin and secretions of toads. More often, chlorinated and non-chlorinated organic solvents or alcohols are used and various techniques have been developed to separate MBG from other solutes, such as classic column chromatography, thin-layer chromatography, preparative-scale high performance liquid chromatography (HPLC) and flash column chromatography [68,73–78].

One of the first extraction techniques to obtain MBG was described by Shimada et al. in 1979. He retrieved this extract by soaking 40 *Bufo marinus* toad skins in ethanol and then dividing them into an ethyl–water acetate system. Later, the aqueous component was broken down via chromatography on Amberlite XAD-4 to split the conjugated steroids. The resulting fractions were purified via HPLC or gel chromatography on Sephadex LH-20 [79]. A different technique used by Bagrov et al. was able to separate MBG from the crystallized poison of Bufo marinus using thin layer chromatography. Today, the most widely used method for chemical characterization is mass spectrometry, allowing us to differentiate these polar molecules based on their mass spectral fragmentation paths [28]. An ELISA enzyme test kit is available for the correct measurement of MBG. Enzymatic reactions can be then quantified with an automatic photometer for microplates [20].

MBG has been extracted from human plasma and urine [8,25,80–83], and there is the possibility of measuring MBG in 24h urine samples in the presence of other steroid hormones, through solid-phase dissociation-enhanced lanthanide fluorescent immunoassay, based on a 4G4 anti-MBG mouse monoclonal antibody [80].

4. Marinobufagenin and Chronic Kidney Disease

CKD is one of the most frequent medical conditions worldwide and, in the general population, the CKD prevalence of all five KDIGO stages is 13.4% [84]. Low estimated glomerular filtration rate (eGFR) is a strong, independent predictor of all-cause mortality and CV diseases [85], which are the first cause of morbidity and mortality in nephropathic patients. Their increased CV risk is related to both traditional (diabetes mellitus, hypertension, etc.) and non-traditional uremia-specific risk factors [86–88]. Given the high social, economic and health impact of CKD worldwide, new possible underlying pathogenetic mechanisms and potential markers that may allow the early identification of the development of this complex and multifaceted disease are always being investigated.

It has been shown that, in both animal models (rats and dogs) [5,89] and in humans [74] with volume-expanding conditions, there are high plasma concentration levels of MBG. Indeed, it has been widely demonstrated that MBG production increases in all conditions of sodium and fluid retention, such as essential hypertension, heart failure, pre-eclampsia (PE), salt-sensitive hypertension in Dahl salt-sensitive (DS) rats on a high NaCl intake [46,90] and CKD.

The influence of MBG in CKD and its complications were initially evaluated in animal models. Originally, the involvement of MBG in cardiac hypertrophy was investigated in a remnant model of CKD [6,7]. In a series of investigations of these remnant kidney models, it has been shown that the development of renal dysfunction is associated with an increase in circulating concentrations of MBG [91]. On the other hand, other studies have shown an increased collagen production through fibroblasts and subsequent fibrosis in experimental uremic cardiomyopathy (UC) [9]. UC is characterized by an association with left ventricular hypertrophy (LVH) and myocardial fibrosis [92]. The etiopathogenesis of UC is extremely complex and involves several factors, such as hemodynamic overload, hypertension, anemia, mineral and bone disorders, endothelial dysfunction, insulin resistance and cardiotonic steroids, as well as several circulating uremic toxins [92,93]. It was assumed that the increase in MBG concentration was secondary to renal failure-dependent volume expansion [58]. Although extracellular volume expansion is thought to be crucial for the development of UC, there is still much debate about the exact pathogenesis [94–96]. Immunization against MBG in partial nephrectomy animals was associated with a substantial attenuation of cardiac hypertrophy, cardiac fibrosis and the oxidant stress state [97].

The fibrotic action of MBG on the kidney was also evaluated through the infusion of MBG in rats, which led to a peritubular and periglomerular accumulation of type I collagen at the renal cortical level [61,98]. This could be triggered by the activation of Transforming Growth Factor Beta type 1 (TGF-β1) via the renin–angiotensin–aldosterone system. In MBG-treated kidneys, the profibrotic transcription factor snail (critical regulator of the epithelial–mesenchymal transition) was expressed in both medullary and cortical tubular epithelial cells. This evidence led to a new hypothesis: MBG can have a key causative role in the epithelial–mesenchymal transition [61]. The administration of MRA occupying endogenous CTS-binding sites prevents pro-fibrotic MBG effects [64]. Since CKD is a complex set of different medical conditions, Na^+/K^+-ATPase alterations may not always be involved in the etiopathogenesis of different causes of CKD and MRA therapy may not be effective in all nephropathic patients. Therefore increased MBG plasma levels could be useful in identifying patients at risk of developing renal fibrosis (and beyond) and CKD progression that could benefit from MRA therapy [19].

Recently, in a single-center study of adults routinely referred for the screening of endocrine hypertension, it was shown that plasma MBG concentrations were significantly associated with albuminuria (a marker of kidney damage) and decline in renal function regardless of pre-existing CKD. These results might indicate that in this cohort of hypertensive patients, MBG could play a role as a potential marker of renal failure at follow-up and that elevated plasma levels of MBG may already precede renal failure rather than being a simple consequence of it [19].

In patients undergoing chronic hemodialysis, the altered MBG plasma values could be due to a compensatory response to the treatment itself [20] and could predict a worsening survival outcome [21]. In this patient population, left ventricular hypertrophy is extremely prevalent and, as mentioned above, contrasts the uremic cardiomyopathy. In experimental models, MBG induces marked hypertrophic changes of adult cardiac myocytes in vitro [10,99] and promotes vascular fibrosis and cardiac hypertrophy in experimental models of salt-sensitive hypertension [91]. For these reasons, we conducted a pilot observational study to investigate a possible relationship between MBG plasma levels, left ventricular (LV) geometry and cardiac dysfunction in end-stage renal disease (ESRD) patients on dialysis [22]. In this cohort of patients with ESRD, we observed that high levels of MBG reflect the structural and functional alterations of the LV. Indeed, MBG plasma levels were higher in the presence of diastolic dysfunction and this molecule demonstrated a strong diagnostic ability to discern patients with normal LV geometry, LV hypertrophy and, above all, eccentric LVH. Circulating MBG plasma levels were significantly higher in ESRD patients than those in healthy controls and were more increased in patients on peritoneal dialysis compared with those undergoing extracorporeal dialysis treatment [22]. This suggests that, in the future, MBG could play the role of biomarker for cardiac evaluation in high-risk populations. Our findings further strengthen the hypothesis that endogenous cardiotonic steroids could substantially contribute to the onset and progression of uremic cardiomyopathy. Of note, there was no correlation between MBG plasma levels and parameters related to volume status in our study [22]. In a recent study, kidney transplant recipients displayed altered MBG levels, which were influenced by sodium balance, renal impairment and the severity of LVH. Thus, MBG might also represent an important missing link between reduced graft function and pathological cardiac remodeling and may hold important prognostic value for improving cardio-renal risk assessment [100].

Moreover, we have demonstrated that higher MBG plasma levels are associated with a lower risk of intradialytic hypotensive events in patients undergoing hemodialysis [20,101,102], who are particularly considered at risk of hypotension. Indeed, about 30% of hemodialysis sessions are characterized by severe symptomatic intra-dialysis hypotension, influencing the morbidity and mortality of patients in chronic treatment. These hypotensive episodes are often due either to an altered ability to mobilize fluids from the interstitial space to the intravascular space during the hemodialysis session or to a removal of a large fluid volume in a short time. It has been noted that, in the cohort of patients on dialysis treatment, patients with lower baseline MBG values showed an approximately five-fold higher risk of severe symptomatic, intradialytic hypotension. There was an initial increase in circulating MBG levels followed by a progressive decrease until the end of treatment. This shows that patients with lower MBG plasma values reflect a lower vascular and hemodynamic tolerance, with a higher number of episodes of severe hypotension, while no significant correlation was found between MBG plasma levels and body weight reduction during dialysis treatment. This could lead to a consideration of MBG as a mediator of a compensatory mechanism, which results in an altered hemodynamic response to plasma volume reduction. Today, it seems that MBG may have an important role in identifying patients at high risk of severe intradialytic hypotensive episodes; this predictive ability has also been found in survival analyses, demonstrating that patients with lower plasma levels of MBG had a higher risk (from four to six times) of severe intra-dialysis episodes during follow-up. MBG plasma levels were the strongest time-dependent predictors of severe intradialytic hypotensive episodes between different variables [20]. The high mobilization of MBG could initially represent a protective response against the hemodynamic changes induced by the extracorporeal treatment but, in the long term, could, in any case, determine the known deleterious effects in the myocardium [20] (Figure 1). However, larger studies with more targeted-oriented surveys are necessary to confirm these data.

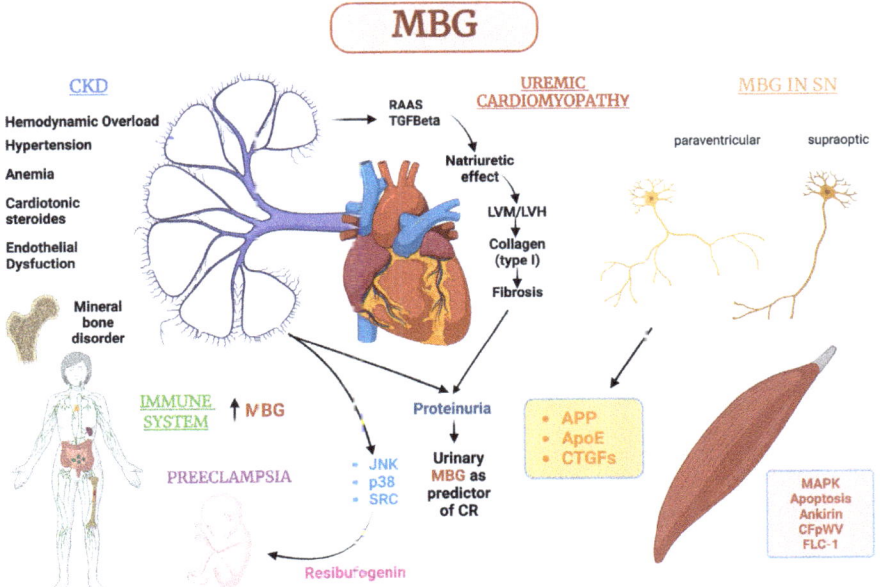

Figure 1. Main known pathways in the interactions between MBG and different organs and systems.

5. Marinobufagenin and CV Diseases

Most of the studies designed to evaluate the pathogenetic mechanisms by which MBG contributes to CV disease risk have been performed in animal models. Increased concentrations of circulating MBG (as a result of sodium loading or via infusion pump) caused several effects: vascular [24,59] and microcirculation [103] alterations, pressor changes [4,46,104,105] and cardiac and renal [8,9,58,61,91] fibrosis. Investigations in humans have shown elevated MBG plasma levels in many pathological conditions: heart failure [8], acute myocardial infarction (elevated urinary MBG levels) [106], primary aldosteronism [107], renal ischemia [108] and CKD [100,109].

There are several scientific pieces of evidence supporting a possible pathogenic role of bufadienolides in hypertensive conditions associated with hydro-saline retention. Firstly, increased plasma and urinary concentration levels of MBG were observed in volume expansion conditions and in hypertensive patients mediated by volume expansion, due to salt accumulation [46,104,105,110]. Secondly, the administration of bufadienolides in experimental animals causes hypertension [11,13,111]. Thirdly, in rats, the hypertension caused by the administration of deoxycorticosterone acetate and salt is reversed through the intraperitoneal injection of an MBG antagonist, resibufogenin (RBG) [12,13,112], which differs from MBG only in the absence of a hydroxyl group in the β 5 position. Finally, the use of anti-MBG antibodies in salt-loaded pregnant rats and in salt-sensitive hypertensive rats, results in the reduction in blood pressure values [113].

In recent years, several evaluations of whether MBG could be used as an early marker of CV risk have been performed. The first study designed to evaluate the possible association between blood pressure values and MBG plasma levels demonstrated an inverse relationship between diastolic blood pressure values and the urinary excretion (24 h) levels of MBG in the case of high sodium intake (16.32 g of salt per day). The natriuretic effects of MBG could represent a homeostatic mechanism to restore blood pressure values to normal, constituting a protective mechanism in healthy subjects [82]. The dietary intervention had a total duration of 12 days; therefore, that effect could represent a homeostatic mechanism in the short term. In contrast, another group has shown that MBG plasma levels are positively associated with systolic blood pressure values during the period of high sodium intake (5 weeks). In that case, it might reflect a long-term homeostatic response in which the vasoconstrictor activity of MBG could superimpose the natriuretic effect [114]. Fedorova et al. showed completely different responses from the above studies. In a cohort of men and women, there was an increase in systolic blood pressure values following dietary sodium loading without changes in both plasma and urinary MBG concentrations [81]. Therefore, the results on the relationship between blood pressure values and circulating and urinary MBG levels in humans are conflicting and require further evaluation.

Recent findings have revealed that in a state of inactivity, sodium can settle in the interstitium between the skin and organs [115]. The alteration of these deposits could also affect blood pressure values. We can say that high sodium intake correlates both with a higher production of MBG and with rigid large arteries, even in healthy subjects. These pieces of evidence were confirmed in laboratory models, as risk factors for dementia and CV events [17]. In addition to MBG, several factors act on peripheral vascular resistance, such as neurohormonal, baroreflexes and myogenic factors [49]. It is also known that sodium regulates the rigidity of endothelial cells and modifies the release of nitric oxide by altering the tone of blood vessels and blood pressure [116]. In the current state of the art, there is still not enough evidence to consider urinary MBG excretion as a predictive value of increased cardiovascular risk before the onset of the disease [24], although numerous studies have confirmed the correlation between plasma MBG levels, sodium and occurrence of arterial hypertension. Furthermore, these results proved to be more applicable to men than to women.

In other parts of the body, such as the arterial vascular smooth muscle cells, MBG generates an increase in cytosolic Ca2+ amount that causes vasoconstriction through the activation of an "ionic pathway" [4]. In addition to this "ionic pathway", MBG can activate different intracellular signaling pathways that trigger cellular effects, such as cell proliferation, ROS genesis or the stimulation of apoptosis, also via the activation of pathways with other molecules, such as Phospholipase C-γ isozyme (PLC-γ), Phosphatidylinositol 3-kinase (PI-3K), IP3 receptor type 3 (IP3R), and ankyrin [117].

Specifically, it has been reported that cardiotonic steroids activate a signal cascade, which is mediated through Src, Ras, ROS, and ERKs, and promote endocytosis of the plasmalemmal Na^+/K^+-ATPase [10,99,118–120]. The activation of this cascade requires that the Na^+/K^+-ATPase to be in caveolae in order to proceed [121,122]. This series of signals is known to cause changes in gene expression, which can be inhibited by antioxidant molecules [7,10,120].

Arterial stiffness is well known to be related to increased CV risk and death in individuals of all ages [123], regardless of blood pressure values. Sodium intake also correlates with arterial stiffness regardless of hypertensive status [124,125], even in healthy subjects. Thus, a possible association between MBG and arterial stiffening was hypothesized. Jablonski et al. have demonstrated, in individuals with high or hypertensive blood pressures, that a positive association between MBG and carotid to femoral pulse wave velocity (cf-PWV) [114] is actually the gold standard measurement of large artery stiffness [126]. The same positive correlation has also been demonstrated in young healthy women, regardless of salt intake [80]. To date, the pathogenetic mechanisms through which MBG is able to determine arterial stiffness are unknown, although MBG has already been shown to promote the development of vascular fibrosis in the aorta of rats [59]. The mechanism by which MBG promotes collagen production and deposition was studied in cultured rat smooth muscle cells and was always dependent on the inhibition of Na$^+$K$^+$-ATPase [58,59]. Collagen-1 production is secondary to the marked downregulation of transcription factor Friend leukemia integration-1 (Fli-1) [58,59]. In fact, it has been shown that MBG could also sub-regulate a negative regulator of collagen-1 synthesis, Fli-1. The phosphorylation of Fli-1 through the active form of Protein Kinase C Delta (PKC-d) induces the activation of a collagen gene promoter. In vitro, MBG was found to be an activator of the Fli-1 pathway in cultured fibroblasts and smooth rat muscle cells.

Another important predictor of both increased CV risk and mortality is the left ventricular mass (LVM) measured using the echocardiogram [127]. In the CARDIA study (Coronary Artery Risk Development in Young Adults), a possible positive association between LVM and sodium in 24h urine levels was shown in young adults, although this relationship was confounded by the presence of obesity [128]. From this observation, it was hypothesized that the increase in MBG plasma levels, induced by sodium intake, may be associated with an increase in LVM. Strauss et al. have observed a significant association between LVM and MBG in young adults: in this case, the relationship was independent on obesity and also on blood pressure values, suggesting a possible pathway through which MBG induces myocardial hypertrophy [25].

To further confirm the correlation between MBG plasma levels and fibrosis, it has been shown that rats with (experimental) renal impairment have increased MBG plasma values, along with cardiac and renal fibrosis. In these mouse models, MBG promotes procollagen-1 expression by cultured cardiac fibroblasts. As procollagen expression increases, collagen and procollagen-1 mRNA increase too. Considering this, MBG probably induces a direct increase in collagen expression by fibroblasts [9]. It has also been observed that in spontaneously hypertensive (SHR) and normotensive Wistar–Kyoto (WKY) mouse models, following a diet rich in sodium, hypertension and left and renal ventricular hypertrophy, due to fibrosis with the overexpression of TGF-β_1 mRNA, were recorded. This has resulted, in both glomerular and peritubular sites, in an increase in collagen type 1 [129]. Interestingly, in animal models characterized by prolonged salt intake, diet-related profibrotic effects were eliminated through treatment with anti-MBG antibodies, without generating hemodynamic effects [130]. The administration of specific antibodies against MBG reduced aortic fibrosis and favored relaxation at the level of aortic fibers. The differences that can be attributed to the vascular component without hemodynamic changes, indicate that the possible vascular stiffening is independent of blood pressure and that the profibrotic factor generated by MBG is responsible for it [131].

Even in laboratory models treated with antibodies to MBG and previously subjected to a diet high in sodium, there was a reduction in systolic blood pressure and also a reduction in the weight of both the heart and kidneys. In these mouse models, TGF-β expression, which had previously been increased, was also downregulated after treatment with anti-MBG antibodies. The immunoneutralization of MBG resulted in the downregulation of genes involved in profibrotic expression. In addition, the normalization of renal function through creatinine clearance was also observed, probably due to the reduction in renal fibrosis, as it was accompanied by a significant decrease in kidney weight for the reduction in type I-III-IV collagen amounts. In mouse models, it has also been observed that treatment with anti-MBG antibodies reduces the development of heart failure. This was established by estimating ventricular weight via ultrasound in hypertensive rats immunoneutralized for MBG, compared with non-immunoneutralized hypertensive rats.

Early vascular damage was also reduced after immunoneutralization. In these models, a reduction in the mRNA expression of TGF-β1, FN1, MAPK1, Col1a2, Col3a1 and Col4a1 was also noted compared with those not treated with antibodies of MBG. This demonstrated how MBG initiates TGFβ-1-signaling in cultured ventricular myocytes, through Na$^+$/K$^+$-ATPase signal transduction and other factors, such as tissue angiotensin II [132]. In humans, sodium restriction also reduces urinary MBG production and excretion, resulting in reduced blood pressure and aortic stiffness. Another factor may impact fibrosis, sodium concentration and MBG plasma levels: it has been observed that the sensitivity of blood pressure dietary salt intake increases with increasing age [23,133,134].

6. MBG in Relation to Sex and Gender Medicine with a Special Focus on Pre-Eclampsia

In the last few years, the concept of gender medicine emerged in relation to the presence of significant and underestimated effects of gender-based differences on clinical evolution and therapeutic outcomes of many diseases [135–137]. Despite CTS, such as MBG, playing a role in human physiopathology, regardless of sex- and gender-related aspects, there is evidence regarding specific actions occurring in sex-specific diseases, such as pregnancy diseases [68], which can be considered a valid example of gender medicine. MBG was identified as a biomarker of angiogenic imbalance in the pathogenesis of PE [47], a relatively common and potentially devastating complication of pregnancy.

PE is a progressive multisystem syndrome that is characterized by the onset, after the 20th week of gestation, of hypertension and proteinuria or by the onset of hypertension with severe organ dysfunction, with or without proteinuria [138–140]. A systematic review stated that 4.6% of pregnancies worldwide were complicated by PE [141], which represents the second leading cause of fetal and maternal morbidity and mortality [142–145]. PE is caused by both maternal and fetal/placental factors. Placental vessels develop abnormally early in pregnancy and result in a placental hypoperfusion with the release of antiangiogenic factors into the maternal circulation. These factors promote endothelial dysfunction, which leads to the development of a vascular leak that enhances the volume expansion. MBG causes endothelial hyperpermeability, activating MAPKs with the disruption of the tight junction. This feature triggers apoptotic mechanisms, resulting in further endothelial dysfunction and leading to edema and the release of angiogenic factors [47,146].

An important element that could make MBG a potential biomarker for the early detection of PE was shown in an animal study, in which circulating MBG was shown to rise earlier than the onset of proteinuria and hypertension [13]. Thus, MBG can represent a predictive marker of PE, opening up new perspectives for its prevention, as well as halting its progression to the severe clinical state of eclampsia. Moreover, the administration of MBG in pregnant rats mimics this syndrome with proteinuria, hypertension and intrauterine growth restriction (IUGR) [12,147].

As well as MBG being involved in the pathophysiology and progression of PE, its antagonist RBG was seen to have a role in the prevention and possible treatment of this disorder [148,149]. The administration of RBG in a rat model of PE leads to the resolution of hypertension and, if given early in pregnancy, it prevents all symptoms of PE, including IUGR [112]. Recently, a relationship between MBG and leptin in a pregnancy model of Sprague Dawley rats was investigated, showing that RBG administration can reverse the leptin-induced increase in systolic blood pressure, proteinuria and endothelial activation and suggesting a link between MBG and leptin signaling during pregnancy [150]. The RBG and, consequently, MBG molecular actions were also related to oxidative stress pathways [151], further amplifying the network of the interactions of CTS.

Similar to the action of RBG, Fedorova at al. investigated the role of antibodies against MBG in reversing the placenta-induced fibrosis of umbilical arteries in PE [152]. Monoclonal anti-MBG antibodies ex vivo reversed the placenta-induced fibrosis of umbilical arteries, indicating an active role of MBG in placental pathology. This represents the starting point on the possible development and use of RBG or monoclonal antibody Fab fragments to MBG [113] for the prevention and/or treatment of this complex syndrome.

Likewise, mineralocorticoid antagonists have been demonstrated to block the development of the fibrosis of umbilical arteries in PE, which is likely related to elevated MGB plasma levels [153].

Increased MBG production in women with PE, compared with physiological pregnancies, has also been demonstrated in humans [14,26]. Indeed, in healthy pregnant women, MBG levels are twice as high as in non-pregnant controls [26], with an increase in up to eight times in patients with PE [27], which leads to an increase in blood pressure values, due to direct vasoconstriction and profibrotic changes that occur at the umbilical and placental level. MBG also alters cytotrophoblast differentiation in the first trimester of gestation [16], suggesting its involvement in the early pathological events leading to PE. Human cytotrophoblast cells cultured in the first trimester and stimulated by MBG have been shown to undergo alterations of proliferation, migration and invasion, caused by the activation of JNKs, p38 and SRC and leading to increased cell apoptosis [15].

The complete and definite role of MBG in the pathogenesis of PE is not yet fully known. In addition, the mechanisms and sites of synthesis of this molecule in mammals are also not completely understood, although it is already known that the placenta is a site for its production.

Beyond sex and gender differences, it was seen that racial differences may contribute to different clinical parameters involving endogenous CTS, such as sodium sensitivity [154], suggesting that these molecules are affected not only by sex- and gender-related factors but also by genetically related ones; further research is needed to define the set of MBG expression-regulating factors. A study by Kantaria et al. showed that salt-sensitivity of blood pressure values, in which CTS are implicated, may vary within the same population [155], suggesting a relevant impact of inter-individual variability on CTS activity.

7. MBG Action on the Nervous System

In addition to CV and renal effects, the action of sodium and MBG also occurs at the level of the central nervous system, through channels in the glial cells of the supraoptic and paraventricular nuclei, where the detection of osmolarity and salt takes place through a new isoform of the sodium Nax channels [156]. MBG also acts on Amyloid Precursor Protein (APP), apolipoprotein E (APOE) and Connective Tissue Growth factors (CTGFs). Specifically, APP triggers a cascade of neurodegenerative events, such as synaptic dysfunctions, the genesis of neurofibrillary tangles and neuronal death. New findings show that, after MBG infusion, downregulation of APP mRNA expression in vivo in DSS rats is present [17,157].

8. MBG Action on Cells of the Immune System

Interestingly, MBG also has an action on some cells of the immune system. For example, in one study [18], the role of MBG in acute inflammation was evaluated in a model of zymosan-induced peritonitis in vivo and in peritoneal macrophages in in vitro culture. Mouse models were treated for three days with either MBG at 0.56 mg/kg, saline or dimethyl sulfoxide, and at one hour after the last treatment, they were treated with 2 mg/mL zymosan. Next, peritoneal exudate was collected, and total and differential leukocyte numbers were evaluated. Among these cells, Zymosan-stimulated peritoneal macrophages showed cytokine changes in IL-6, IL-1β, and TNF-α plasma concentrations compared with the control group. Those treated with MBG at the lowest concentration had reduced plasma levels of IL-1β (45%), IL-6 (17%), and TNF-α (20%) compared to the zymosan group. In the other two groups, cytokine plasma levels remained similar to those of the control group. This demonstrated that MBG pre-treatment reduced neutrophil migration, probably due to alterations in vascular permeability. In addition, MBG showed no cytotoxicity to cultured peritoneal macrophages. As already mentioned, plasma concentrations of MBG that are not able to inhibit the enzyme Na^+/K^+-ATPase, however, can trigger the production of messengers and the activation of intracellular signaling pathways.

9. Conclusions

Altered (circulating or urinary) levels of MBG seem to predict the development of diseases characterized by volume expansion, such as CKD, certain CV diseases and PE, demonstrating its possible preventive, diagnostic or monitoring role. MBG can now probably be observed in a different "light", as a new important target for the prevention/treatment of kidney and CV development and progression.

Author Contributions: Conceptualization, D.B. and G.C.; Methodology, G.C.; Writing—Original Draft Preparation, M.D., G.F., M.T.Z., N.C., A.M., P.P., D.B. and G.C.; Writing—Review and Editing, D.B., M.M., M.A. and G.C. All authors have read and agreed to the published version of the manuscript.

Funding: This research received no external funding.

Institutional Review Board Statement: Not applicable.

Informed Consent Statement: Not applicable.

Data Availability Statement: Not applicable.

Conflicts of Interest: All authors deny any conflict of interest with respect to the present manuscript.

References

1. Schoner, W. Endogenous cardiac glycosides, a new class of steroid hormones. *Eur. J. Biochem.* **2002**, *269*, 2440–24488. [CrossRef] [PubMed]
2. Schoner, W.; Scheiner-Bobis, G. Endogenous cardiac glycosides: Hormones using the sodium pump as signal transducer. *Semin. Nephrol.* **2005**, *25*, 343–351. [CrossRef] [PubMed]
3. Schoner, W.; Scheiner-Bobis, G. Endogenous and exogenous cardiac glycosides: Their roles in hypertension, salt metabolism, and cell growth. *Am. J. Physiol. Cell Physiol.* **2007**, *293*, C509–C536. [CrossRef] [PubMed]
4. Fedorova, O.V.; Lakatta, E.; Bagrov, A.Y. Endogenous Na,K pump ligands are differentially regulated during acute NaCl loading of Dahl rats. *Circulation* **2000**, *102*, 3009–3014. [CrossRef] [PubMed]
5. Bagrov, A.Y.; Fedorova, O.V.; Dmitriev, R.I.; French, A.W.; Anderson, D.E. Plasma marinobufagenin-like and ouabain-like immunoreactivity during saline volume expansion in anesthetized dogs. *Cardiovasc. Res.* **1996**, *31*, 296–305. [CrossRef]
6. Kennedy, D.J.; Elkareh, J.; Shidyak, A.; Shapiro, A.P.; Smaili, S.; Mutgi, K.; Gupta, S.; Tian, J.; Morgan, E.; Khouri, S.; et al. Partial nephrectomy as a model for uremic cardiomyopathy in the mouse. *Am. J. Physiol. Renal Physiol.* **2008**, *294*, F450–F454. [CrossRef] [PubMed]
7. Priyadarshi, S.; Valentine, B.; Han, C.; Fedorova, O.V.; Bagrov, A.Y.; Liu, J.; Periyasamy, S.M.; Kennedy, D.; Malhotra, D.; Xie, Z.; et al. Effect of green tea extract on cardiac hypertrophy following 5/6 nephrectomy in the rat. *Kidney Int.* **2003**, *63*, 1785–1790. [CrossRef] [PubMed]
8. Kennedy, D.J.; Shrestha, K.; Sheehey, B.; Li, X.S.; Guggilam, A.; Wu, Y.; Finucan, M.; Gabi, A.; Medert, C.M.; Westfall, K.M.; et al. Elevated Plasma Marinobufagenin, An Endogenous Cardiotonic Steroid, Is Associated with Right Ventricular Dysfunction and Nitrative Stress in Heart Failure. *Circ. Heart Fail.* **2015**, *8*, 1068–1076. [CrossRef]
9. Elkareh, J.; Kennedy, D.J.; Yashaswi, B.; Vetteth, S.; Shidyak, A.; Kim, E.G.R.; Smaili, S.; Periyasamy, S.M.; Hariri, I.M.; Fedorova, L.; et al. Marinobufagenin Stimulates Fibroblast Collagen Production and Causes Fibrosis in Experimental Uremic Cardiomyopathy. *Hypertension* **2007**, *49*, 215–224. [CrossRef]
10. Xie, Z.; Kometiani, P.; Liu, J.; Li, J.; Shapiro, J.I.; Askari, A. Intracellular reactive oxygen species mediate the linkage of Na+/K+-ATPase to hypertrophy and its marker genes in cardiac myocytes. *J. Biol. Chem.* **1999**, *274*, 19323–19328. [CrossRef]
11. Pamnani, M.B.; Chen, S.; Yuan, C.M.; Haddy, F.J. Chronic blood pressure effects of bufalin, a sodium-potassium ATPase inhibitor, in rats. *Hypertension* **1994**, *23*, I106–I109. [CrossRef] [PubMed]
12. Vu, H.; Ianosi-Irimie, M.; Danchuk, S.; Rabon; Nogawa, T.; Kamano, Y.; Pettit, G.R.; Wiese, T.; Puschett, J.B. Resibufogenin Corrects Hypertension in a Rat Model of Human Preeclampsia. *Exp. Biol. Med.* **2006**, *231*, 215–220. [CrossRef] [PubMed]
13. Vu, H.V.; Ianosi-Irimie, M.R.; Pridjian, C.A.; Whitbred, J.M.; Durst, J.M.; Bagrov, A.Y.; Fedorova, O.V.; Pridjian, G.; Puschett, J.B. Involvement of marinobufagenin in a rat model of human preeclampsia. *Am. J. Nephrol.* **2005**, *25*, 520–528. [CrossRef] [PubMed]
14. Agunanne, E.; Horvat, D.; Harrison, R.; Uddin, M.; Jones, R.; Kuehl, T.; Ghanem, D.; Berghman, L.; Lai, X.; Li, J.; et al. Marinobufagenin Levels in Preeclamptic Patients: A Preliminary Report. *Am. J. Perinatol.* **2011**, *28*, 509–514. [CrossRef] [PubMed]
15. Uddin, M.N.; Horvat, D.; Glaser, S.S.; Mitchell, B.M.; Puschett, J.B. Examination of the Cellular Mechanisms by Which Marinobufagenin Inhibits Cytotrophoblast Function. *J. Biol. Chem.* **2008**, *283*, 17946–17953. [CrossRef]
16. LaMarca, H.; Morris, C.; Pettit, G.; Nagowa, T.; Puschett, J. Marinobufagenin Impairs First Trimester Cytotrophoblast Differentiation. *Placenta* **2006**, *27*, 984–988. [CrossRef] [PubMed]
17. Grigorova, Y.N.; Juhasz, O.; Long, J.M.; Zernetkina, V.I.; Hall, M.L.; Wei, W.; Morrell, C.H.; Petrashevskaya, N.; Morrow, A.; LaNasa, K.H.; et al. Effect of Cardiotonic Steroid Marinobufagenin on Vascular Remodeling and Cognitive Impairment in Young Dahl-S Rats. *Int. J. Mol. Sci.* **2022**, *23*, 4563. [CrossRef]
18. Carvalho, D.C.M.; Cavalcante-Silva, L.H.A.; Lima, D.A.; Galvão, J.G.F.M.; Alves, A.K.D.A.; Feijó, P.R.O.; Quintas, L.E.M.; Rodrigues-Mascarenhas, S. Marinobufagenin Inhibits Neutrophil Migration and Proinflammatory Cytokines. *J. Immunol. Res.* **2019**, *2019*, 1094520. [CrossRef]
19. Keppel, M.H.; Piecha, G.; März, W.; Cadamuro, J.; Auer, S.; Felder, T.K.; Mrazek, C.; Oberkofler, H.; Trummer, C.; Grübler, M.R.; et al. The endogenous cardiotonic steroid Marinobufagenin and decline in estimated glomerular filtration rate at follow-up in patients with arterial hypertension. *PLoS ONE* **2019**, *14*, e0212973. [CrossRef]

20. Bolignano, D.; Greco, M.; Presta, P.; Crugliano, G.; Sabatino, J.; Carullo, N.; Arena, R.; Leo, I.; Comi, A.; Andreucci, M.; et al. Altered circulating marinobufagenin levels and recurrent intradialytic hypotensive episodes in chronic hemodialysis patients: A pilot, prospective study. *Rev. Cardiovasc. Med.* **2021**, *22*, 1577–1587. [CrossRef]
21. Piecha, G.; Kujawa-Szewieczek, A.; Kuczera, P.; Skiba, K.; Sikora-Grabka, E.; Więcek, A. Plasma marinobufagenin immunoreactivity in patients with chronic kidney disease: A case control study. *Am. J. Physiol. Renal Physiol.* **2018**, *315*, F637–F643. [CrossRef] [PubMed]
22. Bolignano, D.; De Rosa, S.; Greco, M.; Presta, P.; Patella, G.; Crugliano, G.; Sabatino, J.; Strangio, A.; Romano, L.R.; Comi, A.; et al. Marinobufagenin, left ventricular geometry and cardiac dysfunction in end-stage kidney disease patients. *Int. Urol. Nephrol.* **2022**, *54*, 2581–2589. [CrossRef] [PubMed]
23. Jablonski, K.L.; Racine, M.L.; Geolfos, C.J.; Gates, P.E.; Chonchol, M.; McQueen, M.B.; Seals, D.R. Seals Faculty Opinions recommendation of Dietary sodium restriction reverses vascular endothelial dysfunction in middle-aged/older adults with moderately elevated systolic blood pressure. *J. Am. Coll. Cardiol.* **2013**, *61*, 335–343. [CrossRef] [PubMed]
24. Strauss, M.; Smith, W.; Fedorova, O.V.; Schutte, A.E. The Na+K+-ATPase Inhibitor Marinobufagenin and Early Cardiovascular Risk in Humans: A Review of Recent Evidence. *Curr. Hypertens. Rep.* **2019**, *21*, 38. [CrossRef] [PubMed]
25. Strauss, M.; Smith, W.; Kruger, R.; Wei, W.; Fedorova, O.V.; Schutte, A.E. Marinobufagenin and left ventricular mass in young adults: The African-PREDICT study. *Eur. J. Prev. Cardiol.* **2018**, *25*, 1587–1595. [CrossRef]
26. Lopatin, D.A.; Ailamazian, E.K.; Dmitrieva, R.I.; Shpen, V.M.; Fedorova, O.V.; Doris, P.A.; Bagrov, A.Y. Circulating bufodienolide and cardenolide sodium pump inhibitors in preeclampsia. *J. Hypertens.* **1999**, *17*, 1179–1187. [CrossRef]
27. Nikitina, E.R.; Mikhailov, A.V.; Nikandrova, E.S.; Frolova, E.V.; Fadeev, A.V.; Shman, V.V.; Shilova, V.Y.; Tapilskaya, N.I.; Shapiro, J.I.; Fedorova, O.V.; et al. In preeclampsia endogenous cardiotonic steroids induce vascular fibrosis and impair relaxation of umbilical arteries. *J. Hypertens.* **2011**, *29*, 769–776. [CrossRef]
28. Lenaerts, C.; Wells, M.; Hambye, S.; Blankert, B. Marinobufagenin extraction from *Rhinella marina* toad glands: Alternative approaches for a systematized strategy. *J. Sep. Sci.* **2019**, *42*, 1384–1392. [CrossRef]
29. Puschett, J.B.; Agunanne, E.; Uddin, M.N. Emerging role of the bufadienolides in cardiovascular and kidney diseases. *Am. J. Kidney Dis. Off. J. Natl. Kidney Found.* **2010**, *56*, 359–370. [CrossRef]
30. Krenn, L.; Kopp, B. Bufadienolides from animal and plant sources. *Phytochemistry* **1998**, *48*, 1–29. [CrossRef]
31. Steyn, P.S.; van Heerden, F.R. Bufadienolides of plant and animal origin. *Nat. Prod. Rep.* **1998**, *15*, 397–413. [CrossRef] [PubMed]
32. Hilton, P.J.; White, R.W.; Lord, G.A.; Garner, G.V.; Gordon, D.B.; Hilton, M.J.; Forni, L.G.; McKinnon, W.; Ismail, F.M.; Keenan, M.; et al. An inhibitor of the sodium pump obtained from human placenta. *Lancet* **1996**, *348*, 303–305. [CrossRef]
33. Dmitrieva, R.I.; Bagrov, A.Y.; Lalli, E.; Sassone-Corsi, P.; Stocco, D.M.; Doris, P.A. Mammalian bufadienolide is synthesized from cholesterol in the adrenal cortex by a pathway that Is independent of cholesterol side-chain cleavage. *Hypertension* **2000**, *36*, 442–448. [CrossRef] [PubMed]
34. Fedorova, O.V.; Zernetkina, V.I.; Shilova, V.Y.; Grigorova, Y.N.; Juhasz, O.; Wei, W.; Marshall, C.A.; Lakatta, E.G.; Bagrov, A.Y. Synthesis of an Endogenous Steroidal Na Pump Inhibitor Marinobufagenin, Implicated in Human Cardiovascular Diseases, Is Initiated by CYP27A1 via Bile Acid Pathway. *Circ. Cardiovasc. Genet.* **2015**, *8*, 736–745. [CrossRef] [PubMed]
35. Lichtstein, D.; Gati, I.; Haver, E.; Katz, U. Digitalis-like compounds in the toad Bufo viridis: Tissue and plasma levels and significance in osmotic stress. *Life Sci.* **1992**, *51*, 119–128. [CrossRef] [PubMed]
36. Bolignano, D.; D'Arrigo, G.; Pisano, A.; Coppolino, G. Pentoxifylline for Anemia in Chronic Kidney Disease: A Systematic Review and Meta-Analysis. *PLoS ONE* **2015**, *10*, e0134104.
37. Jing, J.; Ren, W.C.; Li, C.; Bose, U.; Parekh, H.S.; Wei, M.Q. Rapid identification of primary constituents in parotoid gland secretions of the Australian cane toad using HPLC/MS-Q-TOF. *Biomed. Chromatogr.* **2013**, *27*, 685–687. [CrossRef]
38. Rash, L.D.; Morales, R.A.V.; Vink, S.; Alewood, P.F. De novo sequencing of peptides from the parotid secretion of the cane toad, *Bufo marinus* (Rhinella marina). *Toxicon* **2011**, *57*, 208–216. [CrossRef]
39. Tian, H.-Y.; Luo, S.-L.; Liu, J.-S.; Wang, L.; Wang, Y.; Zhang, D.-M.; Zhang, X.-Q.; Jiang, R.-W.; Ye, W.-C. C23 Steroids from the Venom of Bufo bufo gargarizans. *J. Nat. Prod.* **2013**, *76*, 1842–1847. [CrossRef]
40. Schmeda-Hirschmann, G.; Quispe, C.; Theoduloz, C.; de Sousa, P.T.; Parizotto, C. Antiproliferative activity and new argininyl bufadienolide esters from the "cururú" toad Rhinella (Bufo) schneideri. *J. Ethnopharmacol.* **2014**, *155*, 1076–1085. [CrossRef]
41. Jared, C.; Antoniazzi, M.M.; Jordão, A.E.; Silva, J.R.M.; Greven, H.; Rodrigues, M.T. Parotoid macroglands in toad (Rhinella jimi): Their structure and functioning in passive defence. *Toxicon* **2009**, *54*, 197–207. [CrossRef] [PubMed]
42. Toledo, R.C.; Jared, C. Cutaneous granular glands and amphibian venoms. *Comp. Biochem. Physiol. Part A Physiol.* **1995**, *111*, 1–29. [CrossRef]
43. Mailho-Fontana, P.L.; Antoniazzi, M.M.; Toledo, L.F.; Verdade, V.K.; Sciani, J.M.; Barbaro, K.C.; Pimenta, D.C.; Rodrigues, M.T.; Jared, C. Passive and active defense in toads: The parotoid macroglands in Rhinella marina and Rhaebo guttatus. *J. Exp. Zool. Part A Ecol. Genet. Physiol.* **2014**, *321*, 65–77. [CrossRef]
44. Cher, K.; Chen, A.L. Notes on the poisonous secretions of twelve species of toads. *J. Pharmacol. Exp. Ther.* **1933**, *47*, 281–293
45. Low, B.S. Evidence from parotoid-gland secretions. *Evol. Genus Bufo* **1972**, *55*, 244–254.
46. Fedorova, O.V.; Talan, M.I.; Agalakova, N.I.; Lakatta, E.G.; Bagrov, A.Y. Endogenous ligand of alpha(1) sodium pump, marinobufagenin, is a novel mediator of sodium chloride—Dependent hypertension. *Circulation* **2002**, *105*, 1122–1127. [CrossRef]

47. Uddin, M.N.; Allen, S.R.; Jones, R.O.; Zawieja, D.C.; Kuehl, T.J. Pathogenesis of pre-eclampsia: Marinobufagenin and angiogenic imbalance as biomarkers of the syndrome. *Translational research: J. Lab. Clin. Med.* **2012**, *160*, 99–113. [CrossRef]
48. Schoner, W.; Scheiner-Bobis, G. Endogenous and Exogenous Cardiac Glycosides and their Mechanisms of Action. *Am. J. Cardiovasc. Drugs Drugs Devices Interv.* **2007**, *7*, 173–189. [CrossRef]
49. Paczula, A.; Wiecek, A.; Piecha, G. Cardiotonic Steroids—A Possible Link Between High-Salt Diet and Organ Damage. *Int. J. Mol. Sci.* **2019**, *20*, 590. [CrossRef]
50. Bagrov, A.Y.; Shapiro, J.I.; Fedorova, O.V. Endogenous Cardiotonic Steroids: Physiology, Pharmacology, and Novel Therapeutic Targets. *Pharmacol. Rev.* **2009**, *61*, 9–38. [CrossRef]
51. Liang, M.; Tian, J.; Liu, L.; Pierre, S.; Liu, J.; Shapiro, J.; Xie, Z.-J. Identification of a Pool of Non-pumping Na/K-ATPase. *J. Biol. Chem.* **2007**, *282*, 10585–10593. [CrossRef]
52. Wang, H.; Haas, M.; Liang, M.; Cai, T.; Tian, J.; Li, S.; Xie, Z. Ouabain assembles signaling cascades through the caveolar Na+/K+-ATPase. *J. Biol. Chem.* **2004**, *27*, 17250–17259. [CrossRef] [PubMed]
53. Bolignano, D.; Coppolino, G.; Criseo, M.; Campo, S.; Romeo, A.; Buemi, M. Aquaretic agents: What's beyond the treatment of hyponatremia? *Curr. Pharm. Des.* **2007**, *13*, 865–871. [CrossRef] [PubMed]
54. Bagrov, A.; Dmitrieva, R.; Fedorova, O.V.; Kazakov, G.P.; Roukoyatkina, N.I.; Shpen, V.M. Endogenous marinobufagenin-like immunoreactive substance*A possible endogenous Na,K-ATPase inhibitor with vasoconstrictor activity. *Am. J. Hypertens.* **1996**, *9*, 982–990. [CrossRef] [PubMed]
55. Bagrov, A.Y.; Fedorova, O.V. Effects of two putative endogenous digitalis-like factors, marinobufagenin and ouabain, on the Na+,K+-pump in human mesenteric arteries. *J. Hypertens.* **1998**, *16*, 1953–1958. [CrossRef] [PubMed]
56. Adrogué, H.J.; Madias, N.E. Sodium and Potassium in the Pathogenesis of Hypertension. *N. Engl. J. Med.* **2007**, *356*, 1966–1978. [CrossRef] [PubMed]
57. Coppolino, G.; Leonardi, G.; Andreucci, M.; Bolignano, D. Oxidative Stress and Kidney Function: A Brief Update. *Curr. Pharm. Des.* **2018**, *24*, 4794–4799. [CrossRef] [PubMed]
58. Elkareh, J.; Periyasamy, S.M.; Shidyak, A.; Vetteth, S.; Schroeder, J.; Raju, V.; Hariri, I.M.; El-Okdi, N.; Gupta, S.; Fedorova, L.; et al. Marinobufagenin induces increases in procollagen expression in a process involving protein kinase C and Fli-1: Implications for uremic cardiomyopathy. *Am. J. Physiol. Physiol.* **2009**, *296*, F1219–F1226. [CrossRef]
59. Fedorova, O.V.; Emelianov, I.V.; Bagrov, K.A.; Grigorova, Y.N.; Wei, W.; Juhasz, O.; Frolova, E.V.; Marshall, C.A.; Lakatta, E.G.; Konradi, A.O.; et al. Marinobufagenin-induced vascular fibrosis is a likely target for mineralocorticoid antagonists. *J. Hypertens.* **2015**, *33*, 1602–1610. [CrossRef]
60. Liu, J.; Kesiry, R.; Periyasamy, S.M.; Malhotra, D.; Xie, Z.; Shapiro, J.I. Ouabain induces endocytosis of plasmalemmal Na/K-ATPase in LLC-PK1 cells by a clathrin-dependent mechanism. *Kidney Int.* **2004**, *66*, 227–241. [CrossRef]
61. Fedorova, L.V.; Raju, V.; El-Okdi, N.; Shidyak, A.; Kennedy, D.J.; Vetteth, S.; Giovannucci, D.R.; Bagrov, A.Y.; Fedorova, O.V.; Shapiro, J.I.; et al. The cardiotonic steroid hormone marinobufagenin induces renal fibrosis: Implication of epithelial-to-mesenchymal transition. *Am. J. Physiol. Renal Physiol.* **2009**, *296*, F922–F934. [CrossRef] [PubMed]
62. Fedorova, O.V.; Agalakova, N.I.; Talan, M.I.; Lakatta, E.G.; Bagrov, A.Y. Brain ouabain stimulates peripheral marinobufagenin via angiotensin II signalling in NaCl-loaded Dahl-S rats. *J. Hypertens.* **2005**, *23*, 1515–1523. [CrossRef] [PubMed]
63. Haller, S.T.; Drummond, C.A.; Yan, Y.; Liu, J.; Tian, J.; Malhotra, D.; Shapiro, J.I. Passive Immunization Against Marinobufagenin Attenuates Renal Fibrosis and Improves Renal Function in Experimental Renal Disease. *Am. J. Hypertens.* **2013**, *27*, 603–609. [CrossRef] [PubMed]
64. Tian, J.; Shidyak, A.; Periyasamy, S.M.; Haller, S.; Taleb, M.; El-Okdi, N.; Elkareh, J.; Gupta, S.; Gohara, S.; Fedorova, O.V.; et al. Spironolactone Attenuates Experimental Uremic Cardiomyopathy by Antagonizing Marinobufagenin. *Hypertension* **2009**, *54*, 1313–1320. [CrossRef] [PubMed]
65. Drummond, C.A.; Fan, X.; Haller, S.T.; Kennedy, D.J.; Liu, J.; Tian, J. Na/K-ATPase signaling mediates miR-29b-3p regulation and cardiac fibrosis formation in mice with chronic kidney disease. *PLoS ONE* **2018**, *13*, e0197688. [CrossRef]
66. Drummond, C.A.; Hill, M.C.; Shi, H.; Fan, X.; Xie, J.X.; Haller, S.T.; Kennedy, D.J.; Liu, J.; Garrett, M.R.; Xie, Z.; et al. Na/K-ATPase signaling regulates collagen synthesis through microRNA-29b-3p in cardiac fibroblasts. *Physiol. Genom.* **2016**, *48*, 220–229. [CrossRef]
67. Bolignano, D.; Greco, M.; Presta, P.; Duni, A.; Vita, C.; Pappas, E.; Mirabelli, M.; Lakkas, L.; Naka, K.K.; Brunetti, A.; et al. A small circulating miRNAs signature predicts mortality and adverse cardiovascular outcomes in chronic hemodialysis patients. *Clin. Kidney J.* **2023**, *16*, 868–878. [CrossRef]
68. Lenaerts, C.; Demeyer, M.; Gerbaux, P.; Blankert, B. Analytical aspects of marinobufagenin. *Clin. Chim. Acta Int. J. Clin. Chem.* **2013**, *421*, 193–201. [CrossRef]
69. Komiyama, Y.; Dong, X.H.; Nishimura, N.; Masaki, H.; Yoshika, M.; Masuda, M.; Takahashi, H. A novel endogenous digitalis, telocinobufagin, exhibits elevated plasma levels in patients with terminal renal failure. *Clin. Biochem.* **2005**, *38*, 36–45. [CrossRef]
70. Kerkhoff, J.; Noronha, J.D.C.; Bonfilio, R.; Sinhorin, A.P.; Rodrigues, D.D.J.; Chaves, M.H.; Vieira, G.M. Quantification of bufadienolides in the poisons of *Rhinella marina* and *Rhaebo guttatus* by HPLC-UV. *Toxicon* **2016**, *119*, 311–318. [CrossRef]
71. Jiang, P.; Dou, S.; Liu, L.; Zhang, W.; Chen, Z.; Xu, R.; Ding, J.; Liu, R. Identification of Multiple Constituents in the TCM-Formula Shexiang Baoxin Pill by LC Coupled with DAD-ESI-MS-MS. *Chromatographia* **2009**, *70*, 133–142. [CrossRef]

72. Miyashiro, Y.; Nishio, T.; Shimada, K. Characterization of In Vivo Metabolites of Toad Venom Using Liquid Chromatography-Mass Spectrometry. *J. Chromatogr. Sci.* **2008**, *46*, 534–533. [CrossRef] [PubMed]
73. Cunha-Filho, G.A.; Resck, I.S.; Cavalcanti, B.C.; Pessoa, C.; Moraes, M.O.; Ferreira, J.R.; Rodrigues, F.A.; dos Santos, M.L. Cytotoxic profile of natural and some modified bufadienolides from toad Rhinella schneideri parotoid gland secretion. *Toxicon* **2010**, *56*, 339–348. [CrossRef]
74. Bagrov, A.Y.; Roukoyatkina, N.I.; Pinaev, A.G.; Dmitrieva, R.I.; Fedorova, O.V. Effects of two endogenous Na+,K(+)-ATPase inhibitors, marinobufagenin and ouabain, on isolated rat aorta. *Eur. J. Pharmacol.* **1995**, *274*, 151–158. [CrossRef]
75. Shimada, K.; Kurata, Y.; Oe, T. Utility of Cyclodextrin in Mobile Phase for High-Performance Liquid Chromatographic Separation of Bufadienolides. *J. Liq. Chromatogr.* **1990**, *13*, 493–504. [CrossRef]
76. Cunha Filho, G.A.; Schwartz, C.A.; Resck, I.S.; Murta, M.M.; Lemos, S.S.; Castro, M.S.; Kyaw, C.; Pires, O.R., Jr.; Leite, J.R.; Bloch, C.; et al. Antimicrobial activity of the bufadienolides marinobufagin and telocinobufagin isolated as major components from skin secretion of the toad Bufo rubescens. *Toxicon* **2005**, *45*, 777–782. [CrossRef] [PubMed]
77. Li, X.; Guo, Z.; Wang, C.; Shen, A.; Liu, Y.; Zhang, X.; Zhao, W.; Liang, X. Purification of bufadienolides from the skin of Bufo bufo gargarizans Cantor with positively charged C18 column. *J. Pharm. Biomed. Anal.* **2014**, *92*, 105–113. [CrossRef]
78. Banfi, F.F.; Guedes, K.D.S.; Andrighetti, C.R.; Aguiar, A.C.; Debiasi, B.W.; Noronha, J.D.C.; Rodrigues, D.D.J.; Júnior, G.M.V.; Sanchez, B.A.M. Antiplasmodial and Cytotoxic Activities of Toad Venoms from Southern Amazon, Brazil. *Korean J. Parasitol.* **2016**, *54*, 415–421. [CrossRef]
79. Shimada, K.; Nambara, T. Isolation and characterization of cardiotonic steroid conjugates from the skin of Bufo marinus (L.) Schneider. *Chem. Pharm. Bull.* **1979**, *27*, 1881–1886. [CrossRef]
80. Strauss, M.; Smith, W.; Wei, W.; Bagrov, A.Y.; Fedorova, O.V.; Schutte, A.E. Large artery stiffness is associated with marinobufagenin in young adults: The African-PREDICT study. *J. Hypertens.* **2018**, *36*, 2333–2339. [CrossRef]
81. Fedorova, O.V.; Lakatta, E.G.; Bagrov, A.Y.; Melander, O. Plasma level of the endogenous sodium pump ligand marinobufagenin is related to the salt-sensitivity in men. *J. Hypertens.* **2015**, *33*, 534–541, discussion 541. [CrossRef] [PubMed]
82. Anderson, D.E.; Fedorova, O.V.; Morrell, C.H.; Longo, D.L.; Kashkin, V.A.; Metzler, J.D.; Bagrov, A.Y.; Lakatta, E.G.; Piecha, G.; Kujawa-Szewieczek, A.; et al. Endogenous sodium pump inhibitors and age-associated increases in salt sensitivity of blood pressure in normotensives. *Am. J. Physiol. Integr. Comp. Physiol.* **2008**, *294*, R1248–R1254. [CrossRef] [PubMed]
83. Strauss, M.; Smith, W.; Wei, W.; Fedorova, O.V.; Schutte, A.E. Marinobufagenin is related to elevated central and 24-h systolic blood pressures in young black women: The African-PREDICT Study. *Hypertens. Res. Off. J. Jpn. Soc. Hypertens.* **2018**, *41*, 183–192. [CrossRef]
84. Hill, N.R.; Fatoba, S.T.; Oke, J.L.; Hirst, J.A.; O'Callaghan, C.A.; Lasserson, D.S.; Hobbs, F.D.R. Global Prevalence of Chronic Kidney Disease—A Systematic Review and Meta-Analysis. *PLoS ONE* **2016**, *11*, e0158765. [CrossRef]
85. Go, A.S.; Chertow, G.M.; Fan, D.; McCulloch, C.E.; Hsu, C.-y. Chronic Kidney Disease and the Risks of Death, Cardiovascular Events, and Hospitalization. *N. Engl. J. Med.* **2004**, *351*, 1296–1305. [CrossRef] [PubMed]
86. Provenzano, M.; Coppolino, G.; Faga, T.; Garofalo, C.; Serra, R.; Andreucci, M. Epidemiology of cardiovascular risk in chronic kidney disease patients: The real silent killer. *Rev Cardiovasc. Med.* **2019**, *20*, 209–220. [CrossRef] [PubMed]
87. Provenzano, M.; Coppolino, G.; De Nicola, L.; Serra, R.; Garofalo, C.; Andreucci, M.; Bolignano, D. Unraveling Cardiovascular Risk in Renal Patients: A New Take on Old Tale. *Front. Cell Dev. Biol.* **2019**, *7*, 314. [CrossRef]
88. Bolignano, D.; Pisano, A.; Coppolino, G. The Dark Side of Blocking RAS in Diabetic Patients with Incipient or Manifested Nephropathy. *Exp. Clin. Endocrinol. Diabetes* **2015**, *124*, 350–360. [CrossRef]
89. Fedorova, O.V.; Doris, P.A.; Bagrov, A.Y. Endogenous Marinobufagenin-Like Factor in Acute Plasma Volume Expansion. *Clin. Exp. Hypertens.* **1998**, *20*, 581–591. [CrossRef]
90. Hauck, C.; Frishman, W.H. Systemic hypertension: The roles of salt, vascular Na+/K+ ATPase and the endogenous glycosides, ouabain and marinobufagenin. *Cardiol. Rev.* **2012**, *20*, 130–138. [CrossRef]
91. Kennedy, D.J.; Vetteth, S.; Periyasamy, S.M.; Kanj, M.; Fedorova, L.; Khouri, S.; Kahaleh, M.B.; Xie, Z.; Malhotra, D.; Kolodkin, N.I.; et al. Central role for the cardiotonic steroid marinobufagenin in the pathogenesis of experimental uremic cardiomyopathy. *Hypertension* **2006**, *47*, 488–495. [CrossRef] [PubMed]
92. Wang, X.; Shapiro, J.I. Evolving concepts in the pathogenesis of uraemic cardiomyopathy. *Nat. Rev. Nephrol.* **2019**, *15*, 159–175. [CrossRef] [PubMed]
93. Suassuna, P.G.D.A.; Sanders-Pinheiro, H.; de Paula, R.B. Uremic Cardiomyopathy: A New Piece in the Chronic Kidney Disease-Mineral and Bone Disorder Puzzle. *Front. Med.* **2018**, *5*, 206. [CrossRef] [PubMed]
94. Middleton, R.J.; Parfrey, P.S.; Foley, R.N. Left ventricular hypertrophy in the renal patient. *J. Am. Soc. Nephrol. JASN* **2001**, *12*, 1079–1084. [CrossRef] [PubMed]
95. Rigatto, C.; Parfrey, P.; Foley, R.; Negrijn, C.; Tribula, C.; Jeffery, J. Congestive heart failure in renal transplant recipients: Risk factors, outcomes, and relationship with ischemic heart disease. *J. Am. Soc. Nephrol.* **2002**, *13*, 1084–1090. [CrossRef] [PubMed]
96. Parfrey, P.S. Is renal insufficiency an atherogenic state? Reflections on prevalence, incidence, and risk. *Am. J. Kidney Dis. Off. J. Natl. Kidney Found.* **2001**, *37*, 154–156. [CrossRef]
97. D'Agostino, M.; Mauro, D.; Zicarelli, M.; Carullo, N.; Greco, M.; Andreucci, M.; Coppolino, G.; Bolignano, D. miRNAs in Uremic Cardiomyopathy: A Comprehensive Review. *Int. J. Mol. Sci.* **2023**, *24*, 5425. [CrossRef]

98. Zeisberg, M.; Kalluri, R. Fibroblasts emerge via epithelial-mesenchymal transition in chronic kidney fibrosis. *Front Biosci.* **2008**, *13*, 6991–6998. [CrossRef]
99. Kometiani, P.; Li, J.; Gnudi, L.; Kahn, B.B.; Askari, A.; Xie, Z. Multiple signal transduction pathways link Na+/K+-ATPase to growth-related genes in cardiac myocytes. The roles of Ras and mitogen-activated protein kinases. *J. Biol. Chem.* **1998**, *273*, 15249–15256. [CrossRef]
100. Bolignano, D.; Greco, M.; Presta, P.; Caglioti, A.; Carullo, N.; Zicarelli, M.; Foti, D.P.; Dragone, F.; Andreucci, M.; Coppolino, G. Marinobufagenin, Left Ventricular Hypertrophy and Residual Renal Function in Kidney Transplant Recipients. *J. Clin. Med.* **2023**, *12*, 3072. [CrossRef]
101. Coppolino, G.; Bolignano, D.; Presta, P.; Ferrari, F.F.; Lionetti, G.; Borselli, M.; Randazzo, G.; Andreucci, M.; Bonelli, A.; Errante, A.; et al. Acquisition of optical coherence tomography angiography metrics during hemodialysis procedures: A pilot study. *Front. Med.* **2022**, *9*, 1057165. [CrossRef]
102. Coppolino, G.; Lucisano, G.; Bolignano, D.; Buemi, M. Acute cardiovascular complications of hemodialysis. *Minerva Urol. Nefrol.* **2010**, *62*, 67–80. [PubMed]
103. Uddin, M.N.; Horvat, D.; Childs, E.W.; Puschett, J.B. Marinobufagenin causes endothelial cell monolayer hyperpermeability by altering apoptotic signaling. *Am. J. Physiol. Integr. Comp. Physiol.* **2009**, *296*, R1726–R1734. [CrossRef] [PubMed]
104. Fedorova, O.V.; Kolodkin, N.I.; Agalakova, N.I.; Lakatta, E.G.; Bagrov, A.Y. Marinobufagenin, an endogenous alpha-1 sodium pump ligand, in hypertensive Dahl salt-sensitive rats. *Hypertension* **2001**, *37*, 462–466. [CrossRef] [PubMed]
105. Fedorova, O.V.; Kolodkin, N.I.; Agalakova, N.I.; Namikas, A.R.; Bzhelyansky, A.; St-Louis, J.; Lakatta, E.G.; Bagrov, A.Y. Antibody to marinobufagenin lowers blood pressure in pregnant rats on a high NaCl intake. *J. Hypertens.* **2005**, *23*, 835–842. [CrossRef] [PubMed]
106. Bagrov, A.Y.; Fedorova, O.V.; Dmitrieva, R.I.; Howald, W.N.; Hunter, A.P.; Kuznetsova, E.A.; Shpen, V.M. Characterization of a urinary bufodienolide Na+,K+-ATPase inhibitor in patients after acute myocardial infarction. *Hypertension* **1998**, *31*, 1097–1103. [CrossRef]
107. Tomaschitz, A.; Piecha, G.; Ritz, E.; Meinitzer, A.; Haas, J.; Pieske, B.; Wiecek, A.; Rus-Machan, J.; Toplak, H.; März, W.; et al. Marinobufagenin in essential hypertension and primary aldosteronism: A cardiotonic steroid with clinical and diagnostic implications. *Clin. Exp. Hypertens.* **2014**, *37*, 108–115. [CrossRef]
108. Tian, J.; Haller, S.; Periyasamy, S.; Brewster, P.; Zhang, H.; Adlakha, S.; Fedorova, O.V.; Xie, Z.-J.; Bagrov, A.Y.; Shapiro, J.I.; et al. Renal Ischemia Regulates Marinobufagenin Release in Humans. *Hypertension* **2010**, *56*, 914–919. [CrossRef]
109. Kolmakova, E.V.; Haller, S.T.; Kennedy, D.J.; Isachkina, A.N.; Budny, G.V.; Frolova, E.V.; Piecha, G.; Nikitina, E.R.; Malhotra, D.; Fedorova, O.V.; et al. Endogenous cardiotonic steroids in chronic renal failure. *Nephrol. Dial. Transplant. Off. Publ. Eur. Dial. Transpl. Assoc. Eur. Ren. Assoc.* **2011**, *26*, 2912–2919. [CrossRef]
110. Meneton, P.; Jeunemaitre, X.; de Wardener, H.E.; Macgregor, G.A. Links Between Dietary Salt Intake, Renal Salt Handling, Blood Pressure, and Cardiovascular Diseases. *Physiol. Rev.* **2005**, *85*, 679–715. [CrossRef]
111. Pamnani, M.B.; Chen, S.; Bryant, H.J.; Schooley, J.F.; Eliades, D.C.; Yuan, C.M.; Haddy, F.J. Effects of three sodium-potassium adenosine triphosphatase inhibitors. *Hypertension* **1991**, *18*, 316–324. [CrossRef] [PubMed]
112. Horvat, D.; Severson, J.; Uddin, M.N.; Mitchell, B.; Puschett, J.B. Resibufogenin prevents the manifestations of preeclampsia in an animal model of the syndrome. *Hypertens. Pregnancy* **2010**, *29*, 1–9. [CrossRef] [PubMed]
113. Fedorova, O.V.; Simbirtsev, A.S.; Kolodkin, N.I.; Kotov, A.Y.; Agalakova, N.I.; Kashkin, V.A.; Tapilskaya, N.I.; Bzhelyansky, A.; Reznik, V.A.; Frolova, E.V.; et al. Monoclonal antibody to an endogenous bufadienolide, marinobufagenin, reverses preeclampsia-induced Na/K-ATPase inhibition and lowers blood pressure in NaCl-sensitive hypertension. *J. Hypertens.* **2008**, *26*, 2414–2425. [CrossRef] [PubMed]
114. Jablonski, K.L.; Fedorova, O.V.; Racine, M.L.; Geolfos, C.J.; Gates, P.E.; Chonchol, M.; Fleenor, B.S.; Lakatta, E.G.; Bagrov, A.Y.; Seals, D.R. Dietary Sodium Restriction and Association with Urinary Marinobufagenin, Blood Pressure, and Aortic Stiffness. *Clin. J. Am. Soc. Nephrol.* **2013**, *8*, 1952–1959. [CrossRef]
115. Titze, J. Sodium balance is not just a renal affair. *Curr. Opin. Nephrol. Hypertens.* **2014**, *23*, 101–105. [CrossRef]
116. Oberleithner, H.; Kusche-Vihrog, K.; Schillers, H. Endothelial cells as vascular salt sensors. *Kidney Int.* **2010**, *77*, 490–494. [CrossRef]
117. Liu, J.; Xie, Z.J. The sodium pump and cardiotonic steroids-induced signal transduction protein kinases and calcium-signaling microdomain in regulation of transporter trafficking. *Biochim. Biophys. Acta* **2010**, *1802*, 1237–1245. [CrossRef] [PubMed]
118. Haas, M.; Askari, A.; Xie, Z. Involvement of Src and epidermal growth factor receptor in the signal-transducing function of Na+/K+-ATPase. *J. Biol. Chem.* **2000**, *275*, 27832–27837. [CrossRef]
119. Huang, L.; Li, H.; Xie, Z. Ouabain-induced Hypertrophy in Cultured Cardiac Myocytes is Accompanied by Changes in Expression of Several Late Response Genes. *J. Mol. Cell. Cardiol.* **1997**, *29*, 429–437. [CrossRef]
120. Liu, J.; Tian, J.; Haas, M.; Shapiro, J.I.; Askari, A.; Xie, Z. Ouabain interaction with cardiac Na+/K+-ATPase initiates signal cascades independent of changes in intracellular Na+ and Ca2+ concentrations. *J. Biol. Chem.* **2000**, *275*, 27838–27844. [CrossRef]
121. Liu, L.; Mohammadi, K.; Aynafshar, B.; Wang, H.; Li, D.; Liu, J.; Ivanov, A.V.; Xie, Z.; Askari, A. Role of caveolae in signal-transducing function of cardiac Na+/K+-ATPase. *Am. J. Physiol. Cell Physiol.* **2003**, *284*, C1550–C1560. [CrossRef] [PubMed]
122. Liu, J.; Liang, M.; Liu, L.; Malhotra, D.; Xie, Z.; Shapiro, J.I. Ouabain-induced endocytosis of the plasmalemmal Na/K-ATPase in LLC-PK1 cells requires caveolin-1. *Kidney Int.* **2005**, *67*, 1844–1854. [CrossRef] [PubMed]

123. Vlachopoulos, C.; Aznaouridis, K.; Stefanadis, C. Prediction of Cardiovascular Events and All-Cause Mortality With Arterial Stiffness: A Systematic Review and Meta-Analysis. *J. Am. Coll. Cardiol.* **2010**, *55*, 1318–1327. [CrossRef]
124. Todd, A.S.; MacGinley, R.J.; Schollum, J.B.; Johnson, R.J.; Williams, S.M.; Sutherland, W.H.; Mann, J.I.; Walker, R.J. Dietary salt loading impairs arterial vascular reactivity. *Am. J. Clin. Nutr.* **2010**, *91*, 557–564. [CrossRef] [PubMed]
125. He, F.J.; Marciniak, M.; Visagie, E.; Markandu, N.D.; Anand, V.; Dalton, R.N.; MacGregor, G.A. Effect of Modest Salt Reduction on Blood Pressure, Urinary Albumin, and Pulse Wave Velocity in White, Black, and Asian Mild Hypertensives. *Hypertension* **2009**, *54*, 482–488. [CrossRef]
126. Mitchell, G.F. Arterial Stiffness and Hypertension. *Hypertension* **2014**, *64*, 210–214. [CrossRef]
127. Levy, D.; Garrison, R.J.; Savage, D.D.; Kannel, W.B.; Castelli, W.P. Prognostic Implications of Echocardiographically Determined Left Ventricular Mass in the Framingham Heart Study. *N. Engl. J. Med.* **1990**, *322*, 1561–1566. [CrossRef]
128. Rodriguez, C.J.; Bibbins-Domingo, K.; Jin, Z.; Daviglus, M.L.; Goff, D.C., Jr.; Jacobs, D.R., Jr. Association of sodium and potassium intake with left ventricular mass: Coronary artery risk development in young adults. *Hypertension* **2011**, *58*, 410–416. [CrossRef]
129. Yu, H.C.M.; Burrell, L.M.; Black, M.J.; Wu, L.L.; Dilley, R.J.; Cooper, M.E.; Johnston, C.I. Salt induces myocardial and renal fibrosis in normotensive and hypertensive rats. *Circulation* **1998**, *98*, 2621–2628. [CrossRef]
130. Grigorova, Y.N.; Wei, W.; Petrashevskaya, N.; Zernetkina, V.; Juhasz, O.; Fenner, R.; Gilbert, C.; Lakatta, E.G.; Shapiro, J.I.; Bagrov, A.Y.; et al. Dietary Sodium Restriction Reduces Arterial Stiffness, Vascular TGF-β-Dependent Fibrosis and Marinobufagenin in Young Normotensive Rats. *Int. J. Mol Sci.* **2018**, *19*, 3168. [CrossRef]
131. Grigorova, Y.N.; Juhasz, O.; Zernetkina, V.; Fishbein, K.W.; Lakatta, E.; Fedorova, O.V.; Bagrov, A.Y. Aortic Fibrosis, Induced by High Salt Intake in the Absence of Hypertensive Response, Is Reduced by a Monoclonal Antibody to Marinobufagenin. *Am. J. Hypertens.* **2015**, *29*, 641–646. [CrossRef] [PubMed]
132. Zhang, Y.; Wei, W.; Shilova, V.; Petrashevskaya, N.N.; Zernetkina, V.I.; Grigorova, Y.N.; Marshall, C.A.; Fenner, R.C.; Lehrmann, E.; Wood, W.H., 3rd; et al. Monoclonal Antibody to Marinobufagenin Downregulates TGFbeta Profibrotic Signaling in Left Ventricle and Kidney and Reduces Tissue Remodeling in Salt-Sensitive Hypertension. *J. Am. Heart Assoc.* **2019**, *8*, e012138. [CrossRef] [PubMed]
133. Weinberger, M.H.; Miller, J.Z.; Luft, F.C.; Grim, C.E.; Fineberg, N.S. Definitions and characteristics of sodium sensitivity and blood pressure resistance. *Hypertension* **1986**, *8*, II127–II134. [CrossRef]
134. Pisano, A.; D'arrigo, G.; Coppolino, G.; Bolignano, D. Biotic Supplements for Renal Patients: A Systematic Review and Meta-Analysis. *Nutrients* **2018**, *10*, 1224. [CrossRef]
135. Regitz-Zagrosek, V.; Seeland, U. Sex and Gender Differences in Clinical Medicine. In *Handbook of Experimental Pharmacology*; Springer: Berlin/Heidelberg, Germany, 2012; pp. 3–22. [CrossRef]
136. Grego, S.; Pasotti, E.; Moccetti, T.; Maggioni, A.P. 'Sex and gender medicine": Il principio della medicina di genere. *G. Ital. Cardiol.* **2020**, *21*, 602–606.
137. Tokatli, M.R.; Sisti, L.G.; Marziali, E.; Nachira, L.; Rossi, M.F.; Amantea, C.; Moscato U.; Malorni, W. Hormones and Sex-Specific Medicine in Human Physiopathology. *Biomolecules* **2022**, *12*, 413. [CrossRef]
138. Gestational Hypertension and Preeclampsia: ACOG Practice Bulletin, Number 222. *Obstet. Gynecol.* **2020**, *135*, e237–e260. [CrossRef] [PubMed]
139. Buemi, M.; Bolignano, D.; Barilla, A.; Nostro, L.; Crasci, E.; Campo, S.; Coppolino, G.; D'Anna, R. Preeclampsia and cardiovascular risk: General characteristics, counseling and follow-up. *J. Nephrol.* **2008**, *21*, 663–672.
140. Bolignano, D.; Coppolino, G.; Aloisi, C.; Romeo, A.; Nicocia, G.; Buemi, M. Effect of a Single Intravenous Immunoglobulin Infusion on Neutrophil Gelatinase-Associated Lipocalin Levels in Proteinuric Patients with Normal Renal Function. *J. Investig. Med.* **2008**, *56*, 997–1003. [CrossRef]
141. Abalos, E.; Cuesta, C.; Grosso, A.L.; Chou, D.; Say, L. Global and regional estimates of preeclampsia and eclampsia: A systematic review. *Eur. J. Obstet. Gynecol. Reprod. Biol.* **2013**, *170*, 1–7. [CrossRef]
142. Duley, L. The Global Impact of Pre-eclampsia and Eclampsia. *Semin. Perinatol.* **2009**, *33*, 130–137. [CrossRef] [PubMed]
143. MacKay, A.P.; Berg, C.J.; Liu, X.; Duran, C.; Hoyert, D.L. Changes in pregnancy mortality ascertainment: United States, 1999–2005. *Obstet. Gynecol.* **2011**, *118*, 104–110. [CrossRef] [PubMed]
144. Main, E.K. Maternal mortality: New strategies for measurement and prevention. *Curr. Opin. Obstet. Gynecol.* **2010**, *22*, 511–515. [CrossRef] [PubMed]
145. Chang, J.; Elam-Evans, L.D.; Berg, C.J.; Herndon, J.; Flowers, L.; Seed, K.A.; Syverson, C.J. Pregnancy-related mortality surveillance—United States, 1991–1999. In *Morbidity and Mortality Weekly Report Surveillance Summaries*; Center for Disease Control and Prevention: Washington, DC, USA, 2003; Volume 52, pp. 1–8.
146. Sturiale, A.; Coppolino, G.; Loddo, S.; Criseo, M.; Campo, S.; Crasci, E.; Bolignano, D.; Nostro, L.; Teti, D.; Buemi, M. Effects of Haemodialysis on Circulating Endothelial Progenitor Cell Count. *Blood Purif.* **2007**, *25*, 242–251. [CrossRef] [PubMed]
147. Agunanne, E.; Horvat, D.; Uddin, M.N.; Puschett, J. The Treatment of Preeclampsia in a Rat Model Employing Digibind®. *Am. J. Perinatol.* **2009**, *27*, 299–305. [CrossRef] [PubMed]
148. Puschett, J.B. Marinobufagenin Predicts and Resibufogenin Prevents Preeclampsia: A Review of the Evidence. *Am. J. Perinatol.* **2012**, *29*, 777–786. [CrossRef] [PubMed]
149. Puschett, J.; Agunanne, E.; Uddin, M. Marinobufagenin, resibufogenin and preeclampsia. *Biochim. Biophys. Acta (BBA) Mol. Basis Dis.* **2010**, *1802*, 1246–1253. [CrossRef]

150. Hassan, M.J.M.; Bakar, N.S.; Aziz, M.A.; Basah, N.K.; Singh, H.J. Leptin-induced increase in blood pressure and markers of endothelial activation during pregnancy in Sprague Dawley rats is prevented by resibufogenin, a marinobufagenin antagonist. *Reprod. Biol.* **2020**, *20*, 184–190. [CrossRef]
151. Uddin, M.N.; Agunanne, E.E.; Horvat, D.; Puschett, J.B. Resibufogenin Administration Prevents Oxidative Stress in a Rat Model of Human Preeclampsia. *Hypertens. Pregnancy* **2010**, *31*, 70–78. [CrossRef]
152. Fedorova, O.V.; Ishkaraeva, V.V.; Grigorova, Y.N.; Reznik, V.A.; Kolodkin, N.I.; Zazerskaya, I.E.; Zernetkina, V.; Agalakova, N.I.; Tapilskaya, N.I.; Adair, C.D.; et al. Antibody to Marinobufagenin Reverses Placenta-Induced Fibrosis of Umbilical Arteries in Preeclampsia. *Int. J. Mol. Sci.* **2018**, *19*, 2377. [CrossRef]
153. Agalakova, N.I.; Grigorova, Y.N.; Ershov, I.A.; Reznik, V.A.; Mikhailova, E.V.; Nadei, O.V.; Samuilovskaya, L.; Romanova, L.A.; Adair, C.D.; Romanova, I.V.; et al. Canrenone Restores Vasorelaxation Impaired by Marinobufagenin in Human Preeclampsia. *Int. J. Mol. Sci.* **2022**, *23*, 3336. [CrossRef] [PubMed]
154. Anderson, D.E.; Scuteri, A.; Agalakova, N.; Parsons, D.J.; Bagrov, A. Racial differences in resting end-tidal CO_2 and circulating sodium pump inhibitor. *Am. J. Hypertens.* **2001**, *14*, 761–767. [CrossRef] [PubMed]
155. Kantaria, N.; Pantsulaia, I.; Andronikashvili, I.; Simonia, G. Assosiation of Endogenous Cardiotonic Steroids with Salt-sensitivity of Blood Pressure in Georgian Population. *Georgian Med. News* **2016**, *258*, 33–37.
156. Orlov, S.N.; Mongin, A.A. Salt-sensing mechanisms in blood pressure regulation and hypertension. *Am. J. Physiol. Circ. Physiol.* **2007**, *293*, H2039–H2053. [CrossRef] [PubMed]
157. Reiss, A.B.; Arain, H.A.; Stecker, M.M.; Siegart, N.M.; Kasselman, L.J. Amyloid toxicity in Alzheimer's disease. *Rev. Neurosci.* **2018**, *29*, 613–627. [CrossRef] [PubMed]

Disclaimer/Publisher's Note: The statements, opinions and data contained in all publications are solely those of the individual author(s) and contributor(s) and not of MDPI and/or the editor(s). MDPI and/or the editor(s) disclaim responsibility for any injury to people or property resulting from any ideas, methods, instructions or products referred to in the content.

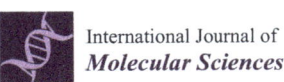

Article

Kidney Injury Causes Accumulation of Renal Sodium That Modulates Renal Lymphatic Dynamics

Jing Liu [1,2], Elaine L. Shelton [2,3], Rachelle Crescenzi [4], Daniel C. Colvin [4], Annet Kirabo [5], Jianyong Zhong [2,6], Eric J. Delpire [7], Hai-Chun Yang [2,6,*], and Valentina Kon [2,*]

1. Department of Nephrology, Tongji University School of Medicine, Shanghai 200070, China; liujing961226@163.com
2. Department of Pediatrics, Vanderbilt University Medical Center, Nashville, TN 37232, USA
3. Department of Pharmacology, Vanderbilt University Medical Center, Nashville, TN 37232, USA; elaine.l.shelton@vumc.org
4. Department of Radiology, Vanderbilt University Medical Center, Nashville, TN 37232, USA; rachelle.crescenzi@vumc.org (R.C.); daniel.colvin@vumc.org (D.C.C.)
5. Department of Medicine, Division of Clinal Pharmacology and Department of Molecular Physiology and Biophysics, Vanderbilt University Medical Center, Nashville, TN 37232, USA; annet.kirabo@vanderbilt.edu (A.K.); jianyong.zhong@vumc.org (J.Z.)
6. Department of Pathology, Microbiology and Immunology, Vanderbilt University Medical Center, Nashville, TN 37232, USA; eric.delpire@vanderbilt.edu
7. Department of Anesthesiology, Vanderbilt University Medical Center, Nashville, TN 37232, USA
* Correspondence: haichun.yang@vumc.org (H.-C.Y.); valentina.kon@vumc.org (V.K.); Tel.: +1-615-343-0110 (H.-C.Y.); +1-615-322-7416 (V.K.)

Abstract: Lymphatic vessels are highly responsive to changes in the interstitial environment. Previously, we showed renal lymphatics express the Na-K-2Cl cotransporter. Since interstitial sodium retention is a hallmark of proteinuric injury, we examined whether renal sodium affects NKCC1 expression and the dynamic pumping function of renal lymphatic vessels. Puromycin aminonucleoside (PAN)-injected rats served as a model of proteinuric kidney injury. Sodium ^{23}Na/^{1}H-MRI was used to measure renal sodium and water content in live animals. Renal lymph, which reflects the interstitial composition, was collected, and the sodium analyzed. The contractile dynamics of isolated renal lymphatic vessels were studied in a perfusion chamber. Cultured lymphatic endothelial cells (LECs) were used to assess direct sodium effects on NKCC1. MRI showed elevation in renal sodium and water in PAN. In addition, renal lymph contained higher sodium, although the plasma sodium showed no difference between PAN and controls. High sodium decreased contractility of renal collecting lymphatic vessels. In LECs, high sodium reduced phosphorylated NKCC1 and SPAK, an upstream activating kinase of NKCC1, and eNOS, a downstream effector of lymphatic contractility. The NKCC1 inhibitor furosemide showed a weaker effect on ejection fraction in isolated renal lymphatics of PAN vs controls. High sodium within the renal interstitium following proteinuric injury is associated with impaired renal lymphatic pumping that may, in part, involve the SPAK-NKCC1-eNOS pathway, which may contribute to sodium retention and reduce lymphatic responsiveness to furosemide. We propose that this lymphatic vessel dysfunction is a novel mechanism of impaired interstitial clearance and edema in proteinuric kidney disease.

Keywords: kidney; lymphatics; sodium; NKCC1 transporter

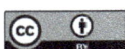

1. Introduction

Sodium retention is a well-documented consequence of many pathophysiological conditions, especially kidney disease, which is clinically recognized as an accumulation of edema [1]. Previous studies found sodium retention in skin and muscle is connected to blood pressure regulation involving lymphatic remodeling [2–4]. Recent research indicates that sodium, along with water, accumulates systemically, including in the lung, liver, muscle, and myocardium [5,6]. While kidneys have a central role in regulating sodium homeostasis, few studies have quantified kidney sodium or water content, including in edema-forming conditions. Such studies have been primarily limited by a lack of methodology for sodium quantification in vivo. Recent developments in noninvasive sodium imaging by ^{23}Na-MRI provide an attractive tool for quantifying kidney sodium content in vivo. Moreover, although kidney disease is regularly accompanied by lymphatic vessel hyperplasia [7–14], whether disease-induced lymphangiogenesis is accompanied by disrupted renal lymphatic vessel dynamics is unknown. Lymphatics are important because unlike blood flow, which relies on the heart as a central pump, lymph flow is propelled by forces in the surrounding tissues and by active rhythmic contractions intrinsic to the lymphatic vessels themselves. These intrinsic mechanisms constitute a major force in lymphatic flow and are exquisitely sensitive to the microenvironment, for example, hydraulic pressure, shear stress, local tissue temperature, and sodium [15]. A recent study provides evidence that lymphangiogenesis accompanying arthritis in TNF-transgenic mice reflects intrinsic dysfunction in popliteal lymphatic vessels that is linked to NOS-dependent as well as independent impairment in lymphatic vessel dynamics that may drive arthritic damage of the joint [16]. Whether intrarenal sodium modulates the renal lymphatic contractions has not been reported.

Lymphatic vessel contractility is driven by action potentials that trigger Ca++ influx generated by ion channels and transporters. We recently showed the Na-K-2Cl cotransporter NKCC1, but not NKCC2, is expressed in renal lymphatic vessels [17]. While NKCC2 is best known for its actions on tubular epithelial cells responsible for the maintenance of sodium homeostasis, NKCC1 is increasingly recognized as a modulator of various unanticipated biological functions, including regulation of vascular tone [18]. Indeed, inhibition of NKCC1 and its activating kinases has become a novel antihypertensive strategy involving direct (non-diuretic) vascular dilation. However, in contrast to blood vessels, little is known about NKCC transporter expression, activity, or function in the lymphatic vascular network and how the microenvironment or disease alters these parameters. This is particularly relevant since the first line of intervention in the treatment of edema and underlying interstitial clearance impairment is NKCC inhibition by furosemide.

Here we assessed whether kidney injury affects renal sodium content, how a high-sodium environment alters the pumping dynamics of renal collecting lymphatic vessels, and the role of NKCC1 in this response.

2. Results

2.1. Proteinuric Kidney Injury Increased Renal Sodium

MRI analysis revealed that puromycin aminonucleoside nephropathy (PAN) injury leads to increased renal sodium content. Both the cortex and medulla in PAN-injured rats had significantly higher sodium than in control rats (Figure 1A). The renal cortex of PAN rats also showed increased water content compared with controls. Although a directionally similar trend occurred in the medulla of PAN-injured rats, the increase did not reach statistical significance (Figure 1B). In companion studies, we measured the sodium concentration in the lymph exiting the kidney, which is thought to reflect the composition within the renal interstitial compartment. These direct measurements revealed that sodium concentration in the renal lymph of PAN rats was significantly higher than in the lymph of control rats (Figure 2A). Sodium concentration in concurrently obtained serum samples was not different between PAN rats and controls (Figure 2B). These results indicate that, in addition to the well-documented proteinuria, hypoalbuminemia, and hyperlipidemia, PAN kidney injury leads to intrarenal sodium and water retention, especially in the renal cortex. Similar to dermal lymphatics of hypertensive animals, which transport excess sodium from the skin [4], our results show for the first time that renal lymphatics are a route for clearing excess sodium from the renal interstitium in the setting of proteinuric kidney injury.

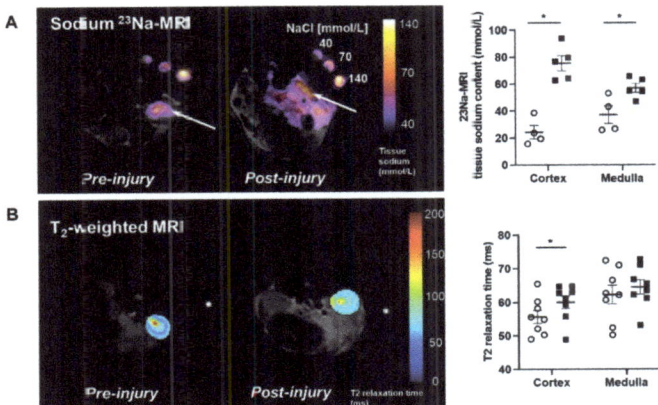

Figure 1. Proteinuric kidney injury increased renal sodium and water content. (**A**) Representative sodium ^{23}Na-MRI in uninjured control (Cont) (open circles) and puromycin (PAN)-injured rats (closed squares). The graph shows mean tissue sodium content localized in the cortex and medulla of the kidneys (arrows). (**B**) Representative T$_2$-weighted MRI images and quantitative T$_2$-relaxation time measurements indicative of renal cortical and medullary water content in Cont and PAN-injured rats. Results are expressed as mean ± SEM. n = 5 to 8 rats per group analyzed by unpaired t test. * $p < 0.05$.

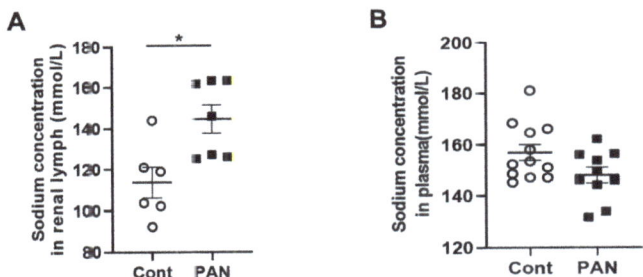

Figure 2. Proteinuric kidney injury increased sodium concentration in renal lymph. (**A**) Analysis of renal lymph showed higher sodium concentration in PAN-injured (closed squares) vs control rats (open circles). (**B**) Analysis of plasma showed no difference in sodium concentration between PAN-injured vs control rats. Results are expressed as mean ± SEM for 6 to 8 rats per group analyzed by unpaired t test. * $p < 0.05$.

2.2. High Sodium Environment Changed Contractility of Renal Lymphatic Vessels Involving the NKCC1 Transporter

To determine the effects of a high-sodium environment on renal lymphatic function, we measured the vasodynamics of renal afferent collecting lymphatic vessels. Similar to studies in afferent skin lymphatics [19], the contractility was assessed in renal afferent vessels isolated from normal rats exposed to normal buffer containing 143 mmol Na+ Krebs solution and compared with dynamics following exposure to Krebs solution containing a sodium concentration of 185 mmol. Compared with the physiologic buffer, a high-sodium environment had little effect on lymphatic contraction frequency. However, although high sodium caused only subtle changes in end diastolic diameter (EDD), a pronounced increase in end systolic diameter (ESD) contributed to reduced contraction amplitude and ejection fraction compared with the physiologic buffer (Figure 3).

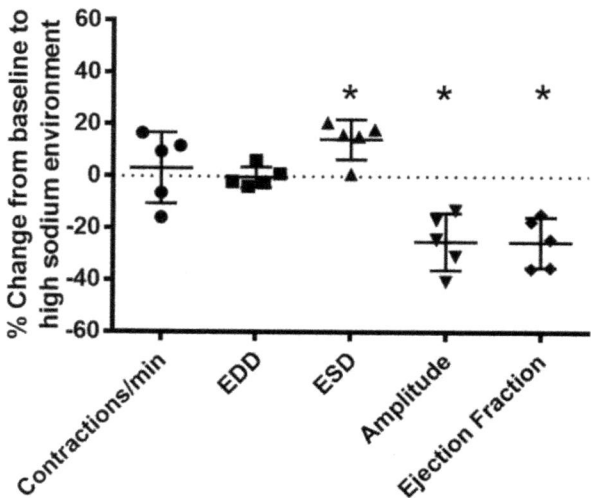

Figure 3. High salt environment altered renal collecting lymphatic vessel pumping function. Extra−renal afferent lymphatic vessels were subjected to a high−sodium buffer (185 mmol Na$^+$ Krebs solution). A digital image capture system was used to measure the following vessel pumping parameters: frequency of spontaneous contractions, end diastolic lumen diameter (EDD), end systolic lumen diameter (ESD), contraction amplitude, and ejection fraction. Exposure to a high−sodium environment caused a significant increase in ESD, resulting in a significant decrease in amplitude and ejection fraction. Data points represent the percent change from measurements captured under baseline conditions (143 mmol Na$^+$ Krebs solution) and are expressed as mean ± SEM. n = 5 individual vessels isolated from 5 rats. Significance was assessed by analyzing raw measurements using an unpaired t test. * $p < 0.05$.

NKCC1 regulates blood vessel dynamics, and our previous study confirmed expression of NKCC1 in lymphatic endothelial cells. However, it is unknown whether NKCC1 has a role in modulating microenvironmental influences on lymphatic vessel dynamics. This is interesting, as lymphatic vessels were recently reported to regulate sodium homeostasis. Renal lymphangiogenesis in mice with kidney-specific overexpression of VEGF-D increased urinary sodium excretion and reduced systemic blood pressure in salt-loaded hypertensive mice but not normotensive basal conditions [20]. The mechanism was linked to downregulation of sodium transporters, namely, total NCC and ENaCα in tubular epithelial cells. NKCC1 expression and renal lymphatic function were not evaluated. Our immunohistochemical staining verified prominent expression of NKCC1 in afferent renal lymphatic vessels (Figure 4A). Moreover, NKCC1 gene expression was increased in vessels from PAN-injured rats compared with controls (Figure 4B). Also, LECs exposed to a high-sodium environment had elevated NKCC1 mRNA compared with cells maintained in media with physiological levels of sodium (Figure 5A). Similar upregulation in NCKK1 mRNA occurred in response to urea that is equimolar to high sodium exposure. Since NKCC activity is determined by phosphorylation, we assessed phosphorated-NKCC1 protein. Our results show that a high-sodium environment significantly reduced expression of phosphorated-NKCC1 protein while the hyperosmolar urea control did not (Figure 5A). Furthermore, as NKCC activity is linked to phosphorylation of WNK-SPAK/OSR1 signaling cascade, we also examined expression of this upstream kinase [21,22]. Our data show that a high-sodium environment also reduced phosphorylated SPAK compared with the baseline sodium control group (Figure 5C) [21]. Among the vasoactive factors, eNOS is a major endothelial-derived mechanism regulating lymphatic dynamics, which is regulated by activity of NKCC1 [23]. Exposing LECs to a high-sodium environment caused a significant reduction in eNOS activity as measured by the amount of phosphorylated eNOS protein (Figure 6A). In contrast, increased osmolarity with urea did not significantly alter the endothelial eNOS activity although the eNOS activity was significantly higher than in cells exposed to a high-sodium environment, echoing reduced p-eNOS levels shown in cardiac tissues of rats fed a high-salt diet [24]. To determine the consequences of reduced NO signaling on renal lymphatic vessel pumping dynamics, we exposed isolated vessels to L-NAME in order to inhibit eNOS activity. This caused a significant increase in contraction frequency, but reduced EDD, magnitude of contraction, and ejection fraction (Figure 6B)

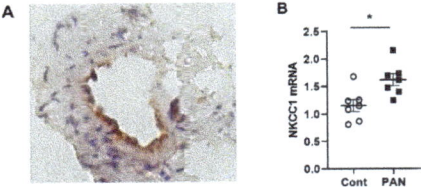

Figure 4. NKCC-1 transporter expression in renal lymphatic vessels and vessels with PAN proteinuric injury. (**A**) Immunostaining of afferent renal lymphatic vessels demonstrated NKCC1 transporter expression, particularly prominent in lymphatic endothelial cells. (**B**) NKCC1 mRNA levels in extra-renal lymphatic vessels were significantly greater in PAN-injured rats vs uninjured controls. Results are mean ± SEM for 7 rats per group analyzed by unpaired t test * $p < 0.05$.

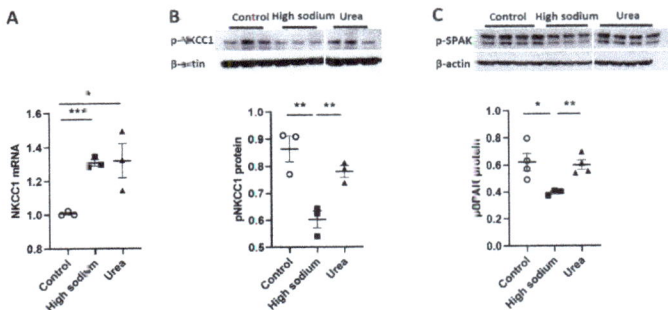

Figure 5. High Na$^+$ environment regulated NKCC-1 signaling pathway in lymphatic endothelial cells (LECs). (**A**) Cultured LECs exposed to a high-sodium environment showed greater expression of NKCC1 mRNA, (**B**) while expression of phosphorated NKCC-1 protein decreased. (**C**) High-sodium environment decreased protein expression of SPaK, an upstream activating kinase of NKCC1. Experiments were performed independently 3 times using 3 wells per treatment and analyzed by ANOVA followed by Dunnett multiple comparisons. * $p < 0.05$, ** $p < 0.01$, *** $p < 0.001$.

2.3. Kidney Injury Diminished the Lymphatic Vascular Response to a High-Sodium Environment and NKCC Inhibition by Furosemide

To gain further insight into the effects of kidney injury on renal lymphatic physiology, we compared the pumping dynamics of control vessels with vessels from a PAN-injured rat in a normal sodium environment (Figure 7). PAN-injured vessels had a significant increase in EDD (Figure 7B), which contributed to a marked decrease in contraction amplitude (Figure 7D) and ejection fraction (Figure 7E) compared with control vessels. Next, to investigate how a high-sodium environment affects vessels in the setting of kidney injury, we compared the lymphatic dynamics in the vessels of PAN-injured rats before and after exposure to a high-sodium environment (Figure 8). PAN-injured lymphatic vessels had a distinct response to a high-sodium environment compared with the response of control vessels (Figure 3), exhibiting a decreased EDD, and a decreased ejection fraction. This suggests that a high-sodium environment and PAN injury both result in reduced ejection fraction, albeit by different mechanisms.

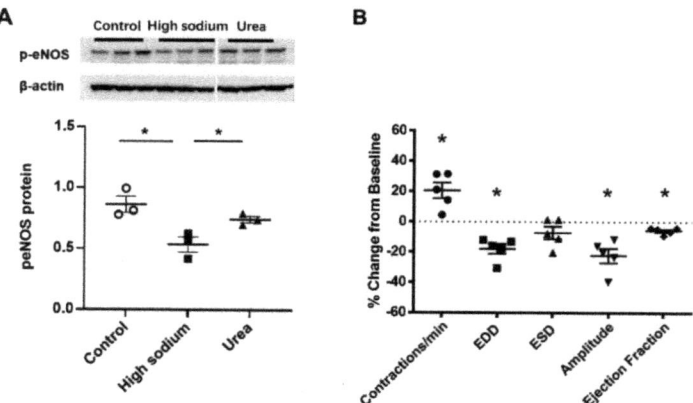

Figure 6. eNOS modulated lymphatic vessel function. (**A**) Cultured LECs exposed to high-sodium, but not high-osmolar environment showed reduced eNOS activity. (**B**) Isolated renal lymphatic vessels challenged with the eNOS inhibitor, L-NAME, exhibited increased contraction frequency and reduced EDD, amplitude, and ejection fraction. EDD, end diastolic diameter; ESD, end systolic diameter. Protein concentration results are expressed as mean ± SEM for 3 samples analyzed by ANOVA followed by Dunnett multiple comparison test. Vessel pumping parameters are expressed as the percent change from measurements captured under baseline conditions (143 mmol Na$^+$ Krebs solution) and are expressed as mean ± SEM for 5 individual vessels isolated from 5 rats. Significance was assessed by analyzing raw measurements using an unpaired t test. * $p < 0.05$.

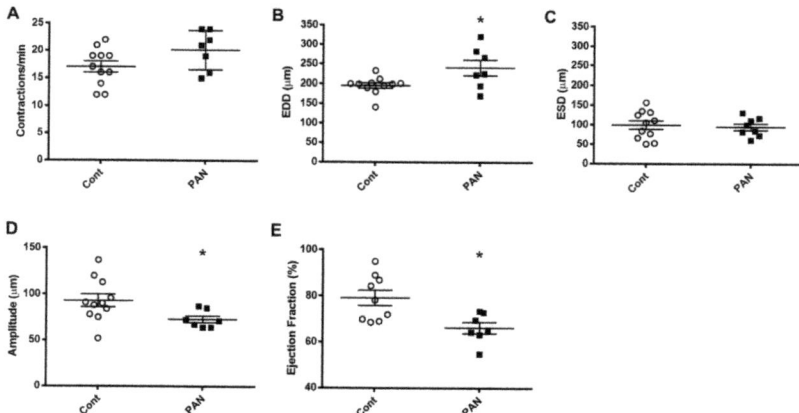

Figure 7. Kidney injury diminishes lymphatic vessel pumping efficiency. Vasodynamic parameters were measured in renal lymphatic vessels isolated from control and PAN-injured rats. Vessels from PAN-injured rats had significantly increased EDD (**B**), resulting in reduced contraction amplitude (**D**) and ejection fraction (**E**), while contraction frequency (**A**) and ESD (**C**) remained unchanged. Datapoints represent raw measurements from individual vessels isolated from 7 to 11 rats per group. Results are expressed as mean ± SEM analyzed by unpaired t test. * $p < 0.05$ EDD, end diastolic diameter; ESD, end systolic diameter.

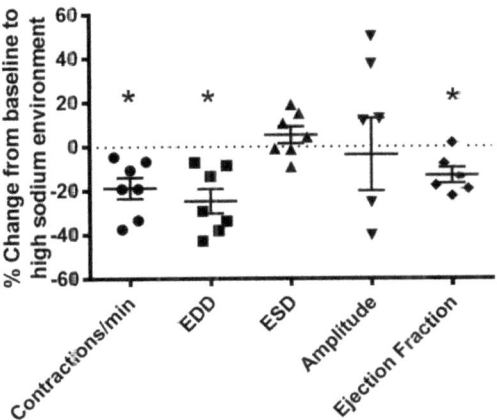

Figure 8. Vasodynamic response of PAN-injured lymphatic vessels exposed to a high-sodium environment. PAN-injured vessels exposed to high sodium had a significant decrease in the frequency of spontaneous contractions, EDD, and ejection compared with PAN-injured vessels in a normal sodium environment. Data points represent the percent change from measurements captured under normal sodium conditions and are expressed as mean ± SEM for 6 to 7 individual vessels isolated from 6 to 7 rats. Significance was assessed by analyzing raw measurements using an unpaired t test. * $p < 0.05$. EDD, end diastolic diameter; ESD, end systolic diameter.

Since injured lymphatic vessels appear to have weaker intrinsic compensatory responses to the high-sodium environment likely prevailing in a disease setting, we examined the effects of the NKCC1 inhibitor furosemide in PAN-injured and control vessels. Control vessels treated with furosemide had a pronounced concentration-dependent decrease in ejection fraction. In contrast, furosemide had more subtle effects on the ejection fraction of PAN-injured vessels, with PAN vessels being significantly less affected by furosemide at physiologically relevant doses (Figure 9). Interestingly, there was no statistical difference in the effects of furosemide on PAN vessels in a normal or high-sodium environment. These results indicate that analogous to a high-sodium environment and PAN-induced kidney injury, furosemide exerts directionally similar moderating effects on lymphatic dynamics that may affect renal interstitial clearance.

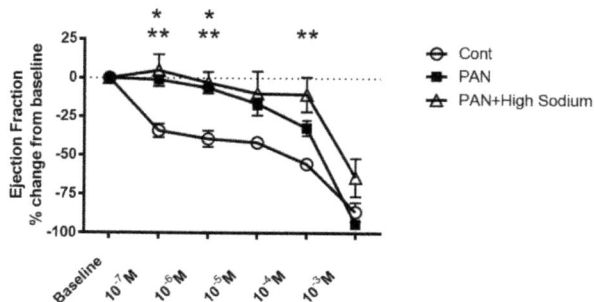

Figure 9. Kidney injury and exposure to elevated sodium blunt lymphatic vessel response to NKCC inhibition by furosemide. Renal lymphatic vessels isolated from PAN-injured rats and normal controls were subjected to increasing concentrations of the NKCC antagonist furosemide. Some PAN vessels were challenged with furosemide in a high-sodium environment. In control vessels, furosemide induces a robust decrease in ejection fraction. In contrast, PAN-injured vessels in normal and high-sodium environments are significantly less sensitive to furosemide. Data points represent the percent change from measurements captured at baseline conditions and are expressed as mean ± SEM for <6 individual vessels isolated from <6 rats. Significance ($p < 0.05$) was analyzed by ANOVA followed by Dunnett multiple comparisons. * PAN vessels compared with control vessels, ** PAN vessels in high sodium compared with control vessels.

3. Discussion

A high-sodium environment is a critical modulator of lymphatic vessels. Although kidneys are central in Na+ homeostasis, little is understood about Na+ effects on renal lymphatics. The current studies provide new insights into regulation of renal lymphatic network by showing (1) proteinuric kidney injury increases renal Na+ by ^{23}Na/1H MRI and direct sampling of renal lymphatic fluid shows elevated Na+ concentration while plasma Na+ is unchanged (2) high Na+ and furosemide inhibition of NKCC1 decrease lymphatic vessel contraction amplitude and ejection fraction in isolated renal lymphatic vessels, (3) a high Na+ environment decreases phosphorated-NKCC1, phosphorylated SPAK, an upstream kinase, and phosphorylated eNOS, a downstream vasoactive factor, and (4) a high Na+ environment together with renal injury contribute to a blunted lymphatic response in PAN-injured kidneys.

Noninvasive imaging by ^{23}Na/1H MRI showed that proteinuric kidney injury leads to accumulation of sodium and water in the in vivo kidneys. This new observation reflects advances in multi-nuclear imaging technology that exploit endogenous ^{23}Na, the second most abundant magnetic nuclei in living systems [25]. Imaging methods are advantageous for longitudinal measurement of tissue sodium before and after intervention, localization of tissue sodium in renal sub-compartments, and comparison of multi-modal data, strategies explored in this study. The findings of this study demonstrate ^{23}Na-MRI quantification of renal sodium as a potential biomarker of renal disease involving lymphatic clearance dysfunction. Imaging results, supported by data, suggest that lymph exiting proteinuric kidneys has significantly higher sodium concertation than the renal lymph of normal, uninjured control rats. Sodium levels in the blood of these proteinuric animals were not different from normal rats. To date, there are only sparse data on the composition of renal lymph, especially in disease settings, although more than 50 years ago, two studies describing partial occlusion of the inferior vena cava model of right heart failure found increased renal lymphatic flow and sodium content [26,27]. More recently, sodium accumulation in the skin of salt-sensitive hypertensive rats was shown to be accompanied by increased sodium concentration in lymph collected from dermal lymphatic vessels, while no change in the circulating level of sodium was observed [4]. These findings reinforce the concept that lymph reflects the composition of the interstitial compartment of the draining organ. Our data make the original observation that kidney injury leads to renal sodium accumulation, although the study did not localize sodium to any specific interstitial compartment [1]. Sodium accumulation in the interstitium has been linked to the modulation of lymphatic vessels, especially lymphangiogenesis. This has been most extensively studied in the skin of hypertensive animals and humans and involves transcription factor tonicity-responsive enhancer protein (TonEBP)-induced macrophage secretion of vascular endothelial growth factor-C (VEGF-C) [4]. Although kidney injury causes renal lymphangiogenesis and modulates sodium reabsorption and excretion, there have been no studies on the possible effects of accumulating interstitial sodium on renal lymphatic function. We now show that direct exposure of renal lymphatic vessels to a high-sodium environment increases the frequency of contraction in the renal collecting lymphatic vessels and reduces the contraction amplitude, and, to a lesser extent, the ejection fraction (Figure 3). These results complement findings that a high-salt diet, or DOCA treatment that increases sodium in skin and muscle, increases contraction frequency while reducing contraction amplitude [19]. These observations are timely, since strategies to improve interstitial clearance currently target lymphatic network growth, although the efficacy appears to be context-dependent. Thus, activation of the VEGF-C–VEGFR-3 pathway to promote lymphangiogenesis can reduce kidney fibrosis and lessen cystic kidney disease in mice and rats [9]. Also, kidney-specific overexpression of VEGF-D before injury increased lymphatic density and amplified recovery from ischemia-reperfusion damage [28]. In contrast, inhibition of VEGFR-3 reduces kidney lymphangiogenesis, glomerulosclerosis, and tubulointerstitial fibrosis in a mouse model of diabetic kidney disease as well as fibrosis following UUO and ischemia-reperfusion [10]. Our data suggest that high interstitial sodium blunts lymphatic dynamics and may be a critical factor contributing to the efficacy of therapeutic intervention.

Currently, the first-line therapy to reduce sodium overload in a variety of diseases, including kidney disease, is inhibition of NKCC cotransporter with furosemide. Immunohistochemical staining clearly demonstrated NKCC1 in endothelial cells of renal collecting lymphatic vessels, and quantitation of mRNA showed increased gene expression in PAN vessels vs collecting vessels of uninjured kidneys (Figure 5). However, a high-sodium environment significantly reduced phosphorylation of NKCC1 in LECs, (Figure 6). Moreover, a high-sodium environment also reduced phosphorylation of SPAK, the upstream kinase of NKCC1, suggesting sodium dampens lymphatic contractility. Previous studies showed high salt downregulated phosphorylation and ubiquitination of WNK [29], which reduced expression of SPAK and NKCC1. Zeniya et al. showed suppressed phosphorylation of NKCC1 on mouse aortae fed a high-salt diet and stimulated phosphorylation of NKCC1 in mice on a low-salt diet [22]. Similar to our results with direct sodium exposure, a high-salt diet caused a divergent effect on the gene and protein expression of upstream kinases. Together, these data fit well with evidence that, aside from maintaining extracellular fluid volume, sodium acts as a signaling molecule.

NKCC1 activity can contribute to both vasoconstriction and vasodilation. Vasoconstrictors such as norepinephrine, endothelin, and angiotensin II directly activate NKCC1 activity in vascular smooth muscle cells, causing constriction, while NO and sodium nitroprusside inhibit NKCC1, resulting in vasodilation [30,31]. High-sodium environments reduce phosphorylated eNOS, which would predict reduced vasodilation but increased contractility. Indeed, inhibiting NO signaling with L-NAME decreased end diastolic and end systolic vessel diameter, the amplitude of contraction, calculated ejection fraction, and increased contraction frequency in renal lymphatic vessels (Figure 6B). Interestingly, previous studies confirm that a high-salt diet and/or direct exposure of lymphatic vessels to a high-sodium environment increases contraction frequency in skin and muscle lymphatics and inguinal lymphatic vessels of mice and rats [19,32,33].

Our data clearly show that a high-sodium environment directly blunts lymphatic dynamics (Figure 3). Since lymphatic vessels are exquisitely sensitive to environmental stimuli, other molecules within the renal interstitial compartment including vasoactive substances, for example, angiotensin II, may also play a role in lymphatic dynamic functions.

However, comparison with vessels from PAN-injured kidneys exposed to a high-sodium environment revealed that renal injury is an additive contributor to lymphatic dysfunction (Figure 7). Thus, injured vessels exposed to high sodium showed diminution in their ability to respond to a pathological shift in their environment. This constellation of findings predicts impaired drainage of the renal interstitium in settings where a high interstitial sodium environment may prevail, such as in congestive heart failure, cirrhosis, and acute and chronic kidney disease. Moreover, these are the very conditions that show relative resistance to interventions that promote sodium excretion by inhibition of NKCC1. Notably, the ejection fraction in PAN-injured vessels is less affected by increasing concentrations of furosemide (Figure 9). Currently, therapeutic resistance to these agents centers on impaired delivery of the therapeutic to the relevant tubular segment. However, based on our data, we propose that dysfunction of renal lymphatic vessels is related to electrolyte abnormalities in the microenvironment of the kidney.

4. Materials and Methods

4.1. Animal Experiments

Male Sprague–Dawley rats (Charles River) weighing 180 g to 250 g were housed in a facility with 1:1 light/dark cycle. The animals were acclimated for at least 7 days and had free access to food and water. The well-established model of puromycin aminonucleoside nephropathy (PAN) was achieved by injecting puromycin aminoglycoside dissolved in 0.9% saline (125 mg/kg body weight i.p.). Rats injected with 0.9% saline served as controls. Eight days later, renal afferent lymphatic vessels were harvested for pressure myography. In a separate subset of PAN and control rats, renal lymph was collected using a glass pipette. The animal protocol was approved by Vanderbilt University Medical Center Institutional Animal Care and Use Committee in accordance with National Institutes of Health guidelines.

4.2. Magnetic Resonance Imaging Acquisition

Imaging experiments were performed in the Vanderbilt University Institute of Imaging Science (VUIIS) Center for Small Animal Imaging. Live animals were anesthetized and respiration and temperature were continuously monitored during imaging. Sodium MRI was acquired with custom-built, single-tuned sodium (^{23}Na) surface coil (approximately 2 cm in diameter) placed over the kidney and the animal positioned prone in a 63 mm quadrature proton (1H) volume coil in a 9.4T scanner (Agilent Technologies, Santa Clara, CA, USA). Sodium standards (NaCl in milli-q water with concentrations 40, 70, 140 mmol/L) were incorporated in the image field-of-view (FOV) to calibrate ^{23}Na signal intensity to standard sodium concentrations. Sodium MRI was acquired using a gradient echo multi-slice sequence with repetition time (TR) = 150 ms, echo time (TE) = 1.45 ms, FOV = 80×80 mm^2, matrix = 32×32 interpolated to 128×128, slice thickness = 20 mm, and the number of experiments (NEX) = 100. Anatomical T1-weighted images were acquired in an identical FOV as sodium MRI with a fast spin-echo sequence (TR/TE = 2000/20 ms, matrix = 128×128, number of slices = 10, slice thickness = 2 mm, and NEX = 4 respiratory-triggered gated acquisitions), sufficient to locate renal compartments.

Quantitative T_2 mapping, which measures the transverse relaxation rate of water protons in tissue, is a commonly used technique both clinically and pre-clinically for identifying and evaluating edema [34,35]. Proton MRI for T_2 relaxation time quantification was acquired at 7T (Bruker Avance III) in live animals with the kidneys centered in a 72 mm quadrature proton (1H) volume coil (Bruker Biospin). A water standard (3 mm NMR tube filled with 5 mM copper sulfate (CuSO$_4$) in distilled water) was placed next to the left kidney. High spatial-resolution T_2-weighted anatomical imaging was performed using a RARE (Rapid Acquisition with Relaxation Enhancement) sequence with TR/TE = 2000/45 ms, FOV = 70×70 mm^2, slice thickness = 1 mm, matrix = 128×128, with 28–36 slices covering the kidneys bilaterally, and NEX = 8. In one axial slice through the center of each kidney, multi-spin-echo imaging was performed for T_2-relaxation time mapping (TR = 2000 ms, echo spacing = 7 ms, 16 echoes, FOV = 70 × 70 mm^2, matrix = 64 × 64, NEX = 4).

Image Analysis

Renal tissue sodium content maps were calculated voxel-wise. First, a calibration curve was calculated as the least-squares linear regression fit of the mean ^{23}Na signal intensity in each standard solution to their known concentrations (40, 70, 140 mmol/L). The calibration curve was applied voxel-wise to calculate tissue sodium content (TSC, mmol/L) in the imaged kidney. T_2 relaxation time maps were calculated voxel-wise for each kidney using a nonlinear least-squares fit of the 1H signal intensity at each echo time, normalized by 1H signal in a standard water phantom, to a monoexponential decay function. Anatomical images were used to segment regions of interest (ROIs) manually in renal compartments consisting of the cortex, medulla, and papilla. Mean TSC (mmol/L) and T_2 relaxation time (ms) metrics were calculated in each ROI and preserved for statistical analyses.

4.3. Serum and Lymph Sodium Analysis

Colorimetric sodium assay kit (Abcam) was used to measure sodium concentration in serum and lymph according to the manufacturers' instructions.

4.4. Measurement of Lymphatic Vessels Contractility

Afferent extra-renal lymphatic collecting vessels were isolated by microdissection and lymphangions mounted on glass pipets in vessel perfusion chambers as reported [17]. A digital image capture system (IonOptix) was used to record pre-valve intraluminal diameters. Vessels were warmed to 37 °C, pressurized to 0.5 mmHg using a column of Krebs buffer, and allowed to equilibrate (20–60 min) before incrementally increasing the intraluminal pressure to 2.5 mmHg. Vessels that failed to contract spontaneously were excluded from further study. For high-sodium environment studies, the vessels were exposed to a modified high-sodium Krebs buffer (see below). Some vessels were also challenged with increasing concentrations of furosemide (10-7-10-3M, Hospira). For each experimental condition, lumen diameters were allowed to plateau (20–40 min) before moving to the next condition. Single vessels were exposed to 1 to 3 compounds over the course of each experiment. We found no difference in response or viability based on the order of compound administration. As previously reported [17,36], the amplitude of contraction was measured as the difference between the end diastolic diameter and end systolic diameter (EDD-ESD). The ejection fraction was calculated as (EDD2-ESD2)/EDD2.

Buffers

Standard Krebs buffer contained the following: 109 mM NaCl, 4.7 mM KCl, 2.5 mM CaCl$_2$, 0.9 mM MgSO$_4$, 1 mM KH$_2$PO$_4$, 11.1 mM glucose, 34 mM NaHCO$_3$. High-sodium Krebs buffer contained the following: 151 mM NaCl, 4.7 mM KCl, 2.5 mM CaCl$_2$, 0.9 mM MgSO$_4$, 1 mM KH$_2$PO$_4$, 11.1 mM glucose, 34 mM NaHCO$_3$.

4.5. Reverse Transcription Quantitative Real-Time PCR

Lymphatic vessels were homogenized in RLT and β-ME buffer using a rotating homogenizer. Cultured cells were harvested directly from culture plates with RLT-β-ME buffer and the RNA extracted using Qiagen RNeasy Mini Kit by standard protocol. Taq-Man Reverse Transcription Kit (Applied Biosystems, Waltham, MA, USA) was used for reverse transcription. β-actin was used as endogenous control and fold difference in gene expression data was calculated by $2^{-\Delta\Delta Ct}$ method. Human and rat NKCC1 and β-actin primers were bought from Thermo Fisher Scientific.

4.6. Immunohistochemical Staining

Renal lymphatic vessels were collected from rats, fixed in the 4% paraformaldehyde, and embedded in paraffin. Three-micron paraffin sections were stained with the standard protocol. For NKCC1 staining, tissues were deparaffinized and then antigen retrieved with citrate buffer (pH = 6.0). After blocking with 2.5% normal horse serum, the tissue was incubated with anti-NKCC1 antibody (Boster Bio, 1:1000, Pleasanton, CA, USA) overnight and then incubated with anti-rabbit secondary antibody. Negative control was prepared by omitting the primary antibody.

4.7. Cell Culture

Adult lymphatic endothelial cells (LECs) (PromoCell) were cultured with endothelial cell growth medium (PromoCell). After starvation with serum-free medium at passage 5–6, LECs were incubated in normal medium (control group, (Na+) = 145 mmol/L) and high-sodium medium ((Na+) = 185 mmol/L) for 24 h. Urea (Sigma–Aldrich, St. Louis, MO, USA) group was used to control for potential osmolarity effects. RT-PCR was performed for *Nkcc1* mRNA quantification. Total protein was extracted for quantitation of NKCC1, SPAK, and eNOS.

4.8. Western Blot

Cells were lysed in RIPA with phosphatase inhibitor and protease inhibitor (Roche). Anti-phospho-NKCC1 antibody (Millipore, 1:5000), anti-phospho-SPAK antibody (Millipore, 1:4000), anti-phospho-eNOS antibody (Millipore, 1:8000), and anti-rabbit secondary antibody were used to detect phosphorate-NKCC1 and phosphorate-SPAK. The two most thoroughly studied sites of phospho-eNOS are the activation site Ser1177 and the inhibitory site Thr495. Several protein kinases, including Akt/PKB, PKA, and AMPK activate eNOS by phosphorylating Ser1177 in response to various stimuli. In our study, we used anti-phospho-eNOS antibody (Ser1177). Sample loading was measured by β-actin (1:30,000) with anti-mouse as secondary antibody.

4.9. Statistical Analysis

Data are presented as mean ± standard error of mean. T-test was used for comparison between the two groups, and the ANOVA analysis was used for the comparison between multiple groups. $p < 0.05$ was considered to be statistically significant.

5. Conclusions

Based on our data, we propose that dysfunction of renal lymphatic vessels is related to electrolyte abnormalities. Furthermore, although lymphangiogenesis has been firmly established to accompany these conditions, our data suggest that sodium-induced lymphatic dysfunction compounds the problem of impaired fluid clearance in the setting of kidney injury. Sodium accumulation suppresses the pumping function of renal lymphatic vessels by inhibiting the SPAK-NKCC1 cascade. These results imply that the lymphatic system should be viewed as a potential target in disease characterized by sodium accumulation, such as various renal diseases or heart failure.

Author Contributions: Conceptualization, V.K.; Methodology, J.L., E.L.S., R.C., D.C.C., J.Z. and H.-C.Y.; Software, J.L, E.L.S., R.C., D.C.C., J.Z. and H.-C.Y.; Validation, J.L., E.L.S., R.C., D.C.C. and H.-C.Y.; Formal Analysis, J.L., E.L.S., R.C., D.C.C. and H.-C.Y.; Resources, J.L., E.L.S., R.C., D.C.C., A.K., E.J.D. and H.-C.Y.; Writing—Original Draft Preparation, J.L., E.L.S. and R.C., Writing—Review & Editing, J.L., E.L.S., R.C., D.C.C., A.K., E.J.D., H.-C.Y. and V.K.; Visualization, J.L., E.L.S., D.C.C., A.K., H.-C.Y. and V.K.; Project Administration, H.-C.Y. and V.K.; Funding Acquisition, V.K. All authors have read and agreed to the published version of the manuscript.

Funding: The work was supported by NIH 1P01HL116263, K01HL13049, R03HL155041 and R01HL144941.

Institutional Review Board Statement: All procedures were approved by the Institutional Animal Care and Use Committee of VUMC and conducted according to the NIH's *Guide for the Care and Use of Laboratory Animals* (National Academies Press, 2011).

Informed Consent Statement: Not applicable.

Data Availability Statement: All data and other materials can be obtained from authors.

Conflicts of Interest: The authors declare no conflict of interest.

References

1. Ellison, D.H.; Welling, P. Insights into Salt Handling and Blood Pressure. *N. Engl. J. Med.* **2021**, *385*, 1981–1993. [CrossRef] [PubMed]
2. Mullins, L.; Ivy, J.; Ward, M.; Tenstad, O.; Wiig, H.; Kitada, K.; Manning, J.; Rakova, N.; Muller, D.; Mullins, J. Abnormal Neonatal Sodium Handling in Skin Precedes Hypertension in the SAME Rat. *Pflugers Arch.* **2021**, *473*, 897–910. [CrossRef] [PubMed]
3. Rabelink, T.J.; Rotmans, J.I. Salt Is Getting Under Our Skin. *Nephrol. Dial. Transplant.* **2009**, *24*, 3282–3283. [CrossRef] [PubMed]
4. Wiig, H.; Schröder, A.; Neuhofer, W.; Jantsch, J.; Kopp, C.; Karlsen, T.V.; Boschmann, M.; Goss, J.; Bry, M.; Rakova, N.; et al. Immune Cells Control Skin Lymphatic Electrolyte Homeostasis and Blood Pressure. *J. Clin. Investig.* **2013**, *123*, 2803–2815. [CrossRef] [PubMed]
5. Matthay, M.A.; Zemans, R.L.; Zimmerman, G.A.; Arabi, Y.M.; Beitler, J.R.; Mercat, A.; Herridge, M.; Randolph, A.G.; Calfee, C.S. Acute Respiratory Distress Syndrome. *Nat. Rev. Dis. Primers* **2019**, *5*, 18. [CrossRef]
6. Rossitto, G.; Mary, S.; Chen, J.Y.; Boder, P.; Chew, K.S.; Neves, K.B.; Alves, R.L.; Montezano, A.C.; Welsh, P.; Petrie, M.C.; et al. Tissue Sodium Excess Is Not Hypertonic and Reflects Extracellular Volume Expansion. *Nat. Commun.* **2020**, *11*, 4222. [CrossRef]
7. Abouelkheir, G.R.; Upchurch, B.D.; Rutkowski, J.M. Lymphangiogenesis: Fuel, Smoke, or Extinguisher of Inflammation's Fire? *Exp. Biol. Med. (Maywood)* **2017**, *242*, 884–895. [CrossRef]
8. Donnan, M.D.; Kenig-Kozlovsky, Y.; Quaggin, S.E. The Lymphatics in Kidney Health and Disease. *Nat. Rev. Nephrol.* **2021**, *17*, 655–675. [CrossRef]
9. Hasegawa, S.; Nakano, T.; Torisu, K.; Tsuchimoto, A.; Eriguchi, M.; Haruyama, N.; Masutani, K.; Tsuruya, K.; Kitazono, T. Vascular Endothelial Growth Factor-C Ameliorates Renal Interstitial Fibrosis through Lymphangiogenesis in Mouse Unilateral Ureteral Obstruction. *Lab. Investig.* **2017**, *97*, 1439–1452. [CrossRef]
10. Hwang, S.D.; Song, J.H.; Kim, Y.; Lim, J.H.; Kim, M.Y.; Kim, E.N.; Hong, Y.A.; Chung, S.; Choi, B.S.; Kim, Y.S.; et al. Inhibition of Lymphatic Proliferation by the Selective VEGFR-3 Inhibitor SAR131675 Ameliorates Diabetic Nephropathy in db/db Mice. *Cell Death Dis.* **2019**, *10*, 219. [CrossRef]
11. Kerjaschki, D.; Huttary, N.; Raab, I.; Regele, H.; Bojarski-Nagy, K.; Bartel, G.; Kröber, S.M.; Greinix, H.; Rosenmaier, A.; Karlhofer, F.; et al. Lymphatic Endothelial Progenitor Cells Contribute to De Novo Lymphangiogenesis in Human Renal Transplants. *Nat. Med.* **2006**, *12*, 230–234. [CrossRef] [PubMed]
12. Pei, G.; Yao, Y.; Yang, Q.; Wang, M.; Wang, Y.; Wu, J.; Wang, P.; Li, Y.; Zhu, F.; Yang, J.; et al. Lymphangiogenesis in Kidney and Lymph Node Mediates Renal Inflammation and Fibrosis. *Sci. Adv.* **2019**, *5*, eaaw5075. [CrossRef] [PubMed]
13. Yazdani, S.; Poosti, F.; Kramer, A.B.; Mirković, K.; Kwakernaak, A.J.; Hovingh, M.; Stagman, M.C.; Sjollema, K.A.; de Borst, M.H.; Navis, G.; et al. Proteinuria Triggers Renal Lymphangiogenesis Prior to the Development of Interstitial Fibrosis. *PLoS ONE* **2012**, *7*, e50209. [CrossRef] [PubMed]
14. Zarjou, A.; Black, L.M.; Bolisetty, S.; Traylor, A.M.; Bowhay, S.A.; Zhang, M.Z.; Harris, R.C.; Agarwal, A. Dynamic Signature of Lymphangiogenesis During Acute Kidney Injury and Chronic Kidney Disease. *Lab. Investig.* **2019**, *99*, 1376–1388. [CrossRef]
15. Solari, E.; Marcozzi, C.; Negrini, D.; Moriondo, A. Lymphatic Vessels and Their Surroundings: How Local Physical Factors Affect Lymph Flow. *Biology* **2020**, *9*, 463. [CrossRef] [PubMed]
16. Scallan, J.P.; Bouta, J.P.; Rahimi, H.; Kenney, H.M.; Ritchlin, C.T.; Davis, C.T.; Schwarz, E.M. Ex vivo Demonstration of Functional Deficiencies in Popliteal Lymphatic Vessels From TNF-Transgenic Mice With Inflammatory Arthritis. *Front. Physiol.* **2021**, *12*, 745096. [CrossRef]
17. Shelton, E.L.; Yang, H.C.; Zhong, J.; Salzman, M.M.; Kon, V. Renal Lymphatic Vessel Dynamics. *Am. J. Physiol. Renal. Physiol.* **2020**, *319*, F1027–F1036. [CrossRef]
18. Dormans, T.P.; Pickkers, P.; Russel, F.G.; Smits, P. Vascular Effects of Loop Diuretics. *Cardiovasc. Res.* **1996**, *32*, 988–997. [CrossRef]
19. Karlsen, T.V.; Nikpey, E.; Han, J.; Reikvam, T.; Rakova, N.; Castorena-Gonzalez, J.A.; Davis, M.J.; Titze, J.M.; Tenstad, O.; Wiig, H. High-Salt Diet Causes Expansion of the Lymphatic Network and Increased Lymph Flow in Skin and Muscle of Rats. *Arter. Thromb. Vasc. Biol.* **2018**, *38*, 2054–2064. [CrossRef]
20. Balasubbramanian, D.; Baranwal, G.; Clark, M.C.; Goodlett, B.L.; Mitchell, B.M.; Rutkowski, J.M. Kidney-specific lymphangiogenesis increases sodium excretion and lowers blood pressure in mice. *J. Hypertens.* **2020**, *38*, 874–885. [CrossRef]
21. Delpire, E.; Gagnon, K.B. Na(+)-K(+)-2cl(−) Cotransporter (Nkcc) Physiological Function in Nonpolarized Cells and Transporting Epithelia. *Compr. Physiol.* **2018**, *8*, 871–901. [CrossRef]
22. Zeniya, M.; Sohara, E.; Kita, S.; Iwamoto, T.; Susa, K.; Mori, T.; Oi, K.; Chiga, M.; Takahashi, D.; Yang, S.S.; et al. Dietary Salt Intake Regulates WNK3-SPAK-NKCC1 Phosphorylation Cascade in Mouse Aorta through Angiotensin II. *Hypertension* **2013**, *62*, 872–878. [CrossRef] [PubMed]
23. Baldwin, S.N.; Sandow, S.L.; Mondéjar-Parreño, G.; Stott, J.B.; Greenwood, I.A. K(V)7 Channel Expression and Function within Rat Mesenteric Endothelial Cells. *Front. Physiol.* **2020**, *11*, 598779. [CrossRef] [PubMed]
24. Li, Y.; Wu, X.; Mao, Y.; Liu, C.; Wu, Y.; Tang, J.; Zhao, K.; Li, P. Nitric Oxide Alleviated High Salt-Induced Cardiomyocyte Apoptosis and Autophagy Independent of Blood Pressure in Rats. *Front. Cell Dev. Biol.* **2021**, *9*, 646575. [CrossRef] [PubMed]

25. Madelin, G.; Lee, J.S.; Regatte, R.R.; Jerschow, A. Sodium MRI: Methods and Applications. *Prog. Nucl. Magn. Reson. Spectrosc.* **2014**, *79*, 14–47. [CrossRef] [PubMed]
26. Katz, Y.J.; Cockett, A.; Moor, R.S. Elevation of Inferior Vena Cava Pressure and Thoracic Lymph and Urine Flow. *Circ. Res.* **1959**, *7*, 118–122. [CrossRef]
27. Lebrie, S.J.; Mayerson, H.S. Influence of Elevated Venous Pressure on Flow and Composition of Renal Lymph. *Am. J. Physiol.* **1960**, *198*, 1037–1040. [CrossRef]
28. Baranwal, G.; Creed, H.A.; Black, L.M.; Auger, A.; Quach, A.M.; Vegiraju, R.; Eckenrode, H.E.; Agarwal, A.; Rutkowski, J.M. Expanded Renal Lymphatics Improve Recovery Following Kidney Injury. *Physiol. Rep.* **2021**, *9*, e15094. [CrossRef]
29. Zhao, X.; Lai, G.; Tu, J.; Liu, S.; Zhao, Y. Crosstalk between Phosphorylation and Ubiquitination Is Involved in High Salt-Induced WNK4 Expression. *Exp. Ther. Med.* **2021**, *21*, 133. [CrossRef]
30. Akar, F.; Jiang, G.; Paul, R.J.; O'Neill, W.C. Contractile Regulation of the Na(+)-K(+)-2cl(−) Cotransporter in Vascular Smooth Muscle. *Am. J. Physiol. Cell Physiol.* **2001**, *281*, C579–C584. [CrossRef]
31. Akar, F.; Skinner, E.; Klein, J.D.; Jena, M.; Paul, R.J.; O'Neill, W.C. Vasoconstrictors and Nitrovasodilators Reciprocally Regulate the Na+-K+-2cl- Cotransporter in Rat Aorta. *Am. J. Physiol.* **1999**, *276*, C1383–C1390. [CrossRef] [PubMed]
32. Kwon, S.; Agollah, G.D.; Sevick-Muraca, E.M.; Chan, W. Altered Lymphatic Function and Architecture in Salt-Induced Hypertension Assessed by Near-Infrared Fluorescence Imaging. *J. Biomed. Opt.* **2012**, *17*, 080504. [CrossRef]
33. Mizuno, R.; Isshiki, M.; Ono, N.; Nishimoto, M.; Fujita, T. A High-Salt Diet Differentially Modulates Mechanical Activity of Afferent and Efferent Collecting Lymphatics in Murine Iliac Lymph Nodes. *Lymphat. Res. Biol.* **2015**, *13*, 85–92. [CrossRef] [PubMed]
34. Hueper, K.; Gutberlet, M.; Brasen, J.H.; Jang, M.S.; Thorenz, A.; Chen, R.; Hertel, B.; Barrmeyer, A.; Schmidbauer, M.; Meier, M.; et al. Multiparametric Functional Mri: Non-Invasive Imaging of Inflammation and Edema Formation after Kidney Transplantation in Mice. *PLoS ONE* **2016**, *11*, e0162705. [CrossRef] [PubMed]
35. Schley, G.; Jordan, J.; Ellmann, S.; Rosen, S.; Eckardt, K.U.; Uder, M.; Willam, C.; Bauerle, T. Multiparametric Magnetic Resonance Imaging of Experimental Chronic Kidney Disease: A Quantitative Correlation Study with Histology. *PLoS ONE* **2018**, *13*, e0200259. [CrossRef]
36. Scallan, J.P.; Zawieja, S.D.; Castorena-Gonzalez, J.A.; Davis, M.J. Lymphatic Pumping: Mechanics, Mechanisms and Malfunction. *J. Physiol.* **2016**, *594*, 5749–5768. [CrossRef]

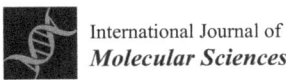

Article

Growth Hormone Improves Adipose Tissue Browning and Muscle Wasting in Mice with Chronic Kidney Disease-Associated Cachexia

Robert H. Mak [1,*], Sujana Gunta [1,2], Eduardo A. Oliveira [1,3] and Wai W. Cheung [1]

1. Division of Pediatric Nephrology, Rady Children's Hospital, University of California, San Diego, CA 92093, USA
2. Pediatric Services, Vista Community Clinic, Vista, CA 92084, USA
3. Department of Pediatrics, Health Sciences Postgraduate Program, School of Medicine, Federal University of Minas Gerais (UFMG), Belo Horizonte 30310-100, Brazil
* Correspondence: romak@health.ucsd.edu; Tel.: +1-858-822-6717; Fax: +1-858-822-6776

Abstract: Cachexia associated with chronic kidney disease (CKD) has been linked to GH resistance. In CKD, GH treatment enhances muscular performance. We investigated the impact of GH on cachexia brought on by CKD. CKD was induced by 5/6 nephrectomy in c57BL/6J mice. After receiving GH (10 mg/kg/day) or saline treatment for six weeks, CKD mice were compared to sham-operated controls. GH normalized metabolic rate, increased food intake and weight growth, and improved in vivo muscular function (rotarod and grip strength) in CKD mice. GH decreased uncoupling proteins (UCP)s and increased muscle and adipose tissue ATP content in CKD mice. GH decreased lipolysis of adipose tissue by attenuating expression and protein content of adipose triglyceride lipase and protein content of phosphorylated hormone-sensitive lipase in CKD mice. GH reversed the increased expression of beige adipocyte markers (UCP-1, CD137, Tmem26, Tbx1, Prdm16, Pgc1α, and Cidea) and molecules implicated in adipose tissue browning (Cox2/Pgf2α, Tlr2, Myd88, and Traf6) in CKD mice. Additionally, GH normalized the molecular markers of processes connected to muscle wasting in CKD, such as myogenesis and muscle regeneration. By using RNAseq, we previously determined the top 12 skeletal muscle genes differentially expressed between mice with CKD and control animals. These 12 genes' aberrant expression has been linked to increased muscle thermogenesis, fibrosis, and poor muscle and neuron regeneration. In this study, we demonstrated that GH restored 7 of the top 12 differentially elevated muscle genes in CKD mice. In conclusion, GH might be an effective treatment for muscular atrophy and browning of adipose tissue in CKD-related cachexia.

Keywords: chronic kidney disease; growth hormone; cachexia; lipolysis; adipose tissue browning; muscle mass; muscle function

1. Introduction

Cachexia in chronic kidney disease (CKD) results in profound loss of adipose tissue and muscle mass [1,2]. Although poor protein-calorie intake is a major factor, growth hormone (GH) resistance has been linked to CKD-associated cachexia [1–4]. GH increases muscle strength in healthy men [5]. Short-term administration of recombinant GH increases muscle protein synthesis and muscle mass as well as improves quality of life in hemodialysis patients [6–10]. However, most studies have used dual energy X-ray absorptiometry (DXA) to measure muscle mass as a surrogate marker for the effect of GH treatment in hemodialysis patients, but the validity of this extrapolation in CKD is questionable since DXA cannot differentiate between a true increase in muscle mass versus fluid overload [11]. Moreover, the effect of GH on muscle function in CKD has not been adequately studied [12]. We have previously described the pathways involved in muscle wasting in a mouse model of CKD [13]. IGF-I and myostatin represent yin-and-yang signaling pathways in the

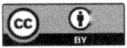

pathogenesis of CKD-associated cachexia muscle wasting [14]. GH resistance in CKD, due to signal transduction defects in JAK-STAT pathways, is associated with upregulated SOCS-2 and downregulated IGF-I in skeletal muscle [15]. Myostatin is overexpressed in CKD-associated wasting and is accompanied by increased protein degradation via FoxOs, Atrogin-1, and MuRF-1, and decreased myogenesis via Pax3 and MyoD [13].

Adipose tissue regulates whole-body energy metabolism. White adipose tissue (WAT) is a key energy reservoir, while brown adipose tissue (BAT) is involved in the regulation of thermogenesis [16]. Recent studies have demonstrated that WAT browning, a process characterized by a phenotypic transition from WAT to thermogenic BAT, is implicated in the pathogenesis of cachexia. Indeed, browning of WAT preceded skeletal muscle atrophy in mouse models of CKD and cancer [17,18]. GH regulates adipose tissue metabolism [19,20]. In this study, we investigate the effects and mechanisms of GH in a mouse model of CKD, with emphasis on adipose tissue browning and muscle wasting.

2. Results

2.1. GH Stimulates Food Intake and Increases Body Weight in CKD Mice

We empirically determined the optimal dose of GH treatments in our mouse model of CKD. Six-week-old c57BL/6J male mice were used for this study. Schematic representation of the experimental design is shown in Figure 1A. CKD in mice was induced by a two-stage subtotal nephrectomy, while a sham procedure was performed in control mice [13]. GH treatment was initiated in eight-week-old CKD or sham mice. CKD or sham mice were treated with recombinant human GH (5 mg/kg/day or 10 mg/kg/day, intraperitoneal) or vehicle for six weeks. During the treatment, all mice were housed in individual cage and fed ad libitum. Dietary intake as well as weight gain for each mouse was recorded weekly. Mice were sacrificed at the age of 14 weeks old. Serum and blood chemistry of CKD and sham mice are listed (Table 1). CKD mice were uremic, as CKD mice had a higher concentration of BUN and serum creatinine than control mice. Over the course of the six-week ad libitum experiment, GH stimulated food intake and improved weight gain in both CKD and sham mice. GH-treated CKD and GH-treated sham mice exhibited significantly more average daily energy intake and weight gain compared to vehicle-treated CKD and vehicle-treated sham mice, respectively (Figure 1B,C). More importantly, we found that CKD mice treated with 10 mg/kg/day demonstrated significantly improved food intake and weight gain relative to CKD mice treated with 5 mg/kg/day or vehicle. As a result, daily dosing of 10 mg/kg of GH for CKD mice was selected for the subsequent food-restrictive study.

Table 1. Serum and blood chemistry of mice from ad libitum study. Eight-week-old CKD and sham mice were treated with GH (5 mg/kg per day or 10 mg/kg per day) or normal saline as a vehicle for six weeks. All mice were fed ad libitum. Data are expressed as mean ± SEM. Results of all five groups of mice were compared to those of Sham + Vehicle mice, respectively. BUN, blood urea nitrogen. [a] $p < 0.05$, significantly higher than Sham + Vehicle mice.

	Sham + Vehicle (n = 9)	Sham + GH (5 mg/kg/day) (n = 9)	Sham + GH (10 mg/kg/day) (n = 9)	CKD + Vehicle (n = 9)	CKD + GH (5 mg/kg/day) (n = 9)	CKD + GH (10 mg/kg/day) (n = 9)
BUN (mg/dL)	34.5 ± 3.5	36.7 ± 4.6	32.6 ± 3.7	65.8 ± 6.9 [a]	75.6 ± 8.1 [a]	65.9 ± 5.8 [a]
Creatinine (mg/dL)	0.32 ± 0.11	0.35 ± 0.14	0.28 ± 0.09	0.57 ± 0.15 [a]	0.65 ± 0.13 [a]	0.75 ± 0.13 [a]

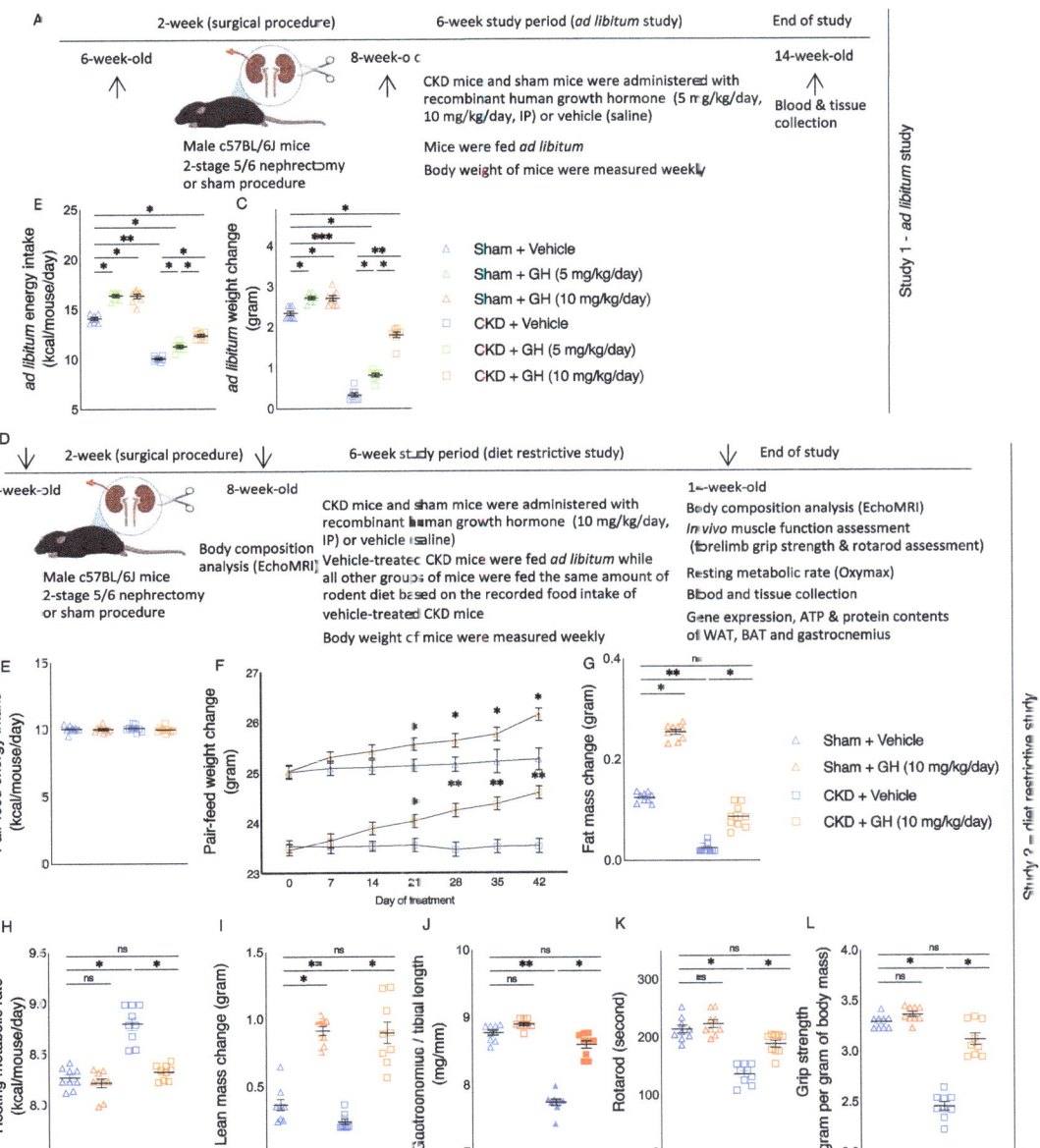

Figure 1. GH attenuates cachexia in CKD mice. We performed two studies. For the first study, we used ad libitum dietary strategy (**A**). CKD and control mice were given GH (5 mg/kg/day or 10 mg/kg/day), or vehicle (normal saline), respectively, for six weeks. All mice were fed ad libitum. We calculated average daily caloric intake (**B**) and recorded final weight change in mice (**C**). Results of Sham + GH (5 mg/kg/day) and Sham + GH (10 mg/kg/day) mice were compared to those of Sham + Vehicle mice, while results of CKD + GH (5 mg/kg/day) and CKD + GH (10 mg/kg/day) mice were compared to those of CKD + Vehicle mice. In addition, results of CKD + GH (5 mg/kg/day) mice were compared to those of CKD + GH (10 mg/kg/day) mice. Furthermore, results of CKD + Vehicle, CKD + GH (5 mg/kg/day), and CKD + GH (10 mg/kg/day) mice were compared to those of Sham + Vehicle,

Sham + GH (5 mg/kg/day), and Sham + GH (10 mg/kg/day) mice, respectively. Data are expressed as mean ± SEM. For comparison of the means between two groups, data were analyzed by Student's 2-tailed t-test. Differences of the means for more than two groups containing two variables were analyzed using two-way ANOVA. Posthoc analysis was performed with Tukey's test. Specific p-values are shown above the bar. * $p < 0.05$, ** $p < 0.01$, *** $p < 0.001$. ns signifies not significant. For the second experiment, we employed a diet-restrictive strategy (**D**). CKD + Vehicle mice were given an ad libitum amount of food, whereas other groups of mice were given an equivalent amount of food (**E**). Weight gain, fat content, resting metabolic rate, lean content, gastrocnemius weight relative to length of tibia, and in vivo muscle function (rotarod and grip strength) were measured (**F–L**). Results of Sham + GH (10 mg/kg/day) mice were compared to those of Sham + Vehicle mice, while results of CKD + GH (10 mg/kg/day) mice were compared to those of CKD + Vehicle mice. Furthermore, results of CKD + Vehicle and CKD + GH (10 mg/kg/day) mice were compared to those of Sham + Vehicle mice, respectively. Data are expressed as mean ± SEM. For comparison of the means between two groups, data were analyzed by Student's 2-tailed t-test. Posthoc analysis was performed with Tukey's test. Specific p-values are shown above the bar. ns signifies not significant, * $p < 0.05$, ** $p < 0.01$.

2.2. GH Improves Energy Homeostasis in CKD Mice

We utilized a food-restrictive strategy to study the pharmacological effects of GH in CKD mice beyond appetite stimulation and their consequent body weight gain (Figure 1D). Two-stage subtotal nephrectomy for CKD mice and a sham procedure for control mice were also performed. Eight-week-old CKD or sham mice were housed individually. Mice were given GH (10 mg/kg/day, intraperitoneal) or vehicle for six weeks. For this diet-restrictive study, vehicle-treated CKD mice were fed ad libitum, while the other mouse groups (GH-treated CKD mice as well as GH-treated or vehicle-treated sham mice) received an energy intake amount equal to that of vehicle-treated CKD mice (Figure 1E). Mice were sacrificed at the age of 14 weeks old. Serum and blood chemistry of mice are listed in Table 2. Vehicle- or GH-treated CKD mice were uremic, as they had a higher concentration of BUN and serum creatinine than sham mice. We verified that daily GH treatments resulted in high circulating concentrations of human GH in mice. Mean circulating human GH was not different between GH-treated CKD (325.3 ± 65.3 μg/L) and GH-treated control mice (364.6 ± 76.4 μg/L), whereas no human GH was detected in CKD or control mice receiving vehicle. A significant increase in weight gain in GH-treated CKD mice relative to vehicle-treated CKD mice was observed at day 21, and the trend remained significant for the rest of the study (Figure 1F). In addition, GH normalized fat and lean mass content, weight of gastrocnemius, resting metabolic rate, and in vivo muscle function (rotarod activity and grip strength) in CKD mice (Figure 1G–L).

Table 2. Serum and blood chemistry in mice from diet-restrictive study. Eight-week-old CKD and sham mice were treated with GH (10 mg/kg per day), or normal saline as a vehicle for six weeks. CKD mice were fed ad libitum. The other mouse groups received an energy intake amount equal to that of CKD + Vehicle mice. BUN, blood urea nitrogen. Results are analyzed and presented as in Table 1. [a] $p < 0.05$, significantly higher than Sham + Vehicle mice.

	Sham + Vehicle ($n = 9$)	Sham + GH (10 mg/kg/day) ($n = 9$)	CKD + Vehicle ($n = 9$)	CKD + GH (10 mg/kg/day) ($n = 9$)
BUN (mg/dL)	36.5 ± 5.8	26.7 ± 4.7	59.8 ± 7.4 [a]	72.8 ± 11.5 [a]
Creatinine (mg/dL)	0.25 ± 0.06	0.31 ± 0.13	0.63 ± 0.21 [a]	0.75 ± 0.25 [a]
Human GH (μg/L)	-	364.6 ± 76.4	-	325.3 ± 65.3

2.3. GH Improves Skeletal Muscle and Adipose Tissue Energy Homeostasis in CKD Mice

For the rest of the investigation, gastrocnemius, WAT, and BAT tissue from the diet-restrictive study were used. We studied the effects of GH on skeletal muscle and adipose tissue energy homeostasis in CKD mice. Protein content of UCPs in gastrocnemius as well as in WAT and BAT was significantly higher in vehicle-treated CKD mice (Figure 2A,C,E). Inversely, ATP content in gastrocnemius, WAT, and BAT was significantly lower in vehicle-treated CKD mice (Figure 2B,D,F). GH decreased UCPs but increased ATP content in muscle and adipose tissue in CKD mice.

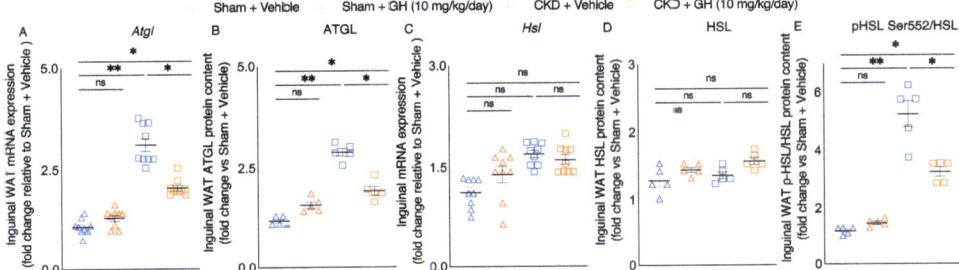

Figure 2. GH enhances energy balance in skeletal muscle and adipose tissue. Measurements were made of the UCP (A,C,E) and ATP contents (B,D,F) in gastrocnemius, WAT, and BAT. CKD mice were fed ad libitum, whereas other mouse groups received an energy intake amount equal to that of CKD + Vehicle mice. Comparisons were made between the outcomes of Sham + GH (10 mg/kg/day) mice and Sham + Vehicle mice, as well as between the outcomes of CKD + GH (10 mg/kg/day) mice and CKD + Vehicle mice. Additionally, the outcomes of the CKD + Vehicle and CKD + GH (10 mg/kg/day) mice were contrasted with those of the Sham + Vehicle mice. Data are expressed as mean ± SEM. For comparison of the means between two groups, data were analyzed by Student's 2-tailed t-test. Posthoc analysis was performed with Tukey's test. Specific p-values are shown above the bar. ns signifies not significant, * $p < 0.05$, ** $p < 0.01$

2.4. GH Mitigates Lipolytic Enzymes in CKD Mice

Elevated lipolysis is important for adipose tissue wasting in cachexia [21]. We investigated the molecular basis for the loss of adipose tissue in CKD mice. Inguinal WAT gene expression and protein content of adipose triglyceride lipase (ATGL) was significantly increased in vehicle-treated CKD mice (Figure 3A,B). Inguinal WAT gene expression and protein content of hormone-sensitive lipase (HSL) was not different among groups of mice (Figure 3C,D). However, phosphorylated HSL Ser552 protein content in inguinal WAT, a surrogate marker for protein kinase A-activated lipolysis, was five-fold higher in vehicle-treated CKD mice compared to control mice (Figure 3E). Importantly, GH significantly decreased inguinal WAT gene expression and protein content of ATGL as well as protein content of phosphorylated HSL in CKD mice.

2.5. GH Mitigates White Adipose Tissue Browning in CKD Mice

Beige adipocyte cell surface markers' (CD137, Tbx1, Tmem26, Prdm16, Pgc1α, and Cidea) mRNA expression in inguinal WAT was normalized or decreased in GH-treated CKD mice relative to vehicle-treated CKD mice (Figure 4A–F). In WAT, de novo browning recruitment is promoted by the activation of Cox2/Pgf2α pathway and toll-like receptor Tlr2 and adaptor molecules, such as Myd88 and Traf6 [22]. GH treatment normalized expression of inguinal WAT Cox2, Pgf2α, Tlr2, Myd88, and Traf6 in CKD mice (Figure 4G–K).

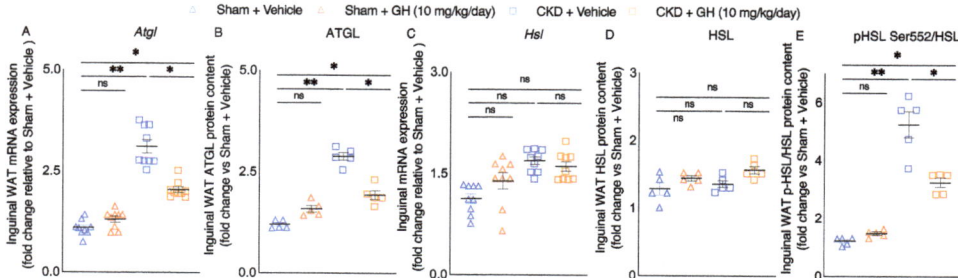

Figure 3. Lipolytic gene expression and protein content in CKD mice. CKD mice were fed ad libitum, whereas other mouse groups received an energy intake amount equal to that of CKD + Vehicle mice. By using qPCR, the expression of lipolytic genes (Atgl and Hsl) in the inguinal WAT was determined (**A**,**C**). In addition, the total protein content of ATGL and HSL as well as the relative phosphorylated HSL/total HSL ratio in the inguinal WAT were evaluated (**B**,**D**,**E**). Results are analyzed and expressed as in Figure 2. Data are expressed as mean ± SEM. For comparison of the means between two groups, data were analyzed by Student's 2-tailed *t*-test. Posthoc analysis was performed with Tukey's test. Specific *p*-values are shown above the bar. ns signifies not significant, * $p < 0.05$, ** $p < 0.01$.

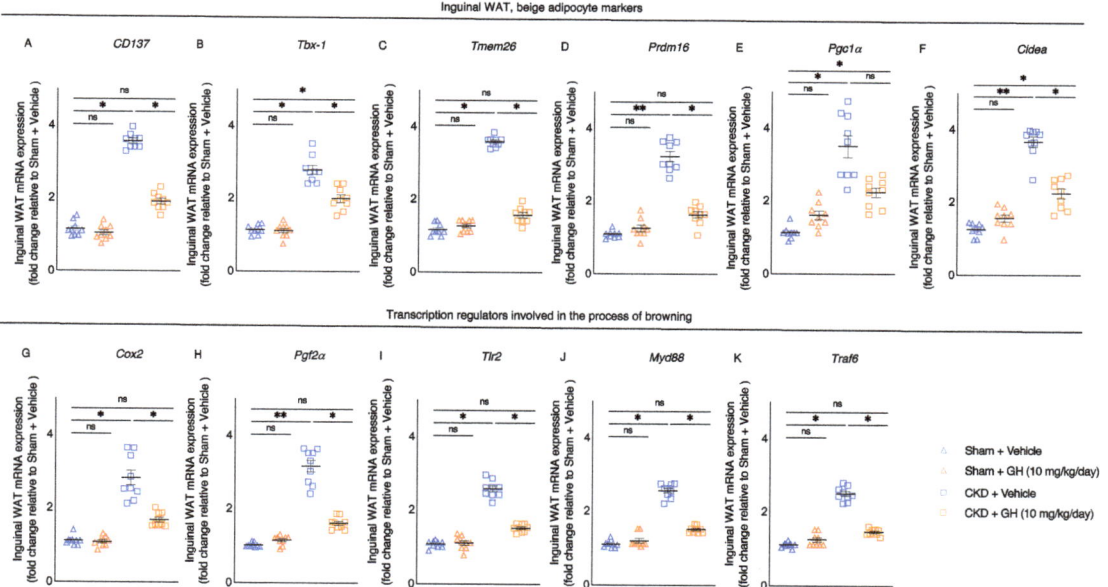

Figure 4. GH reduces browning of adipose tissue in CKD mice. CKD mice were fed ad libitum, whereas other mouse groups received an energy intake amount equal to that of CKD + Vehicle mice. qPCR was used to assess the gene expression of the beige adipocyte markers CD137, Tbx-1, Tmem26, Prdm16, Pgc1α, and Cidea in the inguinal WAT (**A**–**F**). In addition, inguinal WAT was also used to evaluate the gene expression of the Cox2 signaling pathway and the toll-like receptor pathway (Cox2, Pgf2, Tlr2, Myd88, and Traf6) (**G**–**K**). Final results were expressed in arbitrary units, with one unit being the mean level in Sham + Vehicle mice. Results are analyzed and expressed as in Figure 2. Data are expressed as mean ± SEM. For comparison of the means between two groups, data were analyzed by Student's 2-tailed *t*-test. Posthoc analysis was performed with Tukey's test. Specific *p*-values are shown above the bar. ns signifies not significant, * $p < 0.05$, ** $p < 0.01$.

2.6. GH Attenuates Muscle-Wasting Signaling and GH Resistance Pathways in CKD Mice

Perturbations of metabolic pathways lead to skeletal muscle atrophy in the cachexia and sarcopenia. Proinflammatory cytokines induce the catabolic pathways in muscle [1,2]. Treatment of GH attenuated gastrocnemius mRNA expression of inflammatory cytokines (Il1β, Il6, and Tnfα) in CKD mice (Figure 5A–C). GH ameliorated muscle regeneration and myogenesis by decreasing the mRNA expression of negative regulators of skeletal muscle mass (Atrogin-1, Murf-1, Myostatin, and Soc2) while increasing the mRNA expression of promyogenic factors (MyoD, Myogenin, Pax-7, and IGF-I) in CKD mice (Figure 5D–G). In agreement with previous observations [14,15], we also found impaired JAK2/STAT5 signaling in gastrocnemius muscle in CKD mice (Figure 5L,M). GH normalized muscle protein content of phosphorylated JAK2 and STAT5 in CKD mice.

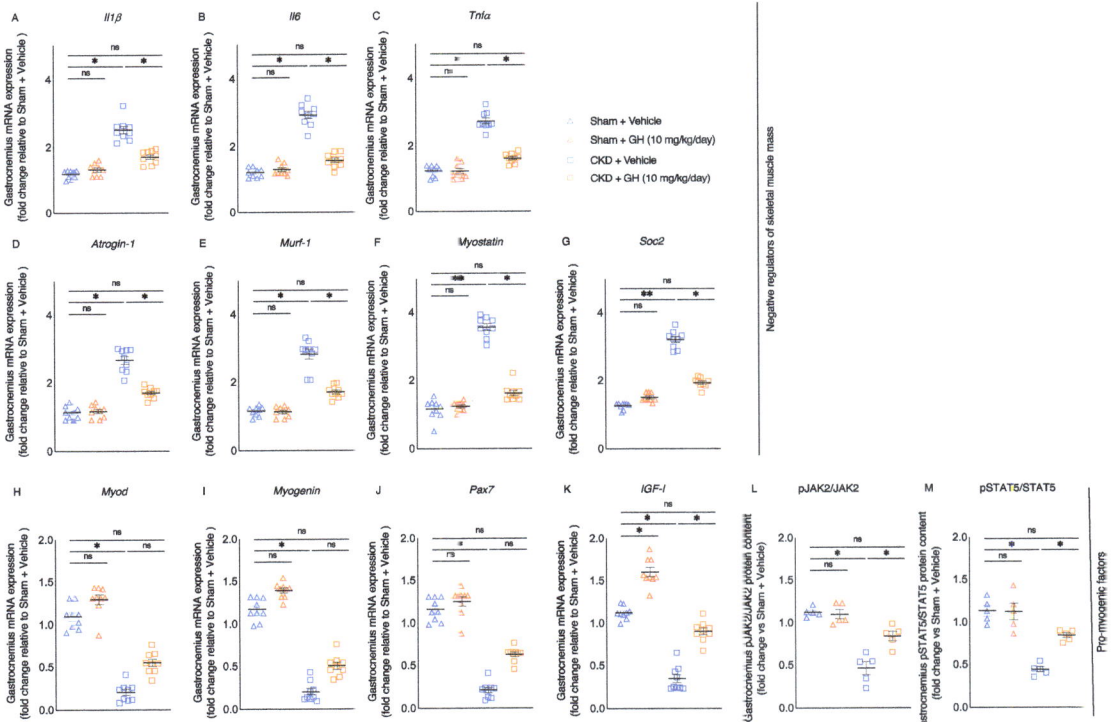

Figure 5. GH reduces muscle-wasting signaling pathways in CKD mice. CKD mice were fed ad libitum, whereas other mouse groups received an energy intake amount equal to that of CKD + Vehicle mice. By using qPCR, the expression of negative regulators of skeletal muscle mass (Il1β, Il6, Tnfα, Atrogin-1, Murf-1, and Socs2) as well as promyogenic factors (MyoD, Myogenin, Pax7, and IGF-I) in the gastrocnemius muscle was determined (A–K). In addition, by using the appropriate ELISA kits, the relative phosphorylated JAK2/total JAK2 ratio and the phosphorylated STAT5/total STAT5 ratio in the gastrocnemius muscle were evaluated (L,M). Results are analyzed and expressed as in Figure 2. Data are expressed as mean ± SEM. For comparison of the means between two groups, data were analyzed by Student's 2-tailed t-test. Posthoc analysis was performed with Tukey's test. Specific p-values are shown above the bar. ns signifies not significant, * $p < 0.05$, ** $p < 0.01$.

2.7. Molecular Mechanism of GH on Muscle Function by RNAseq Analysis

We previously performed transcriptomic profiling of muscle wasting in CKD by RNAseq analysis and identified 12 differentially expressed genes in muscle [23]. Perturbations of these 12 muscle genes are correlated with impaired muscle and neuron regeneration, enhanced muscle thermogenesis, and fibrosis. Hence, we studied the effects of GH on expression of these 12 muscle genes in CKD mice. Notably, GH normalized or attenuated 7 out of those 12 differentially expressed muscle genes identified in CKD mice, while the expression of 5 muscle genes remained different in GH-treated CKD mice (Figure 6A–L).

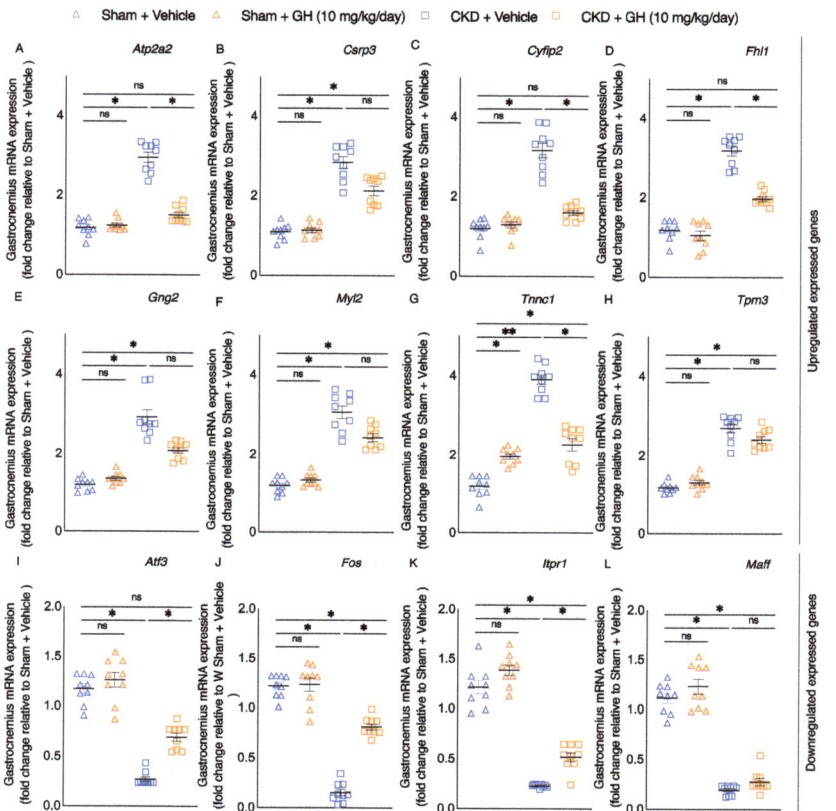

Figure 6. GH reduces the expression of differentially expressed genes in the muscles of CKD mice. CKD mice were fed ad libitum, whereas other mouse groups received an energy intake amount equal to that of CKD + Vehicle mice. The expression of relevant genes in the mouse gastrocnemius muscle was assessed using qPCR (**A–L**). Results are analyzed and expressed as in Figure 2. Data are expressed as mean ± SEM. For comparison of the means between two groups, data were analyzed by Student's 2-tailed *t*-test. Posthoc analysis was performed with Tukey's test. Specific *p*-values are shown above the bar. ns signifies not significant, * $p < 0.05$, ** $p < 0.01$.

3. Discussion

Patients with CKD frequently have cachexia, which has been linked to higher morbidity and mortality rates [1]. We looked into how GH affected cachexia in CKD mice. First, we showed that intraperitoneal administration of GH significantly increased caloric intake and weight growth in CKD mice (Figure 1B,C). We also demonstrated that the beneficial metabolic benefits of GH go beyond appetite stimulation. GH improves organismal metabolism (Figure 1F–L) as well as specific tissue energy balance (skeletal muscle and adipose tissue) in CKD mice (Figure 2). The findings of this study are consistent with those of other, earlier studies. In hemodialysis patients, GH enhances nutrition intake and increases lean body mass [8–10]. With the help of GH, the body's anabolism is stimulated, and protein accretion happens in the muscles and extramuscular tissues [6,7,24].

By increasing muscle mass and improving energy efficiency, GH may improve muscle strength. Anaerobic and aerobic energy sources comprise the continuum of energy needed to fuel muscular function. Anaerobic energy systems are stimulated by GH, which suppresses the aerobic energy system. This increases muscle strength. After six months of GH therapy, healthy males showed a considerable improvement in their lower body muscle strength [5]. By "uncoupling" ATP synthesis, UCPs regulate energy homeostasis by dissipating the mitochondrial proton gradient for ATP synthesis and producing heat [25,26]. UCP3 is expressed in skeletal muscle, and upregulation of UCP3 has been reported in various conditions characterized by skeletal muscle atrophy, including denervation, diabetes, cancer, and sepsis [27]. Gastrocnemius UCP3 protein content along with ATP content was normalized in GH-treated CKD mice (Figure 2A,B). Putative functions of UCP3 are controversial. Interesting evidence for and against UCP3 involvement in thermogenesis has been published [27,28]. Furthermore, increased muscle expression of UCP3 has been postulated to modulate oxidative stress and lipotoxicity in a rat model of cachexic sepsis [29]. GH therapy reduced abnormal UCP1 and ATP content in WAT and BAT in CKD mice (Figure 2C–F). However, the precise role of UCP1 in disease-associated cachexia in humans is still a topic of debate. Several studies have described UCP1 expression, a biomarker of WAT browning, as a critical component of WAT dysfunction in cancer cachexia [17,18,30]. Results also suggested that a UCP-1 independent cascade could also regulate adipocyte homeostasis and influence tumor-induced WAT wasting [31]. Moreover, activation of BAT has been associated with hypermetabolism in cachexia, but information from human studies is scarce. A recent study investigated the relationship between activation of BAT and hypermetabolism in patients with emphysematous COPD (chronic obstructive pulmonary disease). BAT activity and gene expression of beige markers of BAT in WAT (Tmem26, Cidea, CD137, Shox2, and Tnfrsf9) were not different between COPD patients versus controls [32]. Medications may influence the sympathetic nervous system and BAT metabolism. Adrenergic receptor blockers and calcium channel blockers are commonly used by COPD patients. Involvement of β-adrenergic receptor signaling in BAT metabolism was reported in humans and rodents [33,34]. Data also indicated that calcium channel blockers regulated adipogenesis and BAT browning [35,36].

CKD-associated cachexia is a progressive, multifactorial metabolic syndrome that results in significant loss of adipose tissue and skeletal muscle mass. Fat loss from adipose tissue in CKD-associated cachexia may be due to the increased rate of lipolysis. Recent longitudinal studies found that the magnitude of adipose tissue wasting predicts poorer survival in cancer patients [37–39]. The bulk of lipid mobilization from adipose tissue is mediated through lipolysis. In canonical adipose tissue lipolysis, triglycerides stored in lipid droplets are hydrolyzed by ATGL and HSL to produce free glycerol and fatty acids and fuel peripheral tissue metabolism [40]. ATGL is the rate-limiting lipase and hydrolyzes triacylglycerol in lipid droplets to diacylglycerol. GH treatment attenuated inguinal WAT mRNA expression and protein content of ATGL in CKD mice (Figure 3A,B). Previous studies have shown increased ATGL expression in the adipose tissue of cancer-associated cachectic animals and humans [21,41,42]. Inguinal WAT gene expression and protein content of HSL was not different among groups of mice (Figure 3C,D). However, phosphorylated HSL Ser552 protein content in inguinal WAT, a surrogate marker for protein kinase A-activated lipolysis [43], was significantly increased in CKD mice (Figure 3E). Importantly, GH attenuated inguinal WAT protein content of phosphorylated HSL in CKD mice. Evidence of enhanced protein kinase A-activated lipolysis correlated with elevated whole-organism energy expenditure and increased adipose tissue thermogenesis, and increased expression of biomarkers of adipose tissue browning in WAT was reported in a mouse model of cancer cachexia [21]. Moreover, increased WAT protein content of phosphorylated HSL and protein Kinase A was also shown in a mouse model of CKD [44].

Browning of adipose tissue is associated with a hypermetabolic state and cachexia. Adipose tissue browning is evident in animal models of CKD-associated cachexia and cancer as well as in cachectic cancer patients [17,18,30]. We demonstrated that in CKD mice, GH reduced the browning of adipose tissue. The expression of biomarkers of beige adipocyte in WAT (CD137, Tbx-1, Tmem26, Prdm16, Pgc1a, and Cidea) was attenuated in CKD mice treated with GH (Figure 4A–F). Cox2/Pgf2 and inflammatory Tlr2, MyD88, and Traf6 signaling pathways have been associated with the biogenesis of browning [22]. GH treatment restored the expression of inflammatory molecules (Tlr2, MyD88, and Trap6) in the inguinal WAT of CKD mice treated with GH (Figure 4G–K). GH influences the metabolism of adipose tissue by binding to the GH receptor (GHR). Disrupted GH/GHR in mice results in multiple metabolic disorders. Global or adipose-specific GHR-deficient mice fail to demonstrate metabolic adaptability when challenged with a high-fat diet or cold temperature [45].

We looked at how GH affected the expression of molecules that control skeletal muscle metabolism in CKD mice. GH increases the expression of promyogenic factors (MyoD, Myogenin, and Pax-7) while decreasing or normalizing the expression of negative regulators of skeletal muscle mass (Atrogin-1, Murf-1, Myostatin, and Soc2, and inflammatory cytokines IL-1β, IL-6, and TNFα) (Figure 5A–J). Recent research indicates that the immune system and the GH/IGF-I axis interact in complicated and bidirectional ways. For example, the GH/IGF-I axis may be suppressed by inflammatory cytokines such as IL-1, IL-6, and TNFα, while GH/IGF-I may also influence systemic inflammation [46]. In cancer cachectic mice, IL-6 causes a decrease in fat content and stimulates adipose tissue browning [47]. In children with GH deficiency, GH has been found to reduce serum concentrations of IL-1β and TNFα [48]. In addition, GH lowers the serum concentrations of TNFα in adult hemodialysis patients [8]. Skeletal muscle growth and repair are influenced by the transcription factors Pax-3 and Pax-7. Pax-3 and Pax-7 regulate MyoD and myogenin [49]. MyoD and Myogenic Factor 5 (Myf5) are required to promote myogenic precursors. A downstream target of MyoD, myogenin controls the differentiation of myoblasts into myocytes and myotubes [49,50].

Because GH and IGF-I are powerful anabolic hormones that stimulate muscle mass increase and are crucial for maintaining skeletal mass, muscle loss in CKD has been linked to disruptions in the GH/IGF axis. As a result, IGF-I resistance may be a factor in the wasting of muscle in CKD [4]. In fact, GH therapy improved muscle mass compared to height in children with CKD [51]. Patients receiving continuous hemodialysis experienced an increase in blood IGF-I concentration following GH therapy [52–54]. The IGF-I signaling pathway, which promotes the proliferation and differentiation of satellite cells into myoblasts and the development of new myofibers, is one of the mechanisms by which GH affects skeletal muscle metabolism [55]. After a prolonged denervation injury, GH enhances muscle reinnervation, nerve regeneration, and functional outcomes [56]. Furthermore, Gautsch et al. have demonstrated that GH stimulates endocrine IGF-I-stimulated protein accretion, enhancing somatic and skeletal muscle growth in malnourished rats [57]. Interesting findings also point to a possible IGF-I-independent mechanism by which GH may exert anabolic effects in muscle [58]. Muscle wasting associated with CKD is brought on by an impaired JAK-STAT signal [14,15]. We have verified that recombinant human GH treatments resulted in high circulating concentration of human GH in CKD and control mice (Table 2). Muscle expression of IGF-I was decreased in CKD mice, and GH treatments normalized muscle IGF-I expression as well as restored the phosphorylated JAK2 and STAT5 muscle protein levels to normal in CKD mice (Figure 5K–M). Previous studies also showed that GH treatment increased muscle mRNA expression of IGF-I and attenuated JAK-STAT signaling in rodent models of CKD [14].

The GH dose administered to the mice in this study was about 200-fold higher than the dose typically used in humans. The recommended dose approved for treatment of growth failure in children with CKD is 0.35 mg/kg per week [59], whereas we used 10 mg/kg/day in mice for this study. However, our dose was comparable to those commonly used in rodent studies [60], and the observation of increased muscle mRNA expression of IGF-I as well as JAK/STAT phosphorylation after GH treatment in our CKD mice (Figure 5K–M) argues against any effect of GHR saturation.

IGF-I is the most important downstream mediator of GH. Thus, IGF-I is generally considered to be the most important biomarker of GH action, as reflected in the inclusion of serum concentrations of IGF-I in the current guidelines for diagnosis and treatment of GH disorders in humans [61]. We have not measured serum IGF-I concentration in this study, as recent studies suggested that concentration of serum IGF-I is not a reliable marker for exogenous growth hormone activity in mice [60]. Male and female mice from four different strains of mice, including the 57BL/6J mouse strain used in this study, were treated with recombinant human GH (500 ug/day, intraperitoneally, for a period of 14 days). The total amount of GH administrated to mouse is ~7 mg in their study [60], which is comparable to the dose we used for the diet-restrictive study (total amount of GH is ~9.2 mg, presumably 22 g of body weight for CKD mice). In agreement to our observation (serum concentration of human GH in Table 2), GH treatment resulted in high circulating concentrations of human GH in all four strains of mice, whereas no human GH was detectable in control mice receiving isotonic 0.9% NaCl as vehicle. Two weeks of daily GH treatment significantly increased body and organ weight in male and female mice of all four inbred mouse strains when compared with controls. GH treatment failed to affect circulating (total) IGF-I concentrations in all strains and in both sexes. The liver is the main source of circulating IGF-I [62]. Hepatic expression of IGF-I mRNA did not show any difference between GH-treated mice versus control mice in any of these four strains of mice and sexes [60]. List et al. investigated the effects of GH in a mouse model of diet-induced diabetes [63]. Male c57BL/6J mice were fed a high-fat diet to induce obesity and type 2 diabetes. Subsequently, obese and diabetic mice were treated with various doses of GH for a period of six weeks. Comparable to our findings in CKD mice (Figure 1C,F,I), their highest dose of GH (215 µg/day/mouse for their study versus 220 µg/day/mouse in our study, presumable 22 g of body weight for CKD mice) resulted in a significant increment of total body mass and lean mass content. However, in contrast to the findings that the treatment of GH did not influence serum concentration of IGF-I in mice [60], GH treatment led to a significant increase in serum IGF-I in diabetic mice [63]. The mice used by List et al. were obese and hyperinsulinemic and showed impaired glucose tolerance. These factors may account for the difference in the results. Serum concentration of insulin, especially insulin concentration of portal vein, is an important regulator of hepatic GHR expression in rodents [64,65].

In this study, eight-week-old male CKD or sham mice on c57BL/6J background were given GH or vehicle for 6 weeks, and all mice were sacrificed at the age of 14 weeks old. We showed that GH administration elicited beneficial metabolic effects in CKD mice. c57BL/6J mice are the most widely used inbred strain for biomedical research. For c57BL/6J mice, many developmental processes such as T-cell and B-cell immunity, as well as the central nervous system, are still ongoing until 26 weeks of life [66–68]. Furthermore, growth patterns and body composition were evaluated in c57BL/6J mice. Data suggested that cortical bone property and peak bone mass on male c57BL/6J mice are not reached until around 26 weeks of age [69–72]. Thus, the results of our present study are of immense importance, as multiple disturbances in the GH/IGF-I axis have been observed in children with CKD.

We recognize the limitations of this study. Firstly, according to our restrictive study design, vehicle-treated CKD mice were fed ad libitum, whereas other mouse groups received an energy intake amount equal to that of vehicle-treated CKD mice. However, we observed that pair-fed mice consumed their restricted amount of the rodent diet within a short period of time. These pair-fed mice were in an overnight fasting state. Mice, as nocturnal creatures, are active mainly during the dark phase. Circadian rhythm affects adipose tissue metabolism [73–75]. Disruption of circadian regulation has been implicated in cancer-induced WAT wasting [42]. Secondly, our work was performed in male c57BJ/6J mice. Results generated from male mice cannot be unambiguously extrapolated to female mice. Sex hormones influence regional adipose tissue fatty acid storage and BAT function in animals and humans. Disruption of estrogen signaling such as by performing ovariectomy resulted in reduced energy expenditure, gain of fat mass, and loss of BAT activity, and these metabolic phenotypes can be reversed by subsequent estrogen replacement in ovariectomized rodents [76]. The reduction of circulating concentration of estradiol is associated with central obesity and decreased metabolism in menopause [77]. Murine and human brown adipocytes express estrogen receptor α [78,79]. Intracerebral administration of estrogen increased BAT activity in mice [80]. On the other hand, follicle-stimulating hormones, which are elevated with estrogen deficiency, downregulated in vivo BAT function in mice [81]. Currently, there are no published data on the effect of estrogen or estrogen deficiency on in vivo BAT function in humans. Dieudonne et al. investigated the effects of sex hormones on adipogenesis in preadipocytes from male versus female rats. They found that androgens and estrogens did not affect adipogenesis in cultured preadipocytes from male rats. However, opposite effects of androgens and estrogens on adipogenesis have been demonstrated in cultured preadipocytes from female rats. Estrogens increased adipogenesis, while androgens acted as negative effectors of terminal differentiation on rat preadipocytes. Subsequent studies suggest that these opposite effects could be related to differential expression of IGF-IR and Pparγ2 on those cultured preadipocytes [82]. Thirdly, uncertainty remains about the precise role of BAT metabolic responses in the pathogenesis of cachexia, and this is partly due to the lack of BAT-specific pharmacological agents. Currently, there is no convincing evidence to suggest that BAT activity can be selectively modulated by any pharmacological agents without influencing WAT metabolism along with cardiac chronotropic side-effects [83,84]. Moreover, BAT activity is mostly driven by the sympathetic signal mediated by β-adrenergic receptors, namely, ADRB3 in mice and ADRB1/ADRB2 in humans. However, the in vivo BAT metabolic activity is the result of the interaction between sympathetic output signal to BAT and other concomitant signaling processes such as α-adrenergic receptors and adenosine receptors as well as postsignaling modulation of these signaling processes [84]. The complexity and redundancy of the endogenous sympathetic regulation of BAT metabolic activity may explain the lack of an optimal pharmacological approach to modulate BAT in vivo.

Previously, we performed RNAseq analysis in the gastrocnemius muscle in CKD and control mice and identified the top 12 differentially expressed genes that have been associated with energy metabolism, skeletal and muscular system development and function, nervous system development and function, as well as organismal injury and abnormalities [23]. We evaluated the effects of GH treatment on muscle transcriptome in this study. A total of 7 of the 12 muscle genes with variable expression in CKD mice were normalized or reduced by GH (Figure 6). These seven muscle genes—Atp2a2, Cyfip2, Fhl1, Tnnc1, Atf3, Fos, and Itpr1—had aberrant expression patterns that have been linked to enhanced tissue thermogenesis, compromised mechanical muscle properties, poor muscle regeneration, and diminished muscle-neuron regeneration capacity [23].

In conclusion, our findings imply that GH might be a useful treatment for adipose tissue browning and muscular atrophy in CKD-associated cachexia.

4. Materials and Methods

4.1. Study Design

This study was conducted in compliance with established guidelines and the prevailing protocol (S01754) as approved by the Institutional Animal Care and Use Committee (IACUC) at the University of California, San Diego, in accordance with the National Institutes of Health. Recombinant human GH was kindly provided by Genetech (South San Francisco, CA, USA). Six-week-old male c57BL/6J mice were purchased from the Jackson Laboratory (strain: 000664) (Bar Harbor, ME, USA) and used for this study. CKD in mice were induced by 2-stage 5/6 nephrectomy while a sham operation was carried out in control mice [13]. Individual mice were housed in each cage in 12:12 hour light–dark cycles with ad libitum access to mouse diet 5015 (LabDiet, St. Louis, MO, USA, catalog 0001328, with a metabolizable energy value of 3.59 kcal/g) and water prior to the initiation of the experiment. We performed the following two studies. Study 1: We evaluated the dietary effects of GH in CKD and sham mice. CKD and sham mice were administrated with GH (5 mg/kg/day or 10 mg/kg/day, intraperitoneal) or vehicle (normal saline), respectively. The study period was 42 days, and all mice were fed ad libitum. We measured caloric intake and accompanying weight change in CKD and sham mice. The caloric intake for each mouse was calculated by multiplying total mouse diet consumption during the 42 days (in grams) with the metabolizable energy value of the diet (3.59 kcal/g). Average daily energy intake in mice was expressed as kcal/mouse/day. Study 2: We evaluated the effects of GH in CKD mice beyond nutritional stimulation by employing a diet-restrictive strategy. CKD and sham mice were given GH (10 mg/kg/day, intraperitoneal) or vehicle for 42 days. Each mouse was individually housed during the study period. CKD mice treated with vehicle were fed ad libitum. We measured caloric intake in vehicle-treated CKD mice by multiplying total mouse 5015 diet consumption during the 42 days (in grams) with the metabolizable energy value of the diet (3.59 kcal/g). The average daily energy intake for vehicle-treated CKD mice was calculated and expressed as kcal/mouse/day. We then fed the same amount of mouse 5015 diet based on the recorded average daily energy intake for vehicle-treated CKD mice to other groups of mice, i.e., CKD mice treated with GH (10 mg/kg/day, intraperitoneal) as well as sham mice treated with GH (10 mg/kg/day, intraperitoneal) or vehicle. We fed the mice daily during the daytime (0900-1200). We measured weekly weight change for each mouse. The schematic study plan for the ad libitum and diet-restrictive study is illustrated in Figure 1A,D, respectively.

4.2. Body Composition, Metabolic Rate, and In Vivo Muscle Function

Body composition (for lean and fat content) was measured by quantitative magnetic resonance analysis (EchoMRI-100^{TM}, Echo Medical System, Houston, TX, USA) [13,23]. Resting metabolic rate was assessed by using Oxymax calorimetry (Columbus Instruments, Columbus, OH, USA) during the daytime (0900-1700) [13]. At the end of the study, rotarod activity (model RRF/SP, Accuscan Instrument, Columbus, OH, USA) and forelimb grip strength (Model 47106, UGO Basile, Gemonio, Italy) in mice were assessed [13,23].

4.3. Serum and Blood Chemistry

Mice were sacrificed and serum samples were collected within 4 h after the last rhGH or vehicle injection. VetScan® Comprehensive Diagnostic Profile reagent rotor and the VetScan Chemistry Analyzer (Union City, CA, USA) were used for quantitative determination of BUN and serum creatine concentration (Supplemental Table S1). Concentrations of serum GH in mice were analyzed using commercially available ELISA kits according to the manufacturer's protocols (Supplemental Table S1).

4.4. Protein Assay for Muscle and Adipose Tissue

Portions of the right gastrocnemius muscle, inguinal WAT, and interscapular BAT were processed in a tissue homogenizer (Omni International, Kennesaw, GA, USA). Protein concentration of tissue homogenate was assayed using a Pierce BCA Protein Assay Kit (Thermo Scientific, catalog 23227, Waltham, MA, USA). Uncoupling (UCP) protein content in muscle and adipose tissue homogenates were assayed. In addition, adenosine triphosphate (ATP) content of tissue homogenate was assessed by using an ATP Assay Kit which relies on the phosphorylation of glycerol that could be quantified by colorimetric or fluorometric methods (Abcam, catalog ab83355, Cambridge, UK). Protein concentration of phospho-JAK2 and total JAK2, as well as phospho-STAT5 and total STAT5, in muscle homogenates was measured (Supplemental Table S1).

4.5. Muscle RNAseq Analysis

Previously, we performed RNAseq analysis on gastrocnemius muscle mRNA in 12-month-old CKD mice versus age-appropriate sham control mice [23]. Detailed procedures for mRNA extraction, purification, and subsequent construction of cDNA libraries as well as analysis of gene expression were published. We then performed ingenuity pathway analysis enrichment tests for those differentially expressed muscle genes in CKD mice versus control mice, focusing on pathways related to energy metabolism, skeletal and muscle system development and function, and organismal injury and abnormalities. We identified the top 12 differentially expressed muscle genes in CKD versus control mice. In this study, we performed qPCR analysis for those top 12 differentially expressed gastrocnemius muscle genes in the different experimental groups.

4.6. Quantative Real-Time PCR

Portions of the right gastrocnemius muscle of mice, inguinal WAT, and interscapular BAT were processed by using a tissue homogenizer (Omni International, Kennesaw, GA, USA). Total RNA from tissue homogenate was isolated using TriZol (Life Technology, Carlsbad, CA, USA). Total RNA (3 µg) was reverse transcribed to cDNA with SuperScript III Reverse Transcriptase (Invitrogen, Waltham, MA, USA). Quantitative real-time RT-PCR of target genes was performed using KAPA SYBR FAST qPCR kit (KAPA Biosystems, Wilmington, MA, USA) [23]. Glyceraldehyde−3-phosphate dehydrogenase (GAPDH) was used as an internal control. Expression levels were calculated according to the relative $2^{-\Delta\Delta Ct}$ method. All primers are listed (Supplemental Table S2).

4.7. Statistics

Statistical analyses were performed using GraphPad Prism version 9.4.1 (GraphPad Software, San Diego, CA, USA). All data are presented as mean ± S.E.M. For comparison of the means between two groups, data were analyzed by Student's 2-tailed *t*-test. Differences of the means for more than two groups containing two variables were analyzed using 2-way ANOVA. Posthoc analysis was performed with Tukey's test. A *p*-value of less than 0.05 was considered significant.

Supplementary Materials: The following supporting information can be downloaded at: https://www.mdpi.com/article/10.3390/ijms232315310/s1.

Author Contributions: Conceptualization, R.H.M. and W.W.C.; methodology, R.H.M., S.G. and W.W.C.; software, W.W.C.; validation, R.H.M., S.G. and W.W.C.; formal analysis, R.H.M., S.G., E.A.O. and W.W.C.; investigation, S.G. and W.W.C.; resources, R.H.M. and W.W.C.; data curation, S.G. and W.W.C.; writing, R.H.M., S.G., E.A.O. and W.W.C.; project administration, W.W.C.; funding acquisition, R.H.M. and S.G. All authors have read and agreed to the published version of the manuscript.

Funding: This research was funded by a Genentech Fellowship grant to S.G.

Institutional Review Board Statement: This study was conducted in compliance with established guidelines and prevailing protocol (S01754) as approved by the Institutional Animal Care and Use Committee (IACUC) at the University of California, San Diego, in accordance with the National Institutes of Health.

Informed Consent Statement: Not applicable.

Data Availability Statement: The authors confirm that the data supporting the findings of this study are available within the article and its Supplementary Materials. Additional raw data supporting the findings of this study are available from the corresponding author (R.H.M.) on request.

Acknowledgments: We thank Jianhua Shao and the UCSD Pediatric Diabetes Research Center for the use of EchoMRI-100™. We acknowledge contributions from Ping Zhou, Sheng Hao, and Ronghao Zheng in the generation of supplemental data.

Conflicts of Interest: The authors declare no conflict of interest.

References

1. Mak, R.H.; Ikizler, A.T.; Kovesdy, C.P.; Raj, D.S. Wasting in Chronic Kidney Disease. *J. Cachexia Sarcopenia Muscle* **2011**, *2*, 9–25. [CrossRef] [PubMed]
2. Koppe, L.; Fouque, D.; Kalantar-Zadeh, K. Kidney Cachexia or Protein-Energy Wasting in CKD: Facts and Numbers. *J. Cachexia Sarcopenia Muscle* **2019**, *10*, 479–484. [CrossRef]
3. Gungor, O.; Ulu, S.; Hasbal, N.B.; Anker, S.D. Effects of Hormonal Changes on Sarcopenia in Chronic Kidney Disease: Where are we now and what can we do? *J. Cachexia Sarcopenia Muscle* **2021**, *12*, 1380–1392. [CrossRef] [PubMed]
4. Oliveria, E.A.; Carter, C.E.; Mak, R.H. The Role of Growth Hormone in Chronic Kidney Disease. *Semin. Nephrol.* **2021**, *41*, 144–155. [CrossRef] [PubMed]
5. Tavares, A.B.W.; Micmacher, E.; Biesek, S.; Assumpcao, R. Effects of Growth Hormone Administration on Muscle Strength in Men over 50 Years Old. *Int. J. Endocrinol.* **2013**, *2013*, 942030. [CrossRef]
6. Garibotto, G.; Barreca, A.; Russo, R.; Sofia, A. Effects of Recombinant Human Growth Hormone on Muscle Protein Turnover in Malnourished Hemodialysis Patients *J. Clin. Investig.* **1997**, *99*, 97–105. [CrossRef]
7. Hansen, T.B.; Gram, J.; Jensen, P.B.; Kristiansen, J.H. Influence of Growth hormone on Whole Body and Regional Soft Tissue Composition in Adult Patients on Hemodialysis. A Double-Blind, Randomized, Placebo-Controlled Study. *Clin. Nephrol.* **2000**, *53*, 99–107.
8. Feldt-Rasmussen, B.; Lange, M.; Sulcwicz, W.; Gafter, U. Growth Hormone Treatment during Hemodialysis in a Randomized Trial Improves Nutrition, Quality of Life, and Cardiovascular Risk. *J. Am. Soc. Nephrol.* **2007**, *18*, 2161–2171. [CrossRef]
9. Nienczyk, S.; Sikorsk, H.; Wiecek, A.; Zukowska-Szczechowska, E. A Super-Agonist of Growth Hormone-Releasing Hormone Causes Rapid Improvement of Nutritional Status in Patients with Chronic Kidney Disease. *Kidney Int.* **2010**, *77*, 450–458. [CrossRef]
10. Merdias, C.L.; Sibilsky Enselman, E.R.; Olszewski, A.M.; Gumucio, J.P. The Use of Recombinant Human Growth Hormone to Protect Against Muscle Weakness in Patients Undergoing Anterior Cruciate Ligament Reconstruction: A Pilot, Randomized Placebo-Controlled Trial. *Am. J. Sports Med.* **2020**, *48*, 1916–1928. [CrossRef]
11. Tavoian, D.; Ampomah, K.; Amano, S.; Law, T.D. Changes in DXA-Derived Lean Mass and MRI-Derived Cross-Sectional Area of the Thigh are Modestly Associated. *Sci. Rep.* **2019**, *9*, 10028. [CrossRef] [PubMed]
12. Sabatino, A.; D'Alessandro, C.D.; Regolisti, G.; di Mario, F. Muscle Mass Assessment in Renal Disease: The Role of Imaging Techniques. *Quant. Imaging Med. Surg.* **2020**, *10*, 1672–1686. [CrossRef] [PubMed]
13. Cheung, W.W.; Ding, W.; Gunta, S.S.; Gu, Y.; Mak, R.H. A Pegylated Leptin Antagonist Ameliorates CKD-Associated Cachexia in Mice. *J. Am. Soc. Nephrol.* **2014**, *25*, 119–128. [CrossRef] [PubMed]
14. Sun, D.F.; Chen, Y.; Rabkin, R. Work-Induced Changes in Skeletal Muscle IGF-1 and Myostatin Gene Expression in Uremia. *Kidney Int.* **2006**, *70*, 453–459. [CrossRef]
15. Schaefer, F.; Chen, Y.; Tsao, T.; Nouri, P. Impaired JAK-STAT Signal Transduction Contributes to Growth Hormone Resistance in Chronic Uremia. *J. Clin. Investig.* **2001**, *108*, 467–475. [CrossRef]
16. Choe, S.S.; Huh, J.Y.; Hwang, I.J.; Kim, J.I. Adipose Tissue Remodeling: Its Role in Energy Metabolism and Metabolic Disorders. *Front. Endocrinol.* **2016**, *7*, 30. [CrossRef]
17. Kir, S.; White, J.P.; Kleiner, S.; Kazak, L. Tumor-Derived PTHrP Triggers Adipose Tissue Browning and Cancer Cachexia. *Nature* **2014**, *513*, 100–104. [CrossRef]
18. Kir, S.; Komaba, H.; Garcia, A.P.; Economopoulos, K.P. PTH/PTHrP Receptor Mediates Cachexia in Models of Kidney Failure and Cancer. *Cell Metab.* **2016**, *23*, 315–323. [CrossRef]
19. Berryman, D.E.; List, E.O. Growth Hormone's Effect on Adipose Tissue: Quality versus Quantity. *Int. J. Mol. Sci.* **2017**, *18*, 1621. [CrossRef]
20. Kopchick, J.J.; Berryman, D.E.; Puri, V.; Lee, K.Y. The Effects of Growth Hormone on Adipose Tissue: Old Observations, New Mechanisms. *Nat. Rev. Endocrinol.* **2020**, *16*, 135–146. [CrossRef]
21. Kliewer, K.L.; Ke, J.Y.; Tian, M.; Cole, R.M.; Andridge, R.R.; Belury, M.A. Adipose tissue lipolysis and energy metabolism in early cancer cachexia mice. *Cancer Biol. Ther.* **2015**, *16*, 886–897. [CrossRef] [PubMed]
22. Vegiopoulos, A.; Müller-Decker, K.; Strzoda, D.; Schmitt, I. Cyclooxygenase-2 Controls Energy Homeostasis in Mice by de Novo Recruitment of Brown Adipocytes. *Science* **2010**, *328*, 1158–1161. [CrossRef] [PubMed]
23. Cheung, W.W.; Ding, W.; Hoffman, H.M.; Wang, Z.; Mak, R.H. Vitamin D Ameliorates Adipose Browning in Chronic Kidney Disease Cachexia. *Sci. Rep.* **2020**, *10*, 14175. [CrossRef] [PubMed]
24. Pupim, L.B.; Flakoll, P.J.; Yu, C.; Alp Ikizer, T. Recombinant Human Growth Hormone Improves Muscle Amino Acid Uptake and Whole-Body Protein Metabolism in Chronic Hemodialysis Patients. *Am. J. Clin. Nutr.* **2005**, *82*, 1235–1243. [CrossRef] [PubMed]
25. Ricquier, D.; Bouillaud, F. Mitochondrial uncoupling proteins: From mitochondria to the regulation of energy balance. *J. Physiol.* **2000**, *529*, 3–10. [CrossRef] [PubMed]
26. Demine, S.; Renard, P.; Arnould, T. Mitochondrial uncoupling: A key controller of biological processes in physiology and diseases. *Cells* **2019**, *8*, 795. [CrossRef]
27. Sun, X.; Wray, C.; Tian, X.; Hasselgren, P.O.; Lu, J. Expression of uncoupling protein is upregulated in skeletal muscle during sepsis. *Am. J. Physiol. Endocrinol. Metab.* **2003**, *285*, E512–E520. [CrossRef]
28. Pohl, E.E.; Rupprecht, A.; Macher, G.; Hilse, K.E. Important trends in UCP3 investigation. *Front. Physiol.* **2019**, *10*, 470. [CrossRef]

29. Minnaard, R.; Schrauwen, P.; Schaart, G.; Hesselink, M.K.C. UCP3 in muscle wasting, a role in modulating lipotoxicity? *FEBS Lett.* **2006**, *580*, 5172–5176. [CrossRef]
30. Petruzzelli, M.; Schweiger, M.; Schreiber, R.; Campos-Olivas, R.; Tsoli, M.; Allen, J.; Swarbrick, M.; Rose-John, S.; Rincon, M.; Robertson, G.; et al. A switch from white to brown fat increased energy expenditure in cancer-associated cachexia. *Cell Metab.* **2014**, *20*, 443–447. [CrossRef]
31. Rohm, M.; Schafer, M.; Laurent, V.; Ustunel, B.K.; Niopek, K.; Algrire, C.; Hautzinger, O.; Sijmonsma, T.P.; Zota, A.; Medrikova, D.; et al. An AMP-activated protein kinase–stabilizing peptide ameliorates adipose tissue wasting in cancer cachexia in mice. *Nat. Med.* **2016**, *22*, 1120–1130. [CrossRef] [PubMed]
32. Sanders, K.J.C.; Wierts, R.; Lichtenbelt, W.D.V.M.; Vos-Geelen, J.D.; Plasqui, G.; Kelders, M.C.J.M.; Schrauwen-Hinderling, V.B.; Bucerius, J.; Dingemans, A.M.C.; Mottaghy, F.M.; et al. Brown adipose tissue activation is not related to hypermetabolism in emphysematous chronic obstructive pulmonary disease patients. *J. Cachexia Sarcopenia Muscle* **2022**, *13*, 1329–1338. [CrossRef] [PubMed]
33. Wijers, S.L.J.; Schrauwen, P.; van Baak, M.A.; Saris, W.H.M.; Lichtenbelt, W.D.V.M. β-Adrenergic receptor blockade does not inhibit cold-induced thermogenesis in humans: Possible involvement of brown adipose tissue. *J. Clin. Endocrinol. Metab.* **2011**, *96*, E598–E605. [CrossRef] [PubMed]
34. Ootsuka, Y.; Kulasekara, K.; de Menezes, R.C.; Blessing, W.M. SR59230A, a beta-3 adrenergic antagonist, inhibit ultradian brown adipose tissue thermogenesis and interrupts associated episodic brain and body heating. *Am. J. Physiol. Regul. Integr. Comp. Physiol.* **2011**, *301*, R987–R994. [CrossRef]
35. Zhai, M.; Yang, D.; Yi, W.; Sun, W. Involvement of calcium channel in the regulation of adipogenesis. *Adipocyte* **2020**, *9*, 132–141. [CrossRef]
36. Yin, Y.; Mao, Y.; Xiao, L.; Sun, Z.; Liu, J.; Zhou, D.; Xu, Z.; Liu, L.; Fu, T.; Ding, C.; et al. FNIPl regulates adipocyte browning and systemic glucose homeostasis in mice by shaping intracellular calcium dynamics. *J. Exp. Med.* **2022**, *219*, e20212491. [CrossRef]
37. Murphy, R.A.; Wilke, M.S.; Perrine, M.; Pawlowicz, M.; Mourtzakis, M.; Lieffers, J.R.; Maneshgar, M.; Bruera, E.; Clandinin, M.T.; Baracos, V.E.; et al. Loss of adipose tissue and plasma phospholipids: Relationship to survival in advanced cancer patients. *Clin. Nutr.* **2010**, *29*, 482–487. [CrossRef]
38. Dalal, S.; Hui, D.; Bidaut, L.; Lem, K.; Del Fabbro, E.; Crane, C.; Reyes-Gibby, C.C.; Bedi, D.; Bruera, E. Relationships among body mass index, longitudinal body composition alterations, and survival in patients with locally advanced pancreatic cancer receiving chemoradiation: A pilot study. *J. Pain Symptom Manag.* **2012**, *44*, 181–191. [CrossRef]
39. Di Sebastiano, K.M.; Yang, L.; Zbuk, K.; Wong, R.K.; Chow, T.; Koff, D.; Moran, G.R.; Mourtzakis, M. Accelerated muscle and adipose tissue loss may predict survival in pancreatic cancer patients: The relationship with diabetes and anaemia. *Br. J. Nutr.* **2013**, *109*, 302–312. [CrossRef]
40. Miyoshi, H.; Perfield, J.W.; Obin, M.S.; Greenberg, A.S. Adipose triglyceride lipase regulates basal lipolysis and lipid droplet size in adipocytes. *J. Cell. Biochem.* **2008**, *105*, 1430–1436. [CrossRef]
41. Das, S.K.; Eder, S.; Schauer, S.; Diwoky, C.; Temmel, H.; Guertl, B.; Gorkiewicz, G.; Tamilarasan, K.P.; Kumari, P.; Trauner, M.; et al. Adipose triglyceride lipase contributes to cancer-associated cachexia. *Science* **2011**, *33*, 233–238. [CrossRef] [PubMed]
42. Tsoli, M.; Schweiger, M.; Vanniasinghe, A.S.; Painter, A.; Zechner, R.; Clarke, S.; Robertson, G. Depletion of white adipose tissue in cancer cachexia syndrome is associated with inflammatory signaling and disrupted circadian regulation. *PLoS ONE* **2014**, *9*, e92966. [CrossRef] [PubMed]
43. Silverio, R.; Lira, F.S.; Oyama, L.M.; do Nascimento, C.M.O.; Otoch, J.P.; Alcantara, P.S.M.; Batista Jr, M.L.; Seelaender, M. Lipase and lipid droplet-associated protein expression in subcutaneous white adipose tissue of cachectic patients with cancer. *Lipids Health Dis.* **2017**, *16*, 159–169. [CrossRef]
44. Wu, J.; Dong, J.; Verzolaa, D.; Hruska, K.; Garibotto, G.; Hu, Z.; Mithc, W.E.; Thomas, S.S. Signal regulatory protein alpha initiates cachexia through muscle to adipose tissue crosstalk. *J. Cachexia Sarcopenia Muscle* **2019**, *10*, 1210–1227. [CrossRef] [PubMed]
45. Ran, L.; Wang, X.; Mi, A.; Liu, Y. Loss of Adipose Growth Hormone Receptor in Mice Enhances Local Fatty Acid Tapping and Impairs Brown Adipose Tissue Thermogenesis. *iSciences* **2019**, *16*, 106–121. [CrossRef]
46. Witkowska-Sedek, E.; Pyrzak, B. Chronic inflammation and the growth hormone/insulin-like growth factor-1 axis. *Cent. Eur. J. Immunol.* **2020**, *45*, 469–475. [CrossRef]
47. Han, J.; Meng, Q.; Shen, L.; Wu, G. Interleukin-6 induces fat loss in cancer cachexia by promoting white adipose tissue lipolysis and browning. *Lipids Health Dis.* **2018**, *17*, 14. [CrossRef]
48. Bozzola, M.; De Amici, M.; Zecca, M.; Schimpff, R.M.; Rapaport, R. Modulating effect of human growth hormone on tumour necrosis factor-alpha and interleukin-1beta. *Eur. J. Endocrinol.* **1998**, *138*, 640–643. [CrossRef]
49. Buckingham, M.; Relaix, F. PAX3 and PAX7 as Upstream Regulators of Myogenesis. *Semin. Cell Dev. Biol.* **2015**, *44*, 115–125. [CrossRef]
50. Wang, Y.X.; Rudnicki, M. Satellite Cells, the Engines of Muscle Repair. *Nat. Rev. Mol. Cell Biol.* **2011**, *13*, 127–133. [CrossRef]
51. Foster, B.J.; Kalkwarf, H.J.; Shults, J.; Zemel, B.S. Association of Chronic Kidney Disease with Muscle Deficits in Children. *J. Am. Soc. Nephrol.* **2011**, *22*, 377–386. [CrossRef] [PubMed]
52. Ziegler, T.R.; Lazarus, J.M.; Young, L.S.; Hakim, R. Effects of Recombinant Human Growth Hormone in Adults Receiving Maintenance Gemodialysis. *J. Am. Soc. Nephrol.* **1991**, *2*, 1130–1135. [CrossRef] [PubMed]

53. Iglesias, P.; Diez, J.J.; Fernandez-Reyes, M.J.; Aguilera, A. Recombinant Human Growth Hormone Therapy in Malnourished Dialysis Patients: A Randomized Controlled Study. *Am. J. Kidney Dis.* **1998**, *32*, 454–463. [CrossRef] [PubMed]
54. Kotzmann, H.; Yilmaz, N.; Lercher, P.; Riedl, M. Differential Effects of Growth Hormone Therapy in Malnourished Hemodialysis Patients. *Kidney Int.* **2001**, *60*, 1578–1585. [CrossRef] [PubMed]
55. Florini, J.R.; Ewton, D.Z.; Coolican, S.A. Growth Hormone and the Insulin-Like Growth Factor System in Myogenesis. *Endocr. Rev.* **1996**, *15*, 481–517.
56. Lopez, J.; Quan, A.; Budihardjo, J.; Xiang, S. Growth Hormone Improves Nerve Regeneration, Muscle Re-innervation and Functional Outcomes after Chronic Denervation Injury. *Sci. Rep.* **2019**, *9*, 3117. [CrossRef]
57. Gautsch, T.A.; Kandl, S.M.; Donovar, S.M.; Layman, D.K. Growth Hormone Promotes Somatic and Skeletal Muscle Growth Recovery in Rats Following Chronic-Energy Malnutrition. *J. Nutr.* **1999**, *129*, 828–837. [CrossRef]
58. Sotiropoulos, A.; Ohanna, M.; Kedzia, C.; Menon, R.K. Growth Hormone Promotes Skeletal Muscle Cell Fusion Independent of Insulin-Like Growth Factor 1 Upregulation. *Proc. Natl. Acad. Sci. USA* **2006**, *103*, 7315–7320. [CrossRef]
59. Mahan, J.D.; Warady, B.A.; Consensus Committee. Assessment and treatment of short stature in pediatric patients with chronic kidney disease: A consensus statement. *Pediatr. Nephrol.* **2006**, *21*, 917–930. [CrossRef]
60. Bielohuby, M.; Schaab, M.; Kummann, M.; Sawitzky, M.; Gebhardt, R.; Binder, G.; Frystyk, J.; Bjerre, M.; Hoeflich, A.; Kratzsch, J.; et al. Serum IGF-I is not a reliable pharmacodynamic marker of exogenous growth hormone activity in mice. *Endocrinology* **2011**, *152*, 4764–4776. [CrossRef]
61. Ho, K.K.Y.; 2007 GH Deficiency Consensus Workshop Participants. Consensus guidelines for the diagnosis and treatment of adults with GH deficiency II: A statement of the GH Research Society in association with the European Society for Pediatric Endocrinology, Lawson Wilkins Society, European Society of Endocrinology, Japan Endocrine Society, and Endocrine Society of Australia. *Eur. J. Endocrinol.* **2007**, *157*, 695–700. [PubMed]
62. Sjogren, K.; Liu, J.L.; Blad, K.; Skrtic, S.; Vidal, O.; Wallenius, V.; LeRoith, D.; Tornell, J.; Isaksson, O.G.; Jansson, J.O.; et al. Liver-derived insulin-like growth factor I (IGF-I) is the principal source of IGF-I in blood but is not required for postnatal body growth in mice. *Proc. Natl. Acad. Sci. USA* **1999**, *96*, 7088–7092. [CrossRef] [PubMed]
63. List, E.O.; Palmer, A.J.; Berryman, D.E.; Bower, B.; Kelder, B.; Kopchick, J.J. Growth hormone improves body composition, fasting blood glucose, glucose tolerance and liver triacylglycerol in a mouse model of diet-induced obesity and type 2 diabetes. *Diabetologia* **2009**, *52*, 1647–1655. [CrossRef] [PubMed]
64. Leung, K.C.; Doyle, N.; Ballesteros, M.; Waters, M.J.; Ho, K.K. Insulin regulation of human hepatic growth hormone receptors: Divergent effects on biosynthesis and surface translocation. *J. Clin. Endocrinol. Metab.* **2000**, *85*, 4712–4720. [CrossRef]
65. Baxter, R.C.; Turtle, J.R. Regulation of hepatic growth hormone receptors by insulin. *Biochem. Biophys. Res. Commun.* **1978**, *84*, 350–357. [CrossRef] [PubMed]
66. Carnieli, D.S.; Yoshioka, E.; Silva, L.F.F.; Lamcas, T.; Arantes, F.M.; Perini, A.; Martins, M.A.; Saldiva, P.H.N.; Dolhnikoff, M.; Mauad, T. Inflammation and remodeling in infantile, juvenile, and adult allergic sensitized mice. *Pediatr. Pulmonol.* **2011**, *46*, 650–665. [CrossRef] [PubMed]
67. Astori, M.; Finke, D.; Karapetian, O.; Acha-Orbea, H. Development of T–B cell collaboration in neonatal mice. *Int. Immunol.* **1999**, *11*, 445–451. [CrossRef]
68. Fu, Y.; Rusznak, Z.; Herculano-Houzel, S.; Watson, C.; Paxinos, G. Cellular composition characterizing postnatal development and maturation of the mouse brain and spinal cord. *Brain Struct. Funct.* **2013**, *218*, 1337–1354. [CrossRef]
69. Somerville, J.M.; Aspden, R.M.; Armour, K.E.; Armour, K.J.; Reid, D.M. Growth of C57BL/6 mice and the material and mechanical properties of cortical bone from the tibia. *Calcif. Tissue Int.* **2004**, *74*, 469–475. [CrossRef]
70. Brodt, M.D.; Ellis, C.B.; Silva, M.J. Growing C57BL/6 mice increase whole bone mechanical properties by increasing geometric and material properties. *J. Bone Miner. Res.* **1999**, *14*, 2159–2166. [CrossRef]
71. Halloran, B.P.; Ferguson, V.L.; Simske, S.J.; Burghardt, A.; Venton, L.L.; Majumdar, S. Changes in bone structure and mass with advancing age in the male C57BL/6J mouse. *J. Bone Miner. Res.* **2002**, *17*, 1044–1050 [CrossRef] [PubMed]
72. Gargiolo, S.; Gramanzini, M.; Megna, R.; Greco, A.; Albanese, S.; Manfredi, C.; Brunetti, A. Evaluation of growth patterns and body composition in c57BL/6J mice using dual energy X-ray absorptiometry. *Biomed Res. Int.* **2014**, *2014*, 253067. [CrossRef] [PubMed]
73. Loboda, A.; Kraft, W.K.; Fine, B.; Joseph, J.; Nebozhyn, M.; Zhang, C.; He, Y.; Yang, X.; Wright, C.; Morris, M.; et al. Diurnal variation of the human adipose transcriptome and the link to metabolic disease. *BMC Med. Genom.* **2009**, *2*, 7. [CrossRef]
74. Zvonic, S.; Ptitsyn, A.A.; Conrad, S.A.; Scott, L.K.; Floyd, Z.E.; Kilroy, G.; Wu, X.; Goh, B.C.; Mynatt, R.L.; Gimble, J.M. Characterization of peripheral circadian clocks in adipose tissues. *Diabetes* **2006**, *55*, 962–970. [CrossRef] [PubMed]
75. Serin, Y.; Acar, T.N. Effect of circadian rhythm on metabolic processes and the regulation of energy balance. *Ann. Nutr. Metab.* **2019**, *74*, 322–330. [CrossRef] [PubMed]
76. Nadal-Casellas, A.; Proenza, A.M.; Llado, I.; Gianotti, M. Effects of ovariectomy and 17-b edstradiol replacement on rat brown adipose tissue mitochondrial function. *Steroids* **2011**, *76*, 1051–1056. [CrossRef]
77. Abdulnour, J.; Doucet, E.; Brochu, M.; Lavoie, J.M.; Streychar, I.; Rabasa-Lhoret, R.; Oud'homme, D. The effect of the menopausal transition on body composition and cardiometabolic risk factors: A Montreal-Ottawa New Emerging Team group study. *Menopause* **2012**, *19*, 760–767. [CrossRef]

78. Wade, G.N.; Gray, J.M. Cytoplasmic 17 beta-[3H] estradiol binding in rat adipose tissues. *Endocrinology* **1978**, *103*, 1695–1701. [CrossRef]
79. Velickovic, K.; Cvoro, A.; Srdic, B.; Stokic, E.; Markelic, M.; Golic, I.; Otasevic, V.; Stancic, A.; Jankovic, A.; Vucetic, M.; et al. Expression and subcellular localization of estrogen receptors α and β in human fetal brown adipose tissue. *J. Clin. Endocrinol. Metab.* **2014**, *99*, 151–159. [CrossRef]
80. de Morentin, P.B.M.; Gonzalez-Garcia, I.; Martins, L.; Lage, R.; Fernandez-Mallo, D.; Martinez-Sanchez, N.; Ruiz-Pino, F.; Liu, J.; Morgan, D.A.; Pinilla, L.; et al. Estradiol regulates brown adipose tissue thermogenesis via hypothalamic AMPK. *Cell Metab.* **2014**, *20*, 41–53.
81. Liu, P.; Ji, Y.; Yuen, T.; Rendina-Ruedy, E.; DeMambro, V.E.; Dhawan, S.; Abu-Amer, W.; Izadmehr, S.; Zhou, B.; Shin, A.C.; et al. Blocking FSH induces thermogenic adipose tissue and reduces body fat. *Nature* **2017**, *546*, 107–112. [CrossRef] [PubMed]
82. Dieudonne, M.; Pecquery, R.; Leneveu, M.C.; Giudicelli, Y. Opposite Effects of Androgens and Estrogens on Adipogenesis in Rat Preadipocytes: Evidence for Sex and Site-Related Specificities and Possible Involvement of Insulin-Like Growth Factor 1 Receptor and Peroxisome Proliferator-Activated Receptor γ 2. *Endocrinology* **2000**, *141*, 649–656. [CrossRef] [PubMed]
83. O'Mara, A.E.; Johnson, J.W.; Limderman, J.D.; Brychta, R.J.; McGehee, S.; Fletcher, L.A.; Fink, Y.A.; Kapuria, D.; Cassimatis, T.M.; Kelsey, N.; et al. Chronic mirabegron treatment increases human brown fat, HDL cholesterol, and insulin activity. *J. Clin. Investig.* **2020**, *130*, 2209–2219. [CrossRef]
84. Carpentier, A.C.; Blondin, D.P.; Haman, F.; Richard, D. Brown adipose tissue—A translational perspective. *Endocr. Rev.* **2022**, bnac015. [CrossRef] [PubMed]

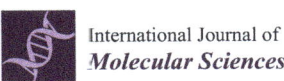 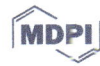

Review

The Potential Modulatory Effects of Exercise on Skeletal Muscle Redox Status in Chronic Kidney Disease

Sara Mendes [1], Diogo V. Leal [1], Luke A. Baker [2], Aníbal Ferreira [3,4], Alice C. Smith [2] and João L. Viana [1,*]

1. Research Center in Sports Sciences, Health Sciences and Human Development, CIDESD, University of Maia, 4475-690 Maia, Portugal; saramendes@umaia.pt (S.M.); diogo.leal@umaia.pt (D.V.L.)
2. Leicester Kidney Lifestyle Team, Department of Health Sciences, University of Leicester, Leicester LE1 7RH, UK; lab69@leicester.ac.uk (L.A.B.); alice.smith@leicester.ac.uk (A.C.S.)
3. Nova Medical School, 1169-056 Lisbon, Portugal; anibalferreira@netcabo.pt
4. NephroCare Portugal SA, 1750-233 Lisbon, Portugal
* Correspondence: jviana@umaia.pt

Abstract: Chronic Kidney Disease (CKD) is a global health burden with high mortality and health costs. CKD patients exhibit lower cardiorespiratory and muscular fitness, strongly associated with morbidity/mortality, which is exacerbated when they reach the need for renal replacement therapies (RRT). Muscle wasting in CKD has been associated with an inflammatory/oxidative status affecting the resident cells' microenvironment, decreasing repair capacity and leading to atrophy. Exercise may help counteracting such effects; however, the molecular mechanisms remain uncertain. Thus, trying to pinpoint and understand these mechanisms is of particular interest. This review will start with a general background about myogenesis, followed by an overview of the impact of redox imbalance as a mechanism of muscle wasting in CKD, with focus on the modulatory effect of exercise on the skeletal muscle microenvironment.

Keywords: chronic kidney disease; skeletal muscle wasting; reactive oxygen species (ROS); oxidative stress; exercise

Citation: Mendes, S.; Leal, D.V.; Baker, L.A.; Ferreira, A.; Smith, A.C.; Viana, J.L. The Potential Modulatory Effects of Exercise on Skeletal Muscle Redox Status in Chronic Kidney Disease. *Int. J. Mol. Sci.* **2023**, *24*, 6017. https://doi.org/10.3390/ijms24076017

Academic Editors: Márcia Carvalho and Luís Belo

Received: 15 February 2023
Revised: 21 March 2023
Accepted: 22 March 2023
Published: 23 March 2023

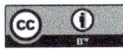

Copyright: © 2023 by the authors. Licensee MDPI, Basel, Switzerland. This article is an open access article distributed under the terms and conditions of the Creative Commons Attribution (CC BY) license (https://creativecommons.org/licenses/by/4.0/).

1. Introduction

Unlike de novo embryonic muscle formation, adult myogenesis or muscle regeneration in higher vertebrates depends on the extracellular matrix (ECM) scaffold remaining (after tissue damage), serving as a template for the muscle fibres [1]. The mechanisms of embryonic myogenesis are to some extent recapitulated during muscle regeneration (see [2,3] for a more detailed description). In brief, it is during embryonic myogenesis that the first muscle fibres are generated [4]. These are derived from mesoderm structures and are the template fibres for the following wave of additionally generated ones [5,6]. Initially, an exponential proliferation occurs up to a degree where the number of fabricated myonuclei starts decreasing, up until a steady state of synthesis rate is reached [7,8]. This leads to the establishment of a matured muscle, followed by quiescence of the progenitor cells and its occupation within the muscle fibres as satellite cells [9,10]. The myogenic rely on the satellite cells' capacity to become activated, and to proliferate and differentiate (including self-renewal), ensuring an efficient muscle repair [11]. Satellite cells exist in a dormant state (i.e., quiescence or reversible G0 state), retaining the ability to reverse to a proliferative state in response to injury, which is essential for satellite cell pool long-term preservation [12–14]. Both timing and extension of satellite cells' activation and subsequent myoblasts' migration, in response to myotraumas to the injury sites, are partly regulated by a plethora of autocrine and paracrine factors [15,16]. These factors are released either from damaged myofibres, by the ECM or secreted by supporting inflammatory (e.g., neutrophils, macrophages) and interstitial cells, present in the niche or that migrate to the site following injury [17]. Moreover, cell-to-cell interactions are fundamental both during developmental (i.e., embryogenesis) and regenerative myogenesis [i.e., in response to physical activity (PA), trauma or disease]. These interactions allow myoblasts to adhere and fuse with myotubes during myogenesis (initial stage) [18] (Figure 1).

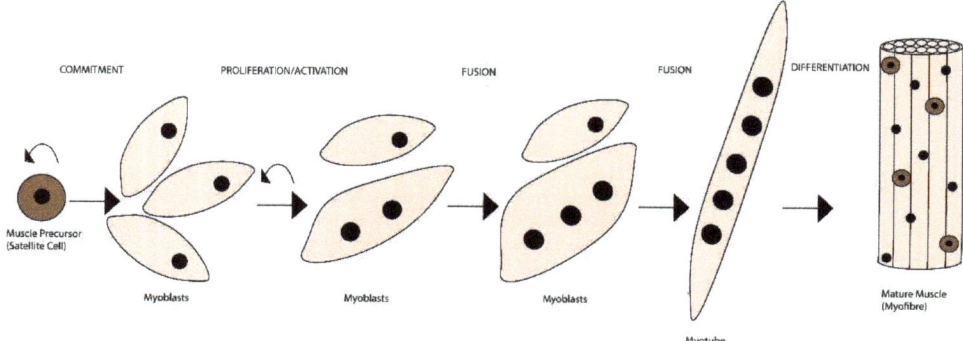

Figure 1. Schematic representation of the mammalian skeletal myogenesis process. Upon muscle injury, a resident population of quiescent skeletal muscle satellite cells can become activated, start to proliferate and differentiate into myoblasts. Over the course of several days, these myoblasts fuse together to form multinucleated myotubes. Further, myoblasts can also fuse to the already existing myotubes to create even larger myotubes, which will eventually align to form muscle fibres. This whole process is regulated by many internal and external cues.

Satellite cells sit closely opposed to the myofibres or near capillaries, facilitating their nutrition, sitting within the ECM, which functions as a scaffold to facilitate their purpose [19,20]. Additionally, activated satellite cells undergo symmetric—give rise to two identical daughter-cells that will self-renew satellite stem cell pools—and asymmetric division—generate one stem cell and one daughter-cell committed to progress through the myogenic lineage and eventually will join the myofibre, ensuring repetitive rounds of regeneration [21,22]. These myofibres are formed by myoblast fusion, producing multinucleated myotubes, further maturing into myofibres (see [23,24] for details). Each myofibre is surrounded by a specialised basal lamina (BL)—endomysium—that harbours a specialised plasma membrane—sarcolemma—allowing neuronal signal transduction and structural stability [25,26]. The sarcolemma is anchor to the BL through transmembrane proteins—dystrophin-associated glycoprotein complex (DGC)—which allow the connection of cytoskeleton to ECM [27].

Muscle fibres are the base of skeletal muscle, being their basic contractile units [28]. These fibres are surrounded by a layer of connective tissue and are grouped in bundles [25,26]. Each myofibre is connected to a single motor neuron and expresses characteristics (e.g., molecules and metabolic enzymes) for contractile function, specifying the myofibre contractile properties, ranging from slow-contracting, fatigue-resistant/oxidative (type I) to fast-contracting, non-fatigue-resistant/glycolytic (type II) fibres. Moreover, the proportion of each fibre type determines overall contractile property within the muscle [29]. The connective tissue that surrounds the skeletal muscle functions as a framework, combining myofibres with myotendinous junctions (i.e., the place where myofibres attach to the skeleton), transforming myofibre contraction into movement [30]. Hence, the skeletal muscle functional properties are dependent on myofibres, motor neurons, blood vessels and ECM.

Skeletal muscle maintenance is accomplished by an interplay between multiple signalling pathways, including two major ones that control protein synthesis, IGF1-PI3K-Akt-mTOR pathway (positive regulator) and myostatin-Smad2/3 pathway (negative regulator) [3,31]. These interconnected pathways control and coordinate hypertrophic and atrophic signalling, creating a balance between protein synthesis and proteolysis [32,33].

Skeletal muscle cells are not isolated elements; they are inserted in their ecological niche, creating a social network with their surroundings. This context consists of interstitial cells, vascular features, ECM proteins and soluble factors, which together constitute the skeletal muscle microenvironment [34]. This microenvironment must be adequate to support skeletal muscle functions and allow a suitable regeneration after assault, such as that imposed by disease (discussed in Sections 3, 4 and 6) or exercise (discussed in Sections 4–6). When this does not occur, we may be confronted with processes leading to muscle wasting.

2. REDOX Imbalance as a Mechanism of Muscle Wasting

Skeletal muscle atrophy is a process that occurs as a result of conditions such as disuse, malnutrition, aging and in certain states of disease. Nonetheless, it is characterized firstly by a decrease in muscle mass (and volume), force production and, on a more detailed perspective, by a diminishment of protein content and fibre diameter [35]. Moreover, the primary loss in muscle strength that occurs with atrophy results from the rapid destruction of myofibrils, the contractile machinery of the muscle, constituting around >70% of the muscle protein [36].

Among all the potential aetiological foundations of muscle wasting, reactive oxygen species (ROS) generation, including the oxidative damage and/or the defective redox signalling, has stood out as the possible main explanation [37–39].

ROS are reactive molecules that contain oxygen, and this family is comprised of free radicals (i.e., species with at least one unpaired electron) and nonradical oxidants (i.e., species with their electronic ground state complete). The chemical reactivity of the various ROS molecules is vastly different; for instance, hydroxyl (•OH), the most unstable, reacts immediately upon formation with biomolecules in its vicinities, whereas hydrogen peroxide (H_2O_2) is capable of crossing cell membranes to exert its effects beyond its original compartment [40–42] (Table 1).

Table 1. The most common reactive oxygen species, antioxidants and respective scavenging reactions.

Reactive Oxygen Species-Oxidants	Antioxidants	Enzymatic Scavenging Reactions
Superoxide radical ($O_2^{-•}$) (Rad)	Superoxide dismutase (Enz), Vit C (Non-Enz)	$2O_2^{-•} + 2H^+ \rightarrow O_2 + H_2O_2$
Hydrogen peroxide (H_2O_2) (Non-Rad)	Catalase (Enz), Glutatione peroxidase (Enz)	$2H_2O_2 \rightarrow 2H_2O + O_2$ $H_2O_2 + 2GSH \rightarrow 2H_2O + GSSG$
Hydroxyl radical (OH•) (Rad)	Glutatione peroxidase (Enz), Vit C (Non-Enz)	$GSH + OH^• \rightarrow GS^• + H_2O$

ROS are generated by various sources, mainly endogenous sources, including mitochondrial respiratory chain enzyme, nicotinamide adenine dinucleotide phosphate oxidase (NOX) activity, microsomal cytochrome P450 and xanthine oxidase; and exogenous sources such as ultraviolet radiation, X- and gamma (γ)-rays, ultrasounds, pesticides, herbicides, and xenobiotics [43]. Superoxide anion ($O_2^{-•}$) is the most frequently generated radical, under physiological conditions. Its main source is the inner mitochondrial membrane, in the complexes I and III, during respiratory chain, by the inevitable electron leakage to O_2 [44,45]. It can also be generated in the short transport chain of endoplasmic reticulum upon electron leakage and during NOX activity, by transferring one electron from nicotinamide adenine dinucleotide phosphate (NADPH) to O_2 [46].

To cope with ROS, the cells have developed control systems to regulate oxidation/reduction balance, since redox balance is critical. A key component is the antioxidant system, which prevents ROS accumulation and deleterious actions. The cells contain both enzymatic and non-enzymatic antioxidants that work by mitigating ROS effects and by drastically delaying/preventing oxidation from happening. Key enzymatic antioxidants are superoxide dismutase (SOD), catalase, glutathione peroxidase (GPx) and thioredoxin (Trx), whereas non-enzymatic are mainly vitamin C (ascorbic acid) and E (tocopherol), zinc and selenium, glutathione, plant polyphenols and carotenoids [47,48]. These act primarily by using three different strategies: (1) scavenging ROS; (2) converting ROS molecules into less reactive ones, and (3) chelation via metal binding proteins. Throughout the cells, antioxidants are compartmentalized in both organelles and cytoplasm, but also exist in the interstitial fluid and blood [49].

ROS are normal products of cell metabolism with significant physiological roles. They regulate signalling pathways (redox signalling) by changing the activity of structural proteins, transcription factors, membrane receptors, ion channels and protein kinases/phosphatases [50,51]. ROS physiological roles depend partly on antioxidant control, establishing a redox balance. When redox homeostasis is disrupted, due to the rising of ROS levels and the unlikely neutralization by the antioxidant defence, a state referred to as oxidative stress (OS) occurs. This leads to an impairment of redox signalling and induces molecular damage to biomolecules [52,53]. Moreover, OS has a graded response, with minor or moderated changes provoking an adaptive response and homeostasis restoration, whereas violent perturbations lead to pathological insults, damage beyond repair and may even lead to cell death [53]. Interestingly, something that is not appreciated often is that our understanding of "low" or "high" response regarding ROS levels is somewhat imprecise, redox time-courses in vivo are scarce and our knowledge is based of immunohistochemical analysis or measuring more stable elements of the family [54,55].

As in other tissues, redox signalling in skeletal muscle has important roles, being the base of skeletal muscle function to elicit exercise adaptation. It supports the neuromuscular development and the long-term remodelling/adaptation of contractile activity [56,57]. Moreover, regulated ROS levels are also involved in skeletal muscle regeneration, regulating the activity of skeletal muscle stem cells, through redox-sensitive signalling pathways [58] (Figure 2).

When an ROS overproduction occurs, cells are capable of maintaining a redox state by activating distinct transcription factors that induce the transcription of antioxidant enzymes to tilt the balance back to homeostasis, protecting them from OS [59,60]. One important transcription factor is the nuclear factor erythroid 2-related factor 2 (Nrf2), which is a ubiquitous protein that modulates OS [61]. In response to elevated ROS levels, Nrf2 triggers the expression of NADPH quinone oxidoreductase (NQO1), heme oxygenease-1 (HO-1), glutamate-cysteine ligase catalytic (GCLC) and glutamate-cysteine ligase modifier (GCLM), which are enzymes involved in redox homeostasis maintenance, cellular defence and detoxification [62,63]. Moreover, enzymes that encapsulate the redox cycling group, mediating the elimination of ROS such as thioredoxin, thioredoxin reductase, sulfiredoxin, peroxiredoxin, gluthatione peroxidase, superoxide dismutase 1 (SOD1), catalase and various glutathione S-transferases, are all of them targeted by Nrf2 [64].

However, during ageing, cells produce even more ROS, mainly from mitochondria and NOX, and even though the activity of antioxidant enzymes in cells and muscle also increases with age, this compensatory adaptation is not sufficient to neutralize ROS levels [37–39]. These increased ROS levels cause deleterious macromolecules oxidative modification, leading not only to various cellular dysfunctions, but also affecting signal transduction pathways that control multiple essential cellular processes, such as protein turnover, mitochondrial homeostasis, energy metabolism, antioxidant gene expression and redox balance (see, for example, [65] for more details). Moreover, the systemic increase in ROS, associated with an OS state, increases proinflammatory transcription factors levels, for instance, nuclear factor kappa B (NF-kB) [66,67]. NF-kB regulates specific UPS genes and leads to the expression of proinflammatory cytokines such as IL-6 and TNF-α that are involved in the development of muscle atrophy [68–70].

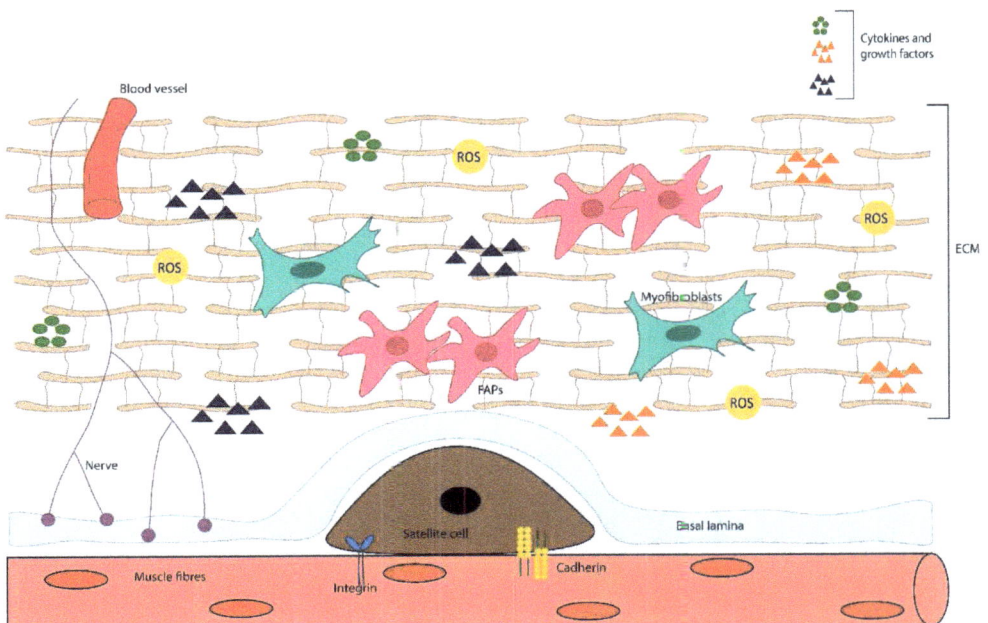

Figure 2. Diagram of the skeletal muscle microenvironment. This niche is composed of various cell types and ECM proteins. In adult skeletal muscle, the quiescent satellite cells stand on the myofiber, under the basal lamina, being surrounded by the ECM, containing blood vessels, nerves, immune cells, fibro-adipogenic progenitors (FAPs), adipocytes and myofibroblast. The satellite cell states are regulated by their interactions with the surrounding microenvironment, direct interaction (e.g., M-cadherin) between muscle fibres and satellite cells; or interact with a variety of components of the ECM and cytokines and growth factors. In addition, stromal cells present can physically interact with satellite cells and release cytokines, growth factors and ECM components, which influence the behaviour of satellite cells, contributing to muscle growth, homeostasis and regeneration.

In summary, ROS load increment and the establishment of an OS state are detrimental to muscle function and are associated with the mechanism of skeletal muscle atrophy [71].

There are two common but distinct conditions that are characterized by skeletal muscle loss, which are sarcopenia and cachexia. In sarcopenia, skeletal muscle loss occurs in a slow and progressive way, being associated with ageing process (in the absence of diseases, whereas, in cachexia, skeletal muscle loss is associated with inflammatory conditions (e.g., AIDS and sepsis) and chronic diseases such as cancer, diabetes, obesity, chronic obstructive pulmonary disease, chronic heart failure, chronic liver disease and chronic kidney disease [72–74].

3. REDOX Imbalance in CKD

CKD consists of a progressive and irreversible loss of kidney function in that, in the more advanced stages of the disease, patients require renal replacement therapy or renal transplantation [75]. The aetiologic factors of the myopathy observed in CKD patients are diverse, from the kidney disease itself, regardless of the need for renal replacement therapy, to the actual dialysis treatment and the typical chronic low-grade inflammation [76,77]. The skeletal muscle fibres of CKD patients present several abnormalities, such as changes in the capillarity, contractile proteins and enzymes [78]. In dialytic patients, this occurs to a greater extent to those who do not undergo dialysis, where atrophy is normally particularly observed in type II fibres [78]. This can be partially explained by the substantial amino acid loss during dialysis, a reduced energy and protein intake and low PA levels, which are recognised to be even lower on dialysis days [79–81]. In fact, these patients present a catabolic environment due to a dysregulated state of energy and protein balance, which includes altered muscle protein metabolism—increased protein degradation (e.g., activation of ubiquitin–proteasome system) (more noticeable) and decreased protein synthesis (e.g., suppressed IGF-1 signalling) (less observed)—and impaired muscle regeneration—satellite cell dysfunction [82]. Furthermore, the haemodialysis procedure itself can stimulate protein degradation and reduce protein synthesis, persisting for 2 h after dialysis [83]. Moreover, even though increasing protein intake (and calories) could enhance protein turnover, the haemodialysis responses were not fully corrected [84–86]. CKD has been previously described as a model of 'premature' or 'accelerated' ageing, associated with a redox imbalance. However, since the mechanisms of age-related muscle loss are similar, but not the same as the CKD-induced, it may be proposed that the two-simile combined amplifies the dysregulated mechanisms [87,88] (Figure 3).

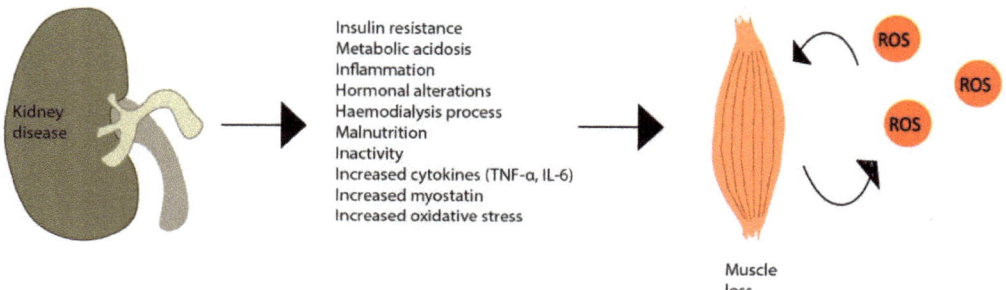

Figure 3. Skeletal muscle wasting induced by chronic kidney disease. Chronic kidney disease creates metabolic changes due to inflammation, haemodialysis increased cytokine production and myostatin and especially oxidative stress, which leads to skeletal muscle atrophy inducing a catabolic program and a vicious cycle of ROS production in site. In CKD patients, this is observed by decreased muscle strength and increased weakness.

Skeletal muscle wasting appears to be a shared feature in the presence of disease, which implies that disease itself can trigger a muscle atrophic response, suggesting that skeletal muscle acts as a source of amino acids providing nourishment for other tissues [89–91].

The dysregulation of skeletal muscle function observed in CKD may also be caused by the presence of uremic toxins, which are normally filtered and excreted by healthy kidneys. However, when kidney function is impaired or inexistent, as in CKD, these uremic toxins are accumulated in the circulation and target other tissues [92,93]. Haemodialysis is in some cases incapable of removing uremic toxins such as protein-bound toxins [i.e., indoxyk sulfate (IS) and p-cresyl sulfate] due to their high affinity to serum albumin [94,95]. The accumulation of these uremic toxins appears to exert negative effects on myoblast proliferation and myotube size (in vitro), skeletal mass (in vivo), reduction of instantaneous muscle strength (loss of fast-twitch myofibres; in vivo) and is accompanied by intramuscular ROS generation [96–98]. High levels of ROS induce the expression of inflammatory cytokines by the muscle, such as tumour necrosis factor (TNF)-α [99,100]. This increase in TNF-α stimulates myostatin expression via NF-kB pathway, which further stimulates myostatin expression accompanied by a rise in IL-6 release [101]. As a result, these activated pathways further increase ROS production by NADPH oxidase [99]. These inflammatory cytokines are known to be elevated in CKD patients, alongside a more pronounced myostatin expression [101,102].

Local high levels of ROS and the subsequent cascade of events (i.e., decreased antioxidant defences and increased inflammatory response) [103] disturb ECM synthesis/degradation homeostasis, favouring excessive collagen deposition, thus promoting tissue fibrosis [104,105]. Additionally, in these more severe CKD stages, skeletal muscle satellite cells and myoblasts are surrounded by an altered microenvironment composed of fibrotic tissue, fat and inflammatory cells [106,107]. The imbalanced crosstalk between resident cells and ECM in the skeletal muscle of CKD patients leads to the production of numerous growth factors, proteolytic enzymes, angiogenic and fibrogenic factors [108,109]. Interestingly, a study by Dong and colleagues [110] observed a differentiation effect of myostatin on fibro-adipogenic progenitors (FAPs), being that myostatin stimulated the proliferation and differentiation of FAPs isolated from EGFP-transgenic mice, leading to fibrosis in the skeletal muscle of CKD mice. An increased α-smooth muscle actin expression was also observed, with the in vivo inhibition of myostatin suppressing both CKD-induced FAP proliferation and muscle fibrosis. This provides a foundation for elucidating what the mechanisms of fibrosis may be in human CKD patients. In a nutshell, these patients present high levels of ROS that increase TNF-α, which stimulates muscle myostatin production. This consequently leads to FAPs proliferation and differentiation, further stimulating muscle fibrosis.

The net consequence of these alterations firstly involves the satellite cell population exhaustion (i.e., loss of activity) or decreased capacity to mediate repair over time, progressively leading to atrophy and loss of individual muscle fibres, associated with concomitant loss of motor units [111]. In fact, it has been already reported that a fibrotic state-derived excess ECM accumulation has a negative impact on muscle force production, thus suggesting that ECM alterations can have significant functional repercussions, with current research highlighting the ECM-cellular interactions as key to better understanding it [112,113]. Keeping this in mind, it has been reported that human-derived muscle cells isolated from CKD patients display and retain CKD-specific cachexia phenotypes in vivo outside of their microenvironment [114]. In addition, there is a reduction in certain muscle properties related to its overall metabolic function (i.e., muscle quality) due to fat infiltration and other non-contractile material [115]. This decrease in overall muscle architecture results in an increased susceptibility to mechanical stress and muscle fibre necrosis. Hence, it is important that ECM microenvironment be actively remodelled to allow ECM cleavage fragments to be released. These "cleaning" programs are activated by endothelial cells sensing mechanical forces such as the ones produced during physical exercise [116,117].

CKD development profoundly linked to OS, in which Nrf2 inactivation seems to be essential. Interestingly, CKD patients appear to have balance between Nrf2 and NF-kB expression; conversely, in CKD patients, under haemodialysis, it has been observed that an Nrf2 expression downregulation was accompanied by NF-kB upregulation [118,119]. Since Nrf2 downregulation contributes to OS and inflammation, it plays a role in causing cardiovascular disease and other complications in CKD patients [120]. Moreover, low levels of Nrf2 increase fibrosis markers, with fibrosis being observed in several tissues in CKD patients, such as kidney, skeletal muscle and heart [121–123].

Additionally, CKD has also been associated with patients with physical inactivity, which is linked with adverse clinical outcomes, increased risk of morbidity and mortality [124].

4. Exercise in Chronic Kidney Disease

Haemodialytic CKD patients are considerably less physically active than their age-matched counterparts [125,126]. Additionally, despite the diverse aetiologic factors of muscle wasting and decreased muscle quality observed in CKD patients, physical inactivity has been proposed as one of the major contributors [127–129]. In fact, a study performed on CKD patients showed similarly low levels of PA between two groups of CKD patients separated depending on disease severity [pre-dialytic (stage 3–4) vs. haemodialytic patients (stage 5)] [130].

Physical inactivity along with the disease itself leads to the patients experiencing skeletal muscle wasting, contributing to frailty, and limiting exercise tolerance [126]. Moreover, considering that CKD patients experience anaemia, hypertension, bone loss and take medications, it is understandable that these patients avoid exercise [131]. This result is unlucky since exercise is beneficial for cardiovascular health and helps with slowing down the progressive skeletal muscle mass loss [132]. Additionally, living a sedentary life and suffering from muscle mass loss negatively affect health [132]. For instance, a single resistance exercise session has been shown to be able to stimulate protein anabolism in haemodialytic patients [133], and 21 weeks of endurance exercise was found to improve protein metabolism markers (e.g., IGF-1 and myostatin). Although it may be demanding of dialysis patients to engage in moderate to vigorous exercise sessions, those who can often experience great benefits. Strategies such as regular resistance and aerobic exercise have shown promising effects in reducing the progression of sarcopenia [102,134–137]. In short, resistance training has shown to be effective in improving skeletal muscle strength and functional capacity and stimulating muscle hypertrophy (e.g., increase in type I, type IIa and type IIx muscle fibre cross sectional areas) [138–142], whereas aerobic training appears to significantly increase aerobic capacity and exercise duration, reduce intra- and interdialytic systolic and diastolic blood pressure, diminish arterial stiffness, increase dialysis efficiency, enhance exercise-induced capillarization in the muscle, improve quality of life (reducing anxiety symptoms), and even exert comparable effects with those of resistance training (i.e., muscle strength) due to poor initial physical state of patients [143–151].

Moreover, CKD is associated with a dysregulated myokine activity and a systemic increase in cytokines [152–154]. In response to exercise, skeletal muscle releases myokines (e.g., IL-15 and IL-6), which exert positive physiological effects on skeletal muscle and bone [155]. This crosstalk through the skeletal muscle secretome (e.g., IGF-1 and myostatin) positively influences bone health [155–157]. In CKD, intradialytic resistance training showed an elevation in osteoprotegerin, which acts by avoiding/protecting excessive bone resorption [158]; bone-specific alkaline phosphatase, another bone resorption inhibitor, showed elevation in resting concentrations after an 8-week intradialytic resistance exercise [159]. For more detailed information about skeletal muscle and bone crosstalk in CKD, see [160].

Connective tissue accumulation (e.g., ECM) has been observed in aged skeletal muscle [161]. A study with aged rats submitted to a resistance exercise protocol—3 times a week for 12 weeks—has shown that training mitigated the age-associated increase of connective tissue. These results can be extrapolated to CKD, since fibrosis is also present in this population [110].

In sum, although there is extensive evidence of the benefits of exercise in CKD, studies showing exercise-induced mechanistic ROS modulation are still lacking.

5. The Impact of Exercise in the REDOX System

Exercise puts pressure on body structures and organs, so blood must be delivered in quantity to the skeletal muscle, heart, lung (among others) rich in oxygen and nutrients to atone for that [162]. However, this stressor leads to an oxygen supply insufficient for the demands of the body, and then, in response to that, many tissues produce ROS [163]. Under normal and healthy conditions, with oxidative levels within a normal range, the available free radicals promote vasodilatation, production of muscle force and maintenance of its content, signal transduction and other related activities [58,164]. In the muscle, contractions during exercise also induce ROS formation, with this upregulating the activity of transcription factors such as NF-kB, activator protein 1 (AP-1) and NRF2, which leads to a more pronounced activity of antioxidants enzymes, inducing muscle adaptations and protecting it from periods of increased OS [165–167]. A study performed in old rats who performed 12 weeks of treadmill-run exercise observed an increased Nrf2 expression [168]. Moreover, a study performed in recreationally active males observed an exercise-induced Nrf2 elevation to 3 h of eccentric contractions of the knee extensors [169].

On this basis, exercise has been shown to enhance ROS detoxifying pathways by increasing the activity of SOD, Gpx, catalase and the master regulator of antioxidant defence, Nrf2 [170,171]. It is the upregulation of these detoxifying pathways that appears to be essential for the adaptive protection developed to work against detrimental effects of OS [172]. For instance, the sarcoplasmic reticulum, which releases Ca2+ necessary for muscle contraction, is highly sensitive to ROS levels, with dysregulated increments in ROS reducing myofibrils sensitivity and therefore affecting muscle contraction [173,174]. Another example that corroborates that ROS effects are dependent on their levels is observed when talking about JNK/SMAD signalling axis, responsible for muscle growth via SMAD2 phosphorylation leading to myostatin inhibition [175]. Low levels of ROS induce JNK phosphorylation, followed by SMAD2 phosphorylation and consequently muscle growth (transient activation of JNK), whereas high levels of ROS also activate JNK but deactivate phosphates, resulting in JNK persistent activation, and were associated with muscle adaptation failure [51,175]. Excess of free radicals, due to intensive exercise or not, may result in OS, putting molecules (i.e., protein, lipids and DNA) at risk for oxidative modifications [53,100]. Proteins are the most susceptible to oxidative modifications, with the more common type of oxidation modification being carbonylation, altering protein conformation leading to partial or total inactivation [176]. The direct consequence is loss of function or structural integrity having wide downstream effects leading to cell dysfunction [177]. PA appears to promote protection against protein carbonylation, which may occur due to antioxidant defence activation or increased protein carbonyls turnover [178]. Other types of oxidation modification that proteins are susceptible to are, for example, tyrosine nitration, S-glutathionylation and advanced glycation end products (AGEs) (see [179,180] for more detailed description of these processes).

Beneficial changes observed in muscle occurs in response to long-term, regular, and moderate training due to muscle adaptation, whereas acute and strenuous exercise provokes excessive free radicals, causing OS damage and fatigue and impacting the body's health and exercise capacity [181,182]. Moreover, exercise modulation through ROS towards muscle provokes different effects on structure and function; this is majorly dependent on the type of training, which leads to activation of different pathways. In general, exercise is divided into two groups: aerobic/endurance exercise and resistance exercise. In endurance (non-exhaustive) training, the source of energy is mainly from the mitochondrial biogenesis, dependent on ROS production by exercise, modulated by peroxisome proliferator-activated receptor gamma coactivator 1-alpha (PGC-1α), the principal pathway to rise oxidative capacity of the muscle [183,184]. Regarding resistance training, the produced ROS activates signalling pathways such as IGF-1 and PI3K/AKT/mTOR, and they are associated with increments in protein synthesis [185]. Additionally, in sprinting, a short-term anaerobic exercise, high levels of ROS are produced mainly by NOXs and xanthine oxidase system; in this case, ROS production by mitochondria is less noticeable [186,187]. Moreover, in general, both resistance and endurance (exhaustive) training are shown to increase ROS levels by the skeletal muscle leading to OS, an increase in cortisol levels and a transitory immunosuppression [39]. In short, together aerobic and resistance training reduces OS, increasing resistance against it, and improves antioxidant status in the long term [188–198].

Finally, it appears that the influence that exercise has on the metabolism and on the redox system may explain the already proven benefits of exercise in health and disease.

6. The Potential Modulatory Effects of Exercise on Skeletal Muscle Redox Status in CKD

It has been already established that exercise is the main stressor that drives skeletal muscle remodelling and metabolic adaptation, and that it achieves that by, in a simple way, stressing the body to produce free radicals and at the same time stimulating it to generate antioxidants to maintain homeostasis, a new homeostasis, being more prepared for the next stress, adapted. However, CKD patients experience elevated OS, and the increase in free radicals induced by acute exercise, especially in unaccustomed patients, could further shift the imbalanced redox status to an even more pro-oxidant state, impairing skeletal muscle metabolism [199]. In response to that, our group has already shown that unaccustomed exercise creates a large inflammatory response in the muscle and that expression of inflammatory cytokines such as IL-6, MCP-1 and TNF-α was upregulated [136]. Still, this is no longer present after a period of training, showing that exercise does not appear to elicit an ongoing and detrimental inflammatory response in the muscle, but an adaptive response instead [136]. Similar to unaccustomed exercise in CKD patients, it can be partially observed with the incidence of the overtraining syndrome (OTS), in which a state of chronic OS is observed due to intensified training/competition and inadequate post-exercise/competition recovery, leading to a persistent fatigue and decline in physical performance [200]. Moreover, a study from our group showed that, after intensified training, leukocyte phagocytic activity decreases and testosterone levels were blunted, showing dysfunction of inflammatory response and at the hypothalamic-pituitary gonadal axis [201]. Interestingly, in OTS are also observed OS blood markers, for example, persistence for more than a month of a reduced glutathione depletion after an ultra-endurance marathon [202]. In these cases, resorting to an antioxidant treatment has been shown to be helpful in restoring muscle weakness and force production [203,204]. In CKD, a systematic review on the use of antioxidants in CKD patients (pre and post dialysis) shows that, in predialysis patients, it may help go prevent end-stage kidney disease, but more powered studies are needed to assess this finding [205].

CKD is considered by some a form of accelerated ageing, so we can withdraw data from older adults. For instance, after 12 weeks of moderate resistance training in elder people, it was observed that ROS generation and OS were decreased [197]. Another study also showed similar results: increase in muscle strength and function associated with decrease in OS markers and enhanced mitochondrial functions [206]. However, one study demonstrated no significant changes in OS biomarkers after aerobic exercise [196]. In sum, it appears that exercise has a positive role in elderly people, with them having OS levels similar to untrained young subjects when exercising [207]. Therefore, it is speculated that decrease in ROS generation, and consequently OS reduction, which could be accompanied by increase in muscle strength and function, may be observed in CKD, despite further evidence still being required. Moreover, like the inflammatory response observed in CKD, aged muscle produces high levels of ROS after acute exercise, while chronic exercise prepares and protects muscle against oxidative damage [208]. In CKD, the majority of studies report disease functional parameters' improvement after a period of training but left out reports about OS markers or investigate mechanisms that cause the exercise benefits observed. A 6-month study performed on haemodialysis patients separated into two groups, intradialytic training (bedside cycling) or no-exercise control group, observed a chronic reduction in various redox status parameters, such as protein carbonylation and lipid oxidation, and an increase in enzymes responsible for ROS detoxification such as catalase and glutathione as an effect of regular exercise [209]. Additionally, this was also accompanied by an increase in aerobic and functional capacity, observed by an elevated peak oxygen consumption, and improved scores on the North Staffordshire Royal Infirmary (NSRI) walk test, and on the 60-s sit-to-stand (STS-60) test [209]. A 4-month intradialytic exercise training (cycling) could reduce plasma lipid peroxidation [210]. The same was observed after 12 weeks of aquatic exercise [211]. Interestingly, a study compared OS parameters in untrained volunteers, CKD patients and professional athletes before and after a strenuous exercise in a rowing cycle ergometer and showed that only athletes presented elevation of antioxidant enzymes due to limited antioxidant capacity in both untrained and dialysis patients, yet the last exhibited increased OS [212]. Moreover, resistance exercises during dialysis appear to be capable of inducing Nrf2 activation [213] (Figure 4).

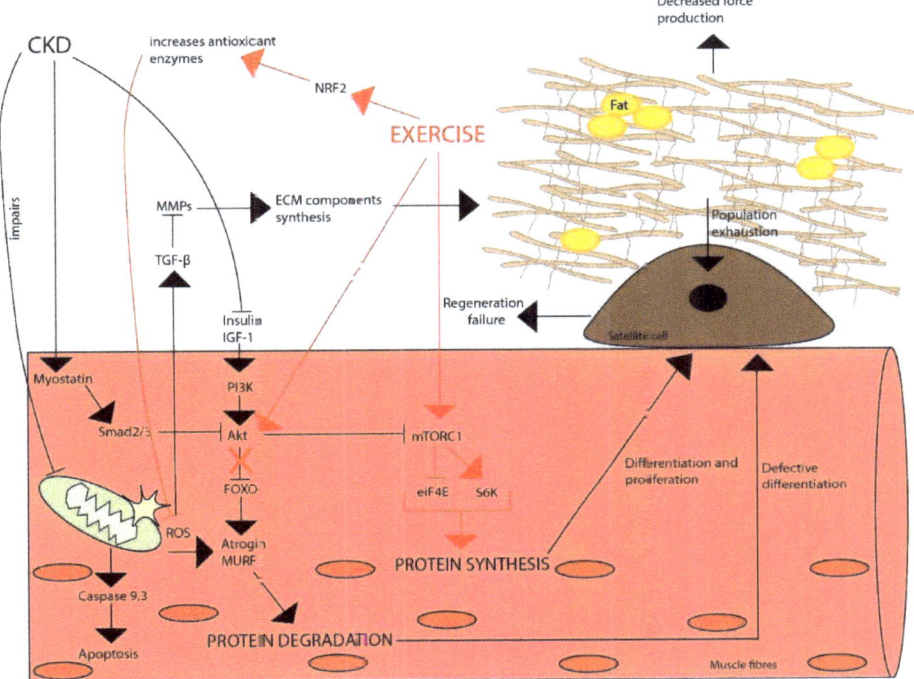

Figure 4. Factors affecting skeletal muscle maintenance in CKD patients. In CKD patients, various factors interact and consequently transduce their effects intracellularly, which affects skeletal muscle maintenance. For instance, insulin and IGF-I positively regulate skeletal muscle due to the activation of mTORC1 through PI3k/Akt, initiating protein synthesis. Later, stimulation of PI3k/Akt by insulin increases FOXO phosphorylation, activates MuRF1 transcription and Atrogin-1, leading to protein degradation via ubiquitin–proteasome pathway. On the other side, myostatin, a negative regulator, leads to SMAD2/3 phosphorylation, reduces Akt activation and consequently FOXO phosphorylation, which inhibits its translocation to nucleus, again accelerating protein degradation. Defective mitochondrial function, due to kidney damage, increases local ROS production, resulting in muscle protein degradation through activation of MuRF1 and Atrogin-1 transcription. These defective mitochondria lead to activation of caspase 9,3 triggering intrinsic apoptotic pathway. Transforming growth factor-β (TGF-β) is activated due to the increased exposure to ROS, while, among other functions, acting as ECM preservatory. It enhances matrix protein synthesis and suppresses ECM degradation proteins such as matrix metalloproteins, which happens in CKD due to an exaggerated activation of TGF-β. Extravagant ECM production leads to fibrosis, impinging on muscle quality, decreasing its force production. This microenvironment affects satellite cells, leading to population exhaustion and regeneration failure; protein degradation also leads to defective differentiation. On the other hand, exercise activates mTORC1, mediating S6k activation, thus promoting protein synthesis and differentiation/proliferation of satellite cells. Additionally, exercise can increase Akt activation, consequently translocating FOXO to the nucleus, blocking protein degradation pathways. Moreover, exercise elicits an increased Nrf2 expression, leading to an elevation in the expression of antioxidant enzymes, therefore decreasing ROS levels.

7. Final Remarks

The balance between muscle mass synthesis/breakdown is essential for the normal function of the muscle, which is partly regulated by ROS. More research is accumulating regarding the impact of redox imbalance in the process of muscle wasting, even though the exact mechanisms are still to be determined. Moreover, the potential influence of exercise on the attenuation of muscle wasting in CKD patients appears to be gaining points. However, it is urgent that worldwide exercise programs be implemented to better solidify the existing results to date. Although numerous dialysis patients may appear too frail and incapable of engaging in exercise sessions, those who do it have experienced the benefits [214]. In these cases, less vigorous exercise offers value, and these types of adaptations will help to gradually lessen some clinicians' misconceptions of exercise as a potential contraindication to the patients' health [214]. Furthermore, besides the compelling evidence of the health benefits, there may also be impactful advantages to the healthcare systems, by reducing collateral costs of CKD patients, such as interventions associated with disease complications. More and more, we believe that the cost savings in the long-term probably overcome the financial limitations that are sometimes still imposed and impede the introduction of exercise programmes as routine in clinical units. Since CKD patients who undergo dialysis experience inevitable sedentary time during treatment, we encourage the implementation of intradialytic exercise interventions as a coadjutant therapeutic strategy to reduce or at least decelerate CKD-associated muscle wasting.

Author Contributions: Conceptualization: S.M., D.V.L. and J.L.V. Writing—Original Draft Preparation: S.M. drafted the manuscript with substantial contributions from D.V.L. and J.L.V. Writing—Review & Editing: D.V.L., L.A.B., A.F., A.C.S. and J.L.V. contributed with important intellectual content during manuscript drafting or revision and accept accountability for the overall work. All authors have read and agreed to the published version of the manuscript.

Funding: SM is supported by a Portuguese Foundation of Science and Technology (FCT) doctoral grant (SFRH/BD/07740/2020). The Research Center in Sports Sciences, Health Sciences and Human Development is funded by FCT (UID/04045/2020).

Institutional Review Board Statement: Not applicable.

Informed Consent Statement: Not applicable.

Data Availability Statement: Not applicable.

Conflicts of Interest: The authors declare that there are no conflict of interest regarding the publication of this paper.

References

1. Ciciliot, S.; Schiaffino, S. Regeneration of mammalian skeletal muscle. Basic mechanisms and clinical implications. *Curr. Pharm. Des.* **2010**, *16*, 906–914. [CrossRef] [PubMed]
2. Bentzinger, C.F.; Wang, Y.X.; Rudnicki, M.A. Building muscle: Molecular regulation of myogenesis. *Cold Spring Harb. Perspect. Biol.* **2012**, *4*, a008342. [CrossRef] [PubMed]
3. Schiaffino, S.; Mammucari, C. Regulation of skeletal muscle growth by the IGF1-Akt/PKB pathway: Insights from genetic models. *Skelet. Muscle* **2011**, *1*, 4. [CrossRef]
4. Tajbakhsh, S. Skeletal muscle stem cells in developmental versus regenerative myogenesis. *J. Intern. Med.* **2009**, *266*, 372–389. [CrossRef]
5. Sambasivan, R.; Tajbakhsh, S. Skeletal muscle stem cell birth and properties. *Semin. Cell Dev. Biol.* **2007**, *18*, 870–882. [CrossRef] [PubMed]
6. Parker, M.H.; Seale, P.; Rudnicki, M.A. Looking back to the embryo: Defining transcriptional networks in adult myogenesis. *Nat. Rev. Genet.* **2003**, *4*, 497–507. [CrossRef]
7. Schultz, E. Satellite cell proliferative compartments in growing skeletal muscles. *Dev. Biol.* **1996**, *175*, 84–94. [CrossRef] [PubMed]
8. Davis, T.A.; Fiorotto, M.L. Regulation of muscle growth in neonates. *Curr. Opin. Clin. Nutr. Metab. Care* **2009**, *12*, 78–85. [CrossRef]
9. Schmalbruch, H.; Lewis, D.M. Dynamics of nuclei of muscle fibers and connective tissue cells in normal and denervated rat muscles. *Muscle Nerve* **2000**, *23*, 617–626. [CrossRef]
10. Pellettieri, J.; Alvarado, A.S. Cell turnover and adult tissue homeostasis: From humans to planarians. *Annu. Rev. Genet.* **2007**, *41*, 83–105. [CrossRef]
11. Zhao, P.; Hoffman, E.P. Embryonic myogenesis pathways in muscle regeneration. *Dev. Dyn.* **2004**, *229*, 380–392. [CrossRef] [PubMed]
12. Bjornson, C.R.R.; Cheung, T.H.; Liu, L.; Tripathi, P.V.; Steeper, K.M.; Rando, T.A. Notch signalling is necessary to maintain quiescence in adult muscle stem cells. *STEM CELLS* **2012**, *30*, 232–242. [CrossRef]

13. Mourikis, P.; Gopalakrishnan, S.; Sambasivan, R.; Tajbakhsh, S. Cell-autonomous Notch activity maintains the temporal specification potential of skeletal muscle stem cells. *Development* **2012**, *139*, 4536–4548. [CrossRef]
14. Forcina, L.; Miano, C.; Pelosi, L.; Musarò, A. An overview about the biology of skeletal muscle satellite cells. *Curr. Genet.* **2019**, *20*, 24–37. [CrossRef] [PubMed]
15. Griffin, C.A.; Apponi, L.H.; Long, K.K.; Pavlath, G.K. Chemokine expression and control of muscle cell migration during myogenesis. *J. Cell Sci.* **2010**, *123 Pt 18*, 3052–3060 [CrossRef]
16. Gonzalez, M.L.; Busse, N.I.; Waits, C.M.; Johnson, S.E. Satellite cells and their regulation in livestock. *J. Anim. Sci.* **2020**, *98*, skaa081. [CrossRef]
17. Tidball, J.G.; Wehling-Henricks, M. Evolving therapeutic strategies for Duchenne muscular dystrophy: Targeting downstream events. *Pediatr. Res.* **2004**, *56*, 831–841 [CrossRef] [PubMed]
18. Pavlath, G.K. Current progress towards understanding mechanisms of myoblast fusion in mammals. In *Cell Fusions: Regulation and Control*; Larsson, L.-I., Ed.; Springer: Dordrecht, The Netherlands, 2011; pp. 249–265.
19. Christov, C.; Chrétien, F.; Abou-Khalil, R.; Bassez, G.; Vallet, G.; Authier, F.J.; Bassaglia, Y.; Shinin, V.; Tajbakhsh, S.; Chazaud, B.; et al. Muscle satellite cells and endothelial cells: Close neighbors and privileged partners. *Mol. Biol. Cell* **2007**, *18*, 1397–1409. [CrossRef]
20. Mauro, A. Satellite cell of skeletal muscle fibers. *J. Biophys. Biochem. Cytol.* **1961**, *9*, 493–495. [CrossRef]
21. Kuang, S.; Kuroda, K.; Le Grand, F.; Rudnicki, M.A. Asymmetric self-renewal and commitment of satellite stem cells in muscle. *Cell* **2007**, *129*, 999–1010. [CrossRef]
22. Troy, A.; Cadwallader, A.B.; Fedorov, Y.; Tyner, K.; Tanaka, K.K.; Olwin, B.B. Coordination of satellite cell activation and self-renewal by Par-complex-dependent asymmetric activation of p38α/β MAPK. *Cell Stem Cell* **2012**, *11*, 541–553. [CrossRef] [PubMed]
23. Abmayr, S.M.; Pavlath, G.K. Myoblast fusion: Lessons from flies and mice. *Development* **2012**, *139*, 641–656. [CrossRef]
24. Lemke, S.B.; Schnorrer, F. Mechanical forces during muscle development. *Mech. Dev.* **2017**, *144*, 92–101. [CrossRef] [PubMed]
25. Bowman, W.; Todd, R.B. XXI. On the minute structure and movements voluntary muscle. *Philos. Trans. R. Soc. Lond.* **1840**, *130*, 457–501. [CrossRef]
26. Sanes, J.R. The basement membrane/basal lamina of skeletal muscle. *J. Biol. Chem.* **2003**, *278*, 12601–12604. [CrossRef] [PubMed]
27. Rahimov, F.; Kunkel, L.M. Cellular and molecular mechanisms underlying muscular dystrophy. *J. Cell Biol.* **2013**, *201*, 499–510. [CrossRef] [PubMed]
28. Sweeney, H.L.; Hammers, D.W. Muscle contraction. *Cold Spring Harb. Perspect. Biol.* **2018**, *10*, a023200. [CrossRef]
29. Kallabis, S.; Abraham, L.; Müller, S.; Dzialas, V.; Türk, C.; Wiederstein, J.L.; Bock, T.; Nolte, H.; Nogara, L.; Blaauw, B.; et al. High-throughput proteomics fiber typing (ProFiT) for comprehensive characterization of single skeletal muscle fibers. *Skelet. Muscle* **2020**, *10*, 7. [CrossRef]
30. Jakobsen, J.R.; Mackey, A.L.; Knudsen, A.B.; Koch, M.; Kjær, M.; Krogsgaard, M.R. Composition and adaptation of human myotendinous junction and neighboring muscle fibers to heavy resistance training. *Scand. J. Med. Sci. Sports* **2017**, *27*, 1547–1559. [CrossRef]
31. Lee, S.-J. Regulation of muscle mass by myostatin. *Annu. Rev. Cell Dev. Biol.* **2004**, *20*, 61–86. [CrossRef]
32. Sugita, H.; Kaneki, M.; Sugita, M.; Yasukawa, T.; Yasuhara, S.; Martyn, J.A. Burn injury impairs insulin-stimulated Akt/PKB activation in skeletal muscle. *Am. J. Physiol. Endocrinol. Metab.* **2005**, *288*, E585–E591. [CrossRef] [PubMed]
33. Latres, E.; Amini, A.R.; Amini, A.A.; Griffiths, J.; Martin, F.J.; Wei, Y.; Lin, H.C.; Yancopoulos, G.D.; Glass, D.J. Insulin-like growth factor-1 (IGF-1) inversely regulates atrophy-induced genes via the phosphatidylinositol 3-kinase/Akt/mammalian target of rapamycin (PI3K/Akt/mTOR) pathway. *J. Biol. Chem.* **2005**, *280*, 2737–2744. [CrossRef] [PubMed]
34. Dinulovic, I.; Furrer, R.; Handschin, C. Plasticity of the Muscle Stem Cell Microenvironment. *Adv. Exp. Med. Biol.* **2017**, *1041*, 141–169. [CrossRef] [PubMed]
35. Jackman, R.W.; Kandarian, S.C. The molecular basis of skeletal muscle atrophy. *Am. J. Physiol. Cell Physiol.* **2004**, *287*, C834–C843. [CrossRef] [PubMed]
36. Cohen, S.; Brault, J.J.; Gygi, S.P.; Glass, D.J.; Valenzuela, D.M.; Gartner, C.; Latres, E.; Goldberg, A.L. During muscle atrophy, thick, but not thin, filament components are degraded by MuRF1-dependent ubiquitylation. *J. Cell Biol.* **2009**, *185*, 1083–1095. [CrossRef] [PubMed]
37. Jackson, M.J. Reactive oxygen species in sarcopenia: Should we focus on excess oxidative damage or defective redox signalling? *Mol. Aspects Med.* **2016**, *50*, 33–40. [CrossRef]
38. Damiano, S.; Muscariello, E.; La Rosa, G.; Di Marco, M.; Mondola, P.; Santillo, M. Dual Role of Reactive Oxygen Species in Muscle Function: Can Antioxidant Dietary Supplements Counteract Age-Related Sarcopenia? *Int. J. Mol. Sci.* **2019**, *20*, 3815. [CrossRef]
39. Ji, L.L. Redox signalling in skeletal muscle: Role of aging and exercise. *Adv. Physiol. Educ.* **2015**, *39*, 352–359. [CrossRef]
40. Halliwell, B.; Cross, C.E. Oxygen-derived species: Their relation to human disease and environmental stress. *Environ. Health Perspect.* **1994**, *102* (Suppl. S10), 5–12. [CrossRef]
41. Kehrer, J.P. The Haber-Weiss reaction and mechanisms of toxicity. *Toxicology* **2000**, *149*, 43–50. [CrossRef]
42. Castro, J.P.; Jung, T.; Grune, T.; Almeida, H. Actin carbonylation: From cell dysfunction to organism disorder. *J. Proteomics* **2013**, *92*, 171–180. [CrossRef] [PubMed]

43. Orient, A.; Donkó, A.; Szabó, A.; Leto, T.L.; Geiszt, M. Novel sources of reactive oxygen species in the human body. *Nephrol. Dial. Transplant.* **2007**, *22*, 1281–1288. [CrossRef] [PubMed]
44. Burton, G.J.; Jauniaux, E. Oxidative stress. *Best Pract. Res. Clin. Obstet. Gynaecol.* **2011**, *25*, 287–299. [CrossRef]
45. Cadenas, E.; Davies, K.J. Mitochondrial free radical generation, oxidative stress, and aging. *Free Radic. Biol. Med.* **2000**, *29*, 222–230. [CrossRef]
46. Tu, B.P.; Weissman, J.S. Oxidative protein folding in eukaryotes: Mechanisms and consequences. *J. Cell Biol.* **2004**, *164*, 341–346. [CrossRef] [PubMed]
47. He, L.; He, T.; Farrar, S.; Ji, L.; Liu, T.; Ma, X. Antioxidants maintain cellular redox homeostasis by elimination of reactive oxygen species. *Cell Physiol. Biochem.* **2017**, *44*, 532–553. [CrossRef] [PubMed]
48. Mirończuk-Chodakowska, I.; Witkowska, A.M.; Zujko, M.E. Endogenous non-enzymatic antioxidants in the human body. *Adv. Med. Sci.* **2018**, *63*, 68–78. [CrossRef]
49. Powers, S.K.; Jackson, M.J. Exercise-induced oxidative stress: Cellular mechanisms and impact on muscle force production. *Physiol. Rev.* **2008**, *88*, 1243–1276. [CrossRef]
50. Marinho, H.S.; Real, C.; Cyrne, L.; Soares, H.; Antunes, F. Hydrogen peroxide sensing, signalling and regulation of transcription factors. *Redox Biol.* **2014**, *2*, 535–562. [CrossRef]
51. Zhang, J.; Wang, X.; Vikash, V.; Ye, Q.; Wu, D.; Liu, Y.; Dong, W. ROS and ROS-mediated cellular signalling. *Oxid. Med. Cell. Longev.* **2016**, *2016*, 4350965. [CrossRef]
52. Sies, H. Oxidative stress: A concept in redox biology and medicine. *Redox Biol.* **2015**, *4*, 180–183. [CrossRef] [PubMed]
53. Sies, H.; Berndt, C.; Jones, D.P. Oxidative stress. *Annu. Rev. Biochem.* **2017**, *86*, 715–748. [CrossRef]
54. Sai, K.K.S.; Chen, X.; Li, Z.; Zhu, C.; Shukla, K.; Forshaw, T.E.; Wu, H.; Vance, S.A.; Pathirannahel, B.L.; Madonna, M.; et al. [(18)F]Fluoro-DCP, a first generation PET radiotracer for monitoring protein sulfenylation in vivo. *Redox Biol.* **2022**, *49*, 102218. [CrossRef]
55. Olowe, R.; Sandouka, S.; Saadi, A.; Shekh-Ahmad, T. Approaches for Reactive Oxygen Species and Oxidative Stress Quantification in Epilepsy. *Antioxidants* **2020**, *9*, 990. [CrossRef]
56. Oswald, M.C.W.; Garnham, N.; Sweeney, S.T.; Landgraf, M. Regulation of neuronal development and function by ROS. *FEBS Lett.* **2018**, *592*, 679–691. [CrossRef] [PubMed]
57. Jackson, M.J. Redox regulation of muscle adaptations to contractile activity and aging. *J. Appl. Physiol. (1985)* **2015**, *119*, 163–171. [CrossRef] [PubMed]
58. Trinity, J.D.; Broxterman, R.M.; Richardson, R.S. Regulation of exercise blood flow: Role of free radicals. *Free Radic. Biol. Med.* **2016**, *98*, 90–102. [CrossRef]
59. Aranda-Rivera, A.K.; Cruz-Gregorio, A.; Aparicio-Trejo, O.E.; Pedraza-Chaverri, J. Mitochondrial Redox Signalling and Oxidative Stress in Kidney Diseases. *Biomolecules* **2021**, *11*, 1144. [CrossRef]
60. Irazabal, M.V.; Torres, V.E. Reactive oxygen species and redox signalling in chronic kidney disease. *Cells* **2020**, *9*, 1342. [CrossRef]
61. He, F.; Ru, X.; Wen, T. NRF2, a Transcription Factor for Stress Response and Beyond. *Int. J. Mol. Sci.* **2020**, *21*, 4777. [CrossRef]
62. Motohashi, H.; Yamamoto, M. Nrf2-Keap1 defines a physiologically important stress response mechanism. *Trends Mol. Med.* **2004**, *10*, 549–557. [CrossRef] [PubMed]
63. Baird, L.; Yamamoto, M. The Molecular Mechanisms Regulating the KEAP1-NRF2 Pathway. *Mol. Cell Biol.* **2020**, *40*, e00099-20. [CrossRef] [PubMed]
64. He, F.; Antonucci, L.; Karin, M. NRF2 as a regulator of cell metabolism and inflammation in cancer. *Carcinogenesis* **2020**, *41*, 405–416. [CrossRef] [PubMed]
65. Foreman, N.A.; Hesse, A.S.; Ji, L.L. Redox Signalling and Sarcopenia: Searching for the Primary Suspect. *Int. J. Mol. Sci.* **2021**, *22*, 9045. [CrossRef]
66. Li, Y.P.; Schwartz, R.J.; Waddell, I.D.; Holloway, B.R.; Reid, M.B. Skeletal muscle myocytes undergo protein loss and reactive oxygen-mediated NF-kappaB activation in response to tumor necrosis factor alpha. *Faseb. J.* **1998**, *12*, 871–880. [CrossRef]
67. Russell, S.T.; Eley, H.; Tisdale, M.J. Role of reactive oxygen species in protein degradation in murine myotubes induced by proteolysis-inducing factor and angiotensin II. *Cell. Signal.* **2007**, *19*, 1797–1806. [CrossRef]
68. Reid, M.B.; Li, Y.P. Tumor necrosis factor-alpha and muscle wasting: A cellular perspective. *Respir. Res.* **2001**, *2*, 269–272. [CrossRef] [PubMed]
69. Li, Y.P.; Reid, M.B. NF-kappaB mediates the protein loss induced by TNF-alpha in differentiated skeletal muscle myotubes. *Am. J. Physiol. Integr. Comp. Physiol.* **2000**, *279*, R1165–R1170. [CrossRef]
70. Pedersen, M.; Bruunsgaard, H.; Weis, N.; Hendel, H.W.; Andreassen, B.U.; Eldrup, E.; Dela, F.; Pedersen, B.K. Circulating levels of TNF-alpha and IL-6 relation to truncal fat mass and muscle mass in healthy elderly individuals and in patients with type-2 diabetes. *Mech. Ageing Dev.* **2003**, *124*, 495–502. [CrossRef]
71. El Assar, M.; Angulo, J.; Rodríguez-Mañas, L. Frailty as a phenotypic manifestation of underlying oxidative stress. *Free Radic. Biol. Med.* **2020**, *149*, 72–77. [CrossRef]
72. Carmeli, E.; Coleman, R.; Reznick, A.Z. The biochemistry of aging muscle. *Exp. Gerontol.* **2002**, *37*, 477–489. [CrossRef] [PubMed]
73. Morley, J.E.; Thomas, D.R.; Wilson, M.M. Cachexia: Pathophysiology and clinical relevance. *Am. J. Clin. Nutr.* **2006**, *83*, 735–743. [CrossRef]

74. von Haehling, S.; Anker, S.D. Prevalence, incidence and clinical impact of cachexia Facts and numbers-update 2014. *J. Cachex-Sarcopenia Muscle* **2014**, *5*, 261–263. [CrossRef] [PubMed]
75. Johnson, C.A.; Levey, A.S.; Coresh, J.; Levin, A.; Lau, J.; Eknoyan, G. Clinical practice guidelines for chronic kidney disease in adults: Part I. Definition, disease stages, evaluation, treatment, and risk factors. *Am. Fam. Physician* **2004**, *70*, 869–876. [PubMed]
76. Workeneh, B.T.; Rondon-Berrios, H.; Zhang, L.; Hu, Z.; Ayehu, G.; Ferrando, A.; Kopple, J.D.; Wang, H.; Storer, T.; Fournier, M.; et al. Development of a diagnostic method for detecting increased muscle protein degradation in patients with catabolic conditions. *J. Am. Soc. Nephrol.* **2006**, *17*, 3233–3239. [CrossRef] [PubMed]
77. Milan, G.; Romanello, V.; Pescatore, F.; Armani, A.; Paik, J.-H.; Frasson, L.; Seydel, A.; Zhao, J.; Abraham, R.; Goldberg, A.L.; et al. Regulation of autophagy and the ubiquitin–proteasome system by the FoxO transcriptional network during muscle atrophy. *Nat. Commun.* **2015**, *6*, 6670. [CrossRef]
78. Diesel, W.; Emms, M.; Knight, B.K.; Noakes, T.D.; Swanepoel, C.R.; van Zyl Smit, R.; Kaschula, R.O.; Sinclair-Smith, C.C. Morphologic features of the myopathy associated with chronic renal failure. *Am. J. Kidney Dis.* **1993**, *22*, 677–684. [CrossRef]
79. Deleaval, P.; Luaire, B.; Laffay, P.; Jambut-Cadon, C.; Stauss-Grabo, M.; Canaud, B.; Chazot, C. Short-term effects of branched-chain amino acids-enriched dialysis fluid on branched-chain amino acids plasma level and mass balance: A randomized cross-over study. *J. Ren. Nutr.* **2020**, *30*, 61–68. [CrossRef]
80. Martins, A.M.; Rodrigues, J.C.D.; de Oliveira Santin, F.G.; Brito, F.D.S.B.; Moreira, A.S.B.; Lourenço, R.A.; Avesani, C.M. Food intake assessment of elderly patients on hemodialysis. *J. Ren. Nutr.* **2015**, *25*, 321–325. [CrossRef]
81. Pike, M.; Taylor, J.; Kabagambe, E.; Stewart, T.G.; Robinson-Cohen, C.; Morse, J.; Akwo, E.; Abdel-Kader, K.; Siew, E.D.; Blot, W.J.; et al. The association of exercise and sedentary behaviours with incident end-stage renal disease: The Southern Community Cohort Study. *BMJ Open* **2019**, *9*, e030661. [CrossRef]
82. Wang, X.H.; Mitch, W.E. Mechanisms of muscle wasting in chronic kidney disease. *Nat. Rev. Nephrol.* **2014**, *10*, 504–516. [CrossRef]
83. Ikizler, T.A.; Pupim, L.B.; Brouillette, J.R.; Leverhagen, D.K.; Farmer, K.; Hakim, R.M.; Flakoll, P.J. Hemodialysis stimulates muscle and whole body protein loss and alters substrate oxidation. *Am. J. Physiol. Metab.* **2002**, *282*, E107–E116. [CrossRef] [PubMed]
84. Pupim, L.B.; Flakoll, P.J.; Brouillette, J.R.; Levenhagen, D.K.; Hakim, R.M.; Ikizler, T.A. Intradialytic parenteral nutrition improves protein and energy homeostasis in chronic hemodialysis patients. *J. Clin. Investig.* **2002**, *110*, 483–492. [CrossRef] [PubMed]
85. Pupim, L.B.; Majchrzak, K.M.; Flakoll, P.J.; Ikizler, T.A. Intradialytic oral nutrition improves protein homeostasis in chronic hemodialysis patients with deranged nutritional status. *J. Am. Soc. Nephrol.* **2006**, *17*, 3149–3157. [CrossRef] [PubMed]
86. Carrero, J.J.; Stenvinkel, P.; Cuppari, L.; Ikizler, T.A.; Kalantar-Zadeh, K.; Kaysen, G.; Mitch, W.E.; Price, S.R.; Wanner, C.; Wang, A.Y.; et al. Etiology of the protein-energy wasting syndrome in chronic kidney disease: A consensus statement from the International Society of Renal Nutrition and Metabolism (ISRNM). *J. Ren. Nutr.* **2013**, *23*, 77–90. [CrossRef]
87. Stenvinkel, P.; Larsson, T.E. Chronic kidney disease: A clinical model of premature aging. *Am. J. Kidney Dis.* **2013**, *62*, 339–351. [CrossRef]
88. Stel, V.S.; Brück, K.; Fraser, S.; Zoccali, C.; Massy, Z.A.; Jager, K.J. International differences in chronic kidney disease prevalence: A key public health and epidemiologic research issue. *Nephrol. Dial. Transplant.* **2017**, *32* (Suppl. S2), ii129–ii135. [CrossRef]
89. Biolo, G.; Fleming, R.Y.; Maggi, S.P.; Nguyen, T.T.; Herndon, D.N.; Wolfe, R.R. Inhibition of muscle glutamine formation in hypercatabolic patients. *Clin. Sci.* **2000**, *99*, 189–194. [CrossRef]
90. Gore, D.; Jahoor, F. Deficiency in Peripheral Glutamine Production in Pediatric Patients With Burns. *J. Burn. Care Rehabil.* **2000**, *21*, 171, discussion 172–177. [CrossRef]
91. Lightfoot, A.; McArdle, A.; Griffiths, R.D. Muscle in defence. *Crit. Care Med.* **2009**, *37* (Suppl. S10), S384–S390. [CrossRef]
92. Thome, T.; Salyers, Z.R.; Kumar, R.A.; Hahn, D.; Berru, F.N.; Ferreira, L.F.; Scali, S.T.; Ryan, T.E. Uremic metabolites impair skeletal muscle mitochondrial energetics through disruption of the electron transport system and matrix dehydrogenase activity. *Am. J. Physiol. Cell Physiol.* **2019**, *317*, C701–C713. [CrossRef] [PubMed]
93. Thome, T.; Kumar, R.A.; Burke, S.K.; Khattri, R.B.; Salyers, Z.R.; Kelley, R.C.; Coleman, M.D.; Christou, D.D.; Hepple, R.T.; Scali, S.T.; et al. Impaired muscle mitochondrial energetics is associated with uremic metabolite accumulation in chronic kidney disease. *JCI Insight* **2020**, *6*, e139826. [CrossRef] [PubMed]
94. Duranton, F.; Cohen, G.; De Smet, R.; Rodriguez, M.; Jankowski, J.; Vanholder, R.; Argiles, A. Normal and pathologic concentrations of uremic toxins. *J. Am. Soc. Nephrol.* **2012**, *23*, 1258–1270. [CrossRef] [PubMed]
95. Vanholder, R.; Schepers, E.; Pletinck, A.; Nagler, E.V.; Glorieux, G. The uremic toxicity of indoxyl sulfate and p-cresyl sulfate: A systematic review. *J. Am. Soc. Nephrol.* **2014**, *25*, 1897–1907. [CrossRef]
96. Enoki, Y.; Watanabe, H.; Arake, R.; Sugimoto, R.; Imafuku, T.; Tominaga, Y.; Ishima, Y.; Kotani, S.; Nakajima, M.; Tanaka, M.; et al. Indoxyl sulfate potentiates skeletal muscle atrophy by inducing the oxidative stress-mediated expression of myostatin and atrogin-1. *Sci. Rep.* **2016**, *6*, 32084. [CrossRef]
97. Rodrigues, G.G.C.; Dellê, H.; Brito, R.B.O.; Cardoso, V.O.; Fernandes, K.P.S.; Mesquita-Ferrari, R.A.; Cunha, R.S.; Stinghen, A.E.M.; Dalboni, M.A.; Barreto, F.C. Indoxyl Sulfate Contributes to Uremic Sarcopenia by Inducing Apoptosis in Myoblasts. *Arch. Med. Res.* **2020**, *51*, 21–29. [CrossRef]
98. Higashihara, T.; Nishi, H.; Takemura, K.; Watanabe, H.; Maruyama, T.; Inagi, R.; Tanaka, T.; Nangaku, M. β2-adrenergic receptor agonist counteracts skeletal muscle atrophy and oxidative stress in uremic mice. *Sci. Rep.* **2021**, *11*, 9130. [CrossRef]

99. Sriram, S.; Subramanian, S.; Sathiakumar, D.; Venkatesh, R.; Salerno, M.S.; McFarlane, C.D.; Kambadur, R.; Sharma, M. Modulation of reactive oxygen species in skeletal muscle by myostatin is mediated through NF-κB. *Aging Cell* **2011**, *10*, 931–948. [CrossRef]
100. Powers, S.K.; Kavazis, A.N.; DeRuisseau, K.C. Mechanisms of disuse muscle atrophy: Role of oxidative stress. *Am. J. Physiol. Regul. Integr. Comp. Physiol.* **2005**, *288*, R337–R344. [CrossRef]
101. Zhang, L.; Pan, J.; Dong, Y.; Tweardy, D.J.; Dong, Y.; Garibotto, G.; Mitch, W.E. Stat3 activation links a C/EBPδ to myostatin pathway to stimulate loss of muscle mass. *Cell Metabol.* **2013**, *18*, 368–379. [CrossRef]
102. Viana, J.L.; Kosmadakis, G.C.; Watson, E.L.; Bevington, A.; Feehally, J.; Bishop, N.C.; Smith, A.C. Evidence for anti-inflammatory effects of exercise in CKD. *J. Am. Soc. Nephrol.* **2014**, *25*, 2121–2130. [CrossRef] [PubMed]
103. Ling, X.C.; Kuo, K.-L. Oxidative stress in chronic kidney disease. *Ren. Replace. Ther.* **2018**, *4*, 53. [CrossRef]
104. Mahdy, M.A.A. Skeletal muscle fibrosis: An overview. *Cell Tissue Res.* **2019**, *375*, 575–588. [CrossRef] [PubMed]
105. Avin, K.G.; Chen, N.X.; Organ, J.M.; Zarse, C.; O'Neill, K.; Conway, R.G.; Konrad, R.J.; Bacallao, R.L.; Allen, M.R.; Moe, S.M. Skeletal muscle regeneration and oxidative stress are altered in chronic kidney disease. *PLoS ONE* **2016**, *11*, e0159411. [CrossRef] [PubMed]
106. Uezumi, A.; Fukada, S.-I.; Yamamoto, N.; Takeda, S.I.; Tsuchida, K. Mesenchymal progenitors distinct from satellite cells contribute to ectopic fat cell formation in skeletal muscle. *Nat. Cell Biol.* **2010**, *12*, 143–152. [CrossRef]
107. Li, Y.; Huard, J. Differentiation of muscle-derived cells into myofibroblasts in injured skeletal muscle. *Am. J. Pathol.* **2002**, *161*, 895–907. [CrossRef]
108. Ahmad, K.; Shaikh, S.; Ahmad, S.S.; Lee, E.J.; Choi, I. Cross-talk between extracellular matrix and skeletal muscle: Implications for myopathies. *Front. Pharmacol.* **2020**, *11*, 142. [CrossRef]
109. Csapo, R.; Gumpenberger, M.; Wessner, B. Skeletal muscle extracellular matrix—What do we know about its composition, regulation, and physiological roles? A narrative review. *Front. Physiol.* **2020**, *11*, 253. [CrossRef]
110. Dong, J.; Dong, Y.; Chen, Z.; Mitch, W.E.; Zhang, L. The pathway to muscle fibrosis depends on myostatin stimulating the differentiation of fibro/adipogenic progenitor cells in chronic kidney disease. *Kidney Int.* **2017**, *91*, 119–128. [CrossRef]
111. Snijders, T.; Verdijk, L.B.; van Loon, L.J. The impact of sarcopenia and exercise training on skeletal muscle satellite cells. *Ageing Res. Rev.* **2009**, *8*, 328–338. [CrossRef]
112. Fry, C.S.; Lee, J.D.; Jackson, J.R.; Kirby, T.J.; Stasko, S.A.; Liu, H.; Dupont-Versteegden, E.E.; McCarthy, J.J.; Peterson, C.A. Regulation of the muscle fiber microenvironment by activated satellite cells during hypertrophy. *FASEB J.* **2014**, *28*, 1654–1665. [CrossRef] [PubMed]
113. Abramowitz, M.K.; Paredes, W.; Zhang, K.; Brightwell, C.R.; Newsom, J.N.; Kwon, H.-J.; Custodio, M.; Buttar, R.S.; Farooq, H.; Zaidi, B.; et al. Skeletal muscle fibrosis is associated with decreased muscle inflammation and weakness in patients with chronic kidney disease. *Am. J. Physiol. Renal. Physiol.* **2018**, *315*, F1658–F1669. [CrossRef]
114. Baker, L.A.; O'Sullivan, T.F.; Robinson, K.A.; Graham-Brown, M.P.M.; Major, R.W.; Ashford, R.U.; Smith, A.C.; Philp, A.; Watson, E.L. Primary skeletal muscle cells from chronic kidney disease patients retain hallmarks of cachexia in vitro. *J. Cachexia Sarcopenia Muscle* **2022**, *13*, 1238–1249. [CrossRef] [PubMed]
115. Ryall, J.G.; Schertzer, J.D.; Lynch, G.S. Cellular and molecular mechanisms underlying age-related skeletal muscle wasting and weakness. *Biogerontology* **2008**, *9*, 213–228. [CrossRef] [PubMed]
116. Yue, Z.; Mester, J. A model analysis of internal loads, energetics, and effects of wobbling mass during the whole-body vibration. *J. Biomech.* **2002**, *35*, 639–647. [CrossRef] [PubMed]
117. Suhr, F. Extracellular matrix, proteases and physical exercise. *Dtsch. Z. Für Sportmed.* **2019**, *70*, 97–104. [CrossRef]
118. Leal, V.O.; Saldanha, J.F.; Stockler-Pinto, M.B.; Cardozo, L.F.M.F.; Santos, F.R.; Albuquerque, A.S.D.; Leite, M., Jr.; Mafra, D. NRF2 and NF-κB mRNA expression in chronic kidney disease: A focus on nondialysis patients. *Int. Urol. Nephrol.* **2015**, *47*, 1985–1991. [CrossRef]
119. Pedruzzi, L.M.; Cardozo, L.F.M.F.; Daleprane, J.B.; Stockler-Pinto, M.B.; Monteiro, E.B.; Leite, M.; Vaziri, N.D.; Mafra, D. Systemic inflammation and oxidative stress in hemodialysis patients are associated with down-regulation of Nrf2. *J. Nephrol.* **2015**, *28*, 495–501. [CrossRef]
120. Nezu, M.; Suzuki, N.; Yamamoto, M. Targeting the KEAP1-NRF2 System to Prevent Kidney Disease Progression. *Am. J. Nephrol.* **2017**, *45*, 473–483. [CrossRef]
121. Wang, J.; Zhu, H.; Huang, L.; Zhu, X.; Sha, J.; Li, G.; Ma, G.; Zhang, W.; Gu, M.; Guo, Y. Nrf2 signalling attenuates epithelial-to-mesenchymal transition and renal interstitial fibrosis via PI3K/Akt signalling pathways. *Exp. Mol. Pathol.* **2019**, *111*, 104296. [CrossRef]
122. Panizo, S.; Barrio-Vázquez, S.; Naves-Díaz, M.; Carrillo-López, N.; Rodríguez, I.; Fernández-Vázquez, A.; Valdivielso, J.M.; Thadhani, R.; Cannata-Andía, J.B. Vitamin D receptor activation, left ventricular hypertrophy and myocardial fibrosis. *Nephrol. Dial. Transplant.* **2013**, *28*, 2735–2744. [CrossRef] [PubMed]
123. Mann, C.J.; Perdiguero, E.; Kharraz, Y.; Aguilar, S.; Pessina, P.; Serrano, A.L.; Muñoz-Cánoves, P. Aberrant repair and fibrosis development in skeletal muscle. *Skelet. Muscle* **2011**, *1*, 21. [CrossRef] [PubMed]
124. Mallamaci, F.; Pisano, A.; Tripepi, G. Physical activity in chronic kidney disease and the EXerCise Introduction To Enhance trial. *Nephrol. Dial. Transplant.* **2020**, *35* (Suppl. S2), ii18–ii22. [CrossRef]
125. Filipčič, T.; Bogataj, Š.; Pajek, J.; Pajek, M. Physical activity and quality of life in hemodialysis patients and healthy controls: A cross-sectional study. *Int. J. Environ. Res.* **2021**, *18*, 1978. [CrossRef]

126. Johansen, K.L.; Chertow, G.M.; Ng, A.V.; Mulligan, K.; Carey, S.; Schoenfeld, P.Y.; Kent-Braun, J.A. Physical activity levels in patients on hemodialysis and healthy sedentary controls. *Kidney Int.* **2000**, *57*, 2564–2570. [CrossRef]
127. Clark, B.C. In vivo alterations in skeletal muscle form and function after disuse atrophy. *Med. Sci. Sports Exerc.* **2009**, *41*, 1869–1875. [CrossRef]
128. Park, H.; Park, S.; Shephard, R.J.; Aoyagi, Y. Yearlong physical activity and sarcopenia in older adults: The Nakanojo Study. *Eur. J. Appl. Physiol.* **2010**, *109*, 953–961. [CrossRef] [PubMed]
129. Johansen, K.L.; Chertow, G.M.; da Silva, M.; Carey, S.; Painter, P. Determinants of physical performance in ambulatory patients on hemodialysis. *Kidney Int.* **2001**, *60*, 1586–1591. [CrossRef] [PubMed]
130. Segura-Ortí, E.; Gordon, P.L.; Doyle, J.W.; Johansen, K.L. Correlates of physical functioning and performance across the spectrum of kidney function. *Clin. Nurs. Res.* **2018**, *27*, 579–596. [CrossRef]
131. Pérez-Sáez, M.J.; Morgado-Pérez, A.; Faura, A.; Muñoz-Redondo, E.; Gárriz, M.; Muns, M.D.; Nogués, X.; Marco, E.; Pascual, J. The FRAILMar Study Protocol: Frailty in Patients with Advanced Chronic Kidney Disease Awaiting Kidney Transplantation. A Randomized Clinical Trial of Multimodal Prehabilitation. *Front. Med.* **2021**, *8*, 675049. [CrossRef]
132. Cho, J.; Choi, Y.; Sajgalik, P.; No, M.H.; Lee, S.H.; Kim, S.; Heo, J.W.; Cho, E.J.; Chang, E.; Kang, J.H.; et al. Exercise as a Therapeutic Strategy for Sarcopenia in Heart Failure: Insights into Underlying Mechanisms. *Cells* **2020**, *9*, 2284. [CrossRef] [PubMed]
133. Majchrzak, K.M.; Pupim, L.B.; Flakoll, P.J.; Ikizler, T.A. Resistance exercise augments the acute anabolic effects of intradialytic oral nutritional supplementation. *Nephrol. Dial. Transplant.* **2008**, *23*, 1362–1369. [CrossRef] [PubMed]
134. Martins, P.; Marques, E.A.; Leal, D.V.; Ferreira, A.; Wilund, K.R.; Viana, J.L. Association between physical activity and mortality in end-stage kidney disease: A systematic review of observational studies. *BMC Nephrol.* **2021**, *22*, 227. [CrossRef]
135. Wilkinson, T.J.; Watson, E.L.; Gould, D.W.; Xenophontos, S.; Clarke, A.L.; Vogt, B.P.; Viana, J.L.; Smith, A.C. Twelve weeks of supervised exercise improves self-reported symptom burden and fatigue in chronic kidney disease: A secondary analysis of the 'ExTra CKD' trial. *Clin. Kidney J.* **2019**, *12*, 113–121. [CrossRef] [PubMed]
136. Watson, E.L.; Viana, J.L.; Wimbury, D.; Martin, N.; Greening, N.J.; Barratt, J.; Smith, A.C. The effect of resistance exercise on inflammatory and myogenic markers in patients with chronic kidney disease. *Front. Physiol.* **2017**, *8*, 541. [CrossRef]
137. Gould, D.W.; Watson, E.L.; Wilkinson, T.J.; Wormleighton, J.; Xenophontos, S.; Viana, J.L.; Smith, A.C. Ultrasound assessment of muscle mass in response to exercise training in chronic kidney disease: A comparison with MRI. *J. Cachexia Sarcopenia Muscle* **2019**, *10*, 748–755. [CrossRef] [PubMed]
138. Chen, J.L.; Godfrey, S.; Ng, T.T.; Moorthi, R.; Liangos, O.; Ruthazer, R.; Jaber, B.L.; Levey, A.S.; Castaneda-Sceppa, C. Effect of intra-dialytic, low-intensity strength training on functional capacity in adult haemodialysis patients: A randomized pilot trial. *Nephrol. Dial. Transplant.* **2010**, *25*, 1936–1943. [CrossRef]
139. Johansen, K.L.; Painter, P.L.; Sakkas, G.K.; Gordon, P.; Doyle, J.; Shubert, T. Effects of resistance exercise training and nandrolone decanoate on body composition and muscle function among patients who receive hemodialysis: A randomized, controlled trial. *J. Am. Soc. Nephrol.* **2006**, *17*, 2307–2314. [CrossRef]
140. Cheema, B.; Abas, H.; Smith, B.; O'Sullivan, A.; Chan, M.; Patwardhan, A.; Kelly, J.; Gillin, A.; Pang, G.; Lloyd, B.; et al. Randomized controlled trial of intradialytic resistance training to target muscle wasting in ESRD: The Progressive Exercise for Anabolism in Kidney Disease (PEAK) study. *Am. J. Kidney Dis.* **2007**, *50*, 574–584. [CrossRef]
141. Kouidi, E.; Albani, M.; Natsis, K.; Megalopoulos, A.; Gigis, P.; Guiba-Tziampiri, O.; Tourkantonis, A.; Deligiannis, A. The effects of exercise training on muscle atrophy in haemodialysis patients. *Nephrol. Dial. Transplant.* **1998**, *13*, 685–699. [CrossRef]
142. Molsted, S.; Andersen, J.L.; Harrison, A.P.; Eidemak, I.; Mackey, A.L. Fiber type-specific response of skeletal muscle satellite cells to high-intensity resistance training in dialysis patients. *Muscle Nerve* **2015**, *52*, 736–745. [CrossRef] [PubMed]
143. Konstantinidou, E.; Koukouvou, G.; Kouidi, E.; Deligiannis, A.; Tourkantonis, A. Exercise training in patients with end-stage renal disease on hemodialysis: Comparison of three rehabilitation programs. *J. Rehabil. Med.* **2002**, *34*, 40–45. [CrossRef] [PubMed]
144. Anderson, J.E.; Boivin, M.R., Jr.; Hatchett, L. Effect of exercise training on interdialytic ambulatory and treatment-related blood pressure in hemodialysis patients. *Ren. Fail.* **2004**, *26*, 539–544. [CrossRef]
145. Mustata, S.; Chan, C.; Lai, V.; Miller, J.A. Impact of an exercise program on arterial stiffness and insulin resistance in hemodialysis patients. *J. Am. Soc. Nephrol.* **2004**, *15*, 2713–2718. [CrossRef]
146. Oh-Park, M.; Fast, A.; Gopal, S.; Lynn, R.; Frei, G.; Drenth, R.; Zohman, L. Exercise for the dialyzed: Aerobic and strength training during hemodialysis. *Am. J. Phys. Med. Rehabil.* **2002**, *81*, 814–821. [CrossRef] [PubMed]
147. Kouidi, E.; Iacovides, A.; Iordanidis, P.; Vassiliou, S.; Deligiannis, A.; Ierodiakonou, C.; Tourkantonis, A. Exercise renal rehabilitation program: Psychosocial effects. *Nephron* **1997**, *77*, 152–158. [CrossRef] [PubMed]
148. Painter, P.; Carlson, L.; Carey, S.; Paul, S.M.; Myll, J. Physical functioning and health-related quality-of-life changes with exercise training in hemodialysis patients. *Am. J. Kidney Dis.* **2000**, *35*, 482–492. [CrossRef]
149. Parsons, T.L.; Toffelmire, E.B.; King-VanVlack, C.E. Exercise training during hemodialysis improves dialysis efficacy and physical performance. *Arch. Phys. Med. Rehabil.* **2006**, *87*, 680–687. [CrossRef]
150. Sakkas, G.K.; Sargeant, A.J.; Mercer, T.H.; Ball, D.; Koufaki, P.; Karatzaferi, C.; Naish, P.F. Changes in muscle morphology in dialysis patients after 6 months of aerobic exercise training. *Nephrol. Dial. Transplant.* **2003**, *18*, 1854–1861. [CrossRef]
151. Storer, T.W.; Casaburi, R.; Sawelson, S.; Kopple, J.D. Endurance exercise training during haemodialysis improves strength, power, fatigability and physical performance in maintenance haemodialysis patients. *Nephrol. Dial. Transplant.* **2005**, *20*, 1429–1437. [CrossRef]

152. Descamps-Latscha, B.; Jungers, P.; Witko-Sarsat, V. Immune system dysregulation in uremia: Role of oxidative stress. *Blood Purif.* **2002**, *20*, 481–484. [CrossRef] [PubMed]
153. Eleftheriadis, T.; Antoniadi, G.; Liakopoulos, V.; Kartsios, C.; Stefanidis, I. Disturbances of acquired immunity in hemodialysis patients. *Semin. Dial.* **2007**, *20*, 440–451. [CrossRef] [PubMed]
154. Kato, S.; Chmielewski, M.; Honda, H.; Pecoits-Filho, R.; Matsuo, S.; Yuzawa, Y.; Tranaeus, A.; Stenvinkel, P.; Lindholm, B. Aspects of immune dysfunction in end-stage renal disease. *Clin. J. Am. Soc. Nephrol.* **2008**, *3*, 1526–1533. [CrossRef]
155. Nielsen, A.R.; Mounier, R.; Plomgaard, P.; Mortensen, O.H.; Penkowa, M.; Speerschneider, T.; Pilegaard, H.; Pedersen, B.K. Expression of interleukin-15 in human skeletal muscle effect of exercise and muscle fibre type composition. *J. Physiol.* **2007**, *584 Pt 1*, 305–312. [CrossRef] [PubMed]
156. Pedersen, B.K.; Febbraio, M.A. Muscles, exercise and obesity: Skeletal muscle as a secretory organ. *Nat. Rev. Endocrinol.* **2012**, *8*, 457–465. [CrossRef] [PubMed]
157. Huh, J.Y. The role of exercise-induced myokines in regulating metabolism. *Arch. Pharm. Res.* **2018**, *41*, 14–29. [CrossRef]
158. Marinho, S.; Lasmar, R.; Mafra, D. Effect of a resistance exercise training program on bone markers in hemodialysis patients. *Sci. Sport.* **2017**, *32*, 99–105. [CrossRef]
159. Marinho, S.M.; Mafra, D.; Pelletier, S.; Hage, V.; Teuma, C.; Laville, M.; Eduardo, J.C.C.; Fouque, D. In Hemodialysis Patients, Intradialytic Resistance Exercise Improves Osteoblast Function: A Pilot Study. *J. Ren. Nutr.* **2016**, *26*, 341–345. [CrossRef]
160. Leal, D.V.; Ferreira, A.; Watson, E.L.; Wilund, K.R.; Viana, J.L. Muscle-bone crosstalk in chronic kidney disease: The potential modulatory effects of exercise. *Calcif. Tissue Int.* **2021**, *108*, 461–475. [CrossRef]
161. Wood, L.K.; Kayupov, E.; Gumucio, J.P.; Mendias, C.L.; Claflin, D.R.; Brooks, S.V. Intrinsic stiffness of extracellular matrix increases with age in skeletal muscles of mice. *J. Appl. Physiol.* **2014**, *117*, 363–369. [CrossRef]
162. Nystoriak, M.A.; Bhatnagar, A. Cardiovascular Effects and Benefits of Exercise. *Front. Cardiovasc. Med.* **2018**, *5*, 135. [CrossRef] [PubMed]
163. Powers, S.K.; Deminice, R.; Ozdemir, M.; Yoshihara, T.; Bomkamp, M.P.; Hyatt, H. Exercise-induced oxidative stress: Friend or foe? *J. Sport Health Sci.* **2020**, *9*, 415–425. [CrossRef] [PubMed]
164. Thirupathi, A.; Pinho, R.A.; Chang, Y.Z. Physical exercise: An inducer of positive oxidative stress in skeletal muscle aging. *Life Sci.* **2020**, *252*, 117630. [CrossRef]
165. Done, A.J.; Gage, M.J.; Nieto, N.C.; Traustadóttir, T. Exercise-induced Nrf2-signalling is impaired in aging. *Free. Radic. Biol. Med.* **2016**, *96*, 130–138. [CrossRef]
166. Vasilaki, A.; McArdle, F.; Iwanejko, L.M.; McArdle, A. Adaptive responses of mouse skeletal muscle to contractile activity: The effect of age. *Mech. Ageing Dev.* **2006**, *127*, 830–839. [CrossRef] [PubMed]
167. Yamada, M.; Iwata, M.; Warabi, E.; Oishi, H.; Lira, V.A.; Okutsu, M. p62/SQSTM1 and Nrf2 are essential for exercise-mediated enhancement of antioxidant protein expression in oxidative muscle. *Faseb. J.* **2019**, *33*, 8022–8032. [CrossRef] [PubMed]
168. George, L.; Lokhandwala, M.F.; Asghar, M. Exercise activates redox-sensitive transcription factors and restores renal D1 receptor function in old rats. *Am. J. Physiol.* **2009**, *297*, F1174–F1180. [CrossRef]
169. Macneil, L.; Safdar, A.; Baker, S.; Melov, S.; Tarnopolsky, M. Eccentric Exercise Affects NRF2-mediated Oxidative Stress Response in Skeletal Muscle by Increasing Nuclear NRF2 Content. *Med. Sci. Sport. Exerc.* **2011**, *43*, 383. [CrossRef]
170. Miyata, M.; Kasai, H.; Kawai, K.; Yamada, N.; Tokudome, M.; Ichikawa, H.; Goto, C.; Tokudome, Y.; Kuriki, K.; Hoshino, H.; et al. Changes of urinary 8-hydroxydeoxyguanosine levels during a two-day ultramarathon race period in Japanese non-professional runners. *Int. J. Sports Med.* **2008**, *29*, 27–33. [CrossRef]
171. Done, A.J.; Traustadóttir, T. Nrf2 mediates redox adaptations to exercise. *Redox Biol.* **2016**, *10*, 191–199. [CrossRef]
172. Shally, A.; McDonagh, B. The redox environment and mitochondrial dysfunction in age-related skeletal muscle atrophy. *Biogerontology* **2020**, *21*, 461–473. [CrossRef] [PubMed]
173. Magherini, F.; Fiaschi, T.; Marzocchini, R.; Mannelli, M.; Gamberi, T.; Modesti, P.A.; Modesti, A. Oxidative stress in exercise training: The involvement of inflammation and peripheral signals. *Free Radic. Res.* **2019**, *53*, 1155–1165. [CrossRef] [PubMed]
174. Cheng, A.J.; Yamada, T.; Rassier, D.E.; Andersson, D.C.; Westerblad, H.; Lanner, J.T. Reactive oxygen/nitrogen species and contractile function in skeletal muscle during fatigue and recovery. *J. Physiol.* **2016**, *594*, 5149–5160. [CrossRef] [PubMed]
175. Lessard, S.J.; MacDonald, T.L.; Pathak, P.; Han, M.S.; Coffey, V.G.; Edge, J.; Rivas, D.A.; Hirshman, M.F.; Davis, R.J.; Goodyear, L.J. JNK regulates muscle remodelling via myostatin/SMAD inhibition. *Nat. Commun.* **2018**, *9*, 3030. [CrossRef] [PubMed]
176. Dalle-Donne, I.; Rossi, R.; Giustarini, D.; Milzani, A.; Colombo, R. Protein carbonyl groups as biomarkers of oxidative stress. *Clin. Chim. Acta* **2003**, *329*, 23–38. [CrossRef] [PubMed]
177. Aldini, G.; Dalle-Donne, I.; Facino, R.M.; Milzani, A.; Carini, M. Intervention strategies to inhibit protein carbonylation by lipoxidation-derived reactive carbonyls. *Med. Res. Rev.* **2007**, *27*, 817–868. [CrossRef]
178. Gorini, G.; Gamberi, T.; Fiaschi, T.; Mannelli, M.; Modesti, A.; Magherini, F. Irreversible plasma and muscle protein oxidation and physical exercise. *Free Radic. Res.* **2019**, *53*, 126–138. [CrossRef]
179. Cai, Z.; Yan, L.J. Protein Oxidative Modifications: Beneficial Roles in Disease and Health. *J. Biochem. Pharmacol. Res.* **2013**, *1*, 15–26.
180. Rungratanawanich, W.; Qu, Y.; Wang, X.; Essa, M.M.; Song, B.-J. Advanced glycation end products (AGEs) and other adducts in aging-related diseases and alcohol-mediated tissue injury. *Exp. Mol. Med.* **2021**, *53*, 168–188. [CrossRef]

181. Neubauer, O.; König, D.; Wagner, K.H. Recovery after an Ironman triathlon: Sustained inflammatory responses and muscular stress. *Eur. J. Appl. Physiol.* **2008**, *104*, 417–426. [CrossRef]
182. Suzuki, K.; Peake, J.; Nosaka, K.; Okutsu, M.; Abbiss, C.R.; Surriano, R.; Bishop, D.; Quod, M.J.; Lee, H.; Martin, D.T.; et al. Changes in markers of muscle damage, inflammation and HSP70 after an Ironman Triathlon race. *Eur. J. Appl. Physiol.* **2006**, *98*, 525–534. [CrossRef] [PubMed]
183. Bassel-Duby, R.; Olson, E.N. Signalling pathways in skeletal muscle remodelling. *Annu. Rev. Biochem.* **2006**, *75*, 19–37. [CrossRef] [PubMed]
184. St-Pierre, J.; Drori, S.; Uldry, M.; Silvaggi, J.M.; Rhee, J.; Jäger, S.; Handschin, C.; Zheng, K.; Lin, J.; Yang, W.; et al. Suppression of reactive oxygen species and neurodegeneration by the PGC-1 transcriptional coactivators. *Cell* **2006**, *127*, 397–408. [CrossRef]
185. Bouviere, J.; Fortunato, R.S.; Dupuy, C.; Werneck-de-Castro, J.P.; Carvalho, D.P.R.A. Louzada Exercise-Stimulated ROS Sensitive Signalling Pathways in Skeletal Muscle. *Antioxidants* **2021**, *10*, 537. [CrossRef] [PubMed]
186. Sakellariou, G.K.; Vasilaki, A.; Palomero, J.; Kayani, A.; Zibrik, L.; McArdle, A.; Jackson, M.J. Studies of mitochondria and nonmitochondrial sources implicate nicotinamide adenine dinucleotide phosphate oxidase(s) in the increased skeletal muscle superoxide generation that occurs during contractile activity. *Antioxid. Redox Signal.* **2013**, *18*, 603–621. [CrossRef]
187. Kang, C.; O'Moore, K.M.; Dickman, J.R.; Ji, L.L. Exercise activation of muscle peroxisome proliferator-activated receptor-gamma coactivator-1alpha signalling is redox sensitive. *Free Radic. Biol. Med.* **2009**, *47*, 1394–1400. [CrossRef]
188. Ferraro, E.; Giammarioli, A.M.; Chiandotto, S.; Spoletini, I.; Rosano, G. Exercise-induced skeletal muscle remodelling and metabolic adaptation: Redox signalling and role of autophagy. *Antioxid. Redox Signal.* **2014**, *21*, 154–176. [CrossRef]
189. Done, A.J.; Traustadóttir, T. Aerobic exercise increases resistance to oxidative stress in sedentary older middle-aged adults. A pilot study. *Age* **2016**, *38*, 505–512. [CrossRef]
190. Parise, G.; Phillips, S.M.; Kaczor, J.J.; Tarnopolsky, M.A. Antioxidant enzyme activity is up-regulated after unilateral resistance exercise training in older adults. *Free Radic. Biol. Med.* **2005**, *39*, 289–295. [CrossRef]
191. Peters, P.G.; Alessio, H.M.; Hagerman, A.E.; Ashton, T.; Nagy, S.; Wiley, R.L. Short-term isometric exercise reduces systolic blood pressure in hypertensive adults: Possible role of reactive oxygen species. *Int. J. Cardiol.* **2006**, *110*, 199–205. [CrossRef]
192. da Silva, E.P.; Soares, E.O.; Malvestiti, R.; Hatanaka, E.; Lambertucci, R.H. Resistance training induces protective adaptation from the oxidative stress induced by an intense-strength session. *Sport Sci. Health* **2016**, *12*, 321–328. [CrossRef]
193. Ammar, A.; Trabelsi, K.; Boukhris, O.; Glenn, J.M.; Bott, N.; Masmoudi, L.; Hakim, A.; Chtourou, H.; Driss, T.; Hoekelmann, A.; et al. Effects of Aerobic-, Anaerobic- and Combined-Based Exercises on Plasma Oxidative Stress Biomarkers in Healthy Untrained Young Adults. *Int. J. Environ. Res. Public Health* **2020**, *17*, 2601. [CrossRef] [PubMed]
194. Zarrindast, S.; Ramezanpour, M.R.; Moghaddam, M.G. Effects of eight weeks of moderate intensity aerobic training and training in water on DNA damage, lipid peroxidation and total antioxidant capacity in sixty years sedentary women. *Sci. Sport.* **2021**, *36*, e81–e85. [CrossRef]
195. Leelarungrayub, D.; Saidee, K.; Pothongsunun, P.; Pratanaphon, S.; YanKai, A.; Bloomer, R.J. Six weeks of aerobic dance exercise improves blood oxidative stress status and increases interleukin-2 in previously sedentary women. *J. Bodyw. Mov. Ther.* **2011**, *15*, 355–362. [CrossRef] [PubMed]
196. Estébanez, B.; Rodriguez, A.L.; Visavadiya, N.P.; Whitehurst, M.; Cuevas, M.J.; González-Gallego, J.; Huang, C.J. Aerobic Training Down-Regulates Pentraxin 3 and Pentraxin 3/Toll-Like Receptor 4 Ratio, Irrespective of Oxidative Stress Response, in Elderly Subjects. *Antioxidants* **2020**, *9*, 110. [CrossRef] [PubMed]
197. Vezzoli, A.; Mrakic-Sposta, S.; Montorsi, M.; Porcelli, S.; Vago, P.; Cereda, F.; Longo, S.; Maggio, M.; Narici, M. Moderate Intensity Resistive Training Reduces Oxidative Stress and Improves Muscle Mass and Function in Older Individuals. *Antioxidants* **2019**, *8*, 431. [CrossRef]
198. El Abed, K.; Ammar, A.; Boukhris, O.; Trabelsi, K.; Masmoudi, L.; Bailey, S.J.; Hakim, A.; Bragazzi, N.L. Independent and Combined Effects of All-Out Sprint and Low-Intensity Continuous Exercise on Plasma Oxidative Stress Biomarkers in Trained Judokas. *Front. Physiol.* **2019**, *10*, 842. [CrossRef]
199. Jamurtas, A.Z. Exercise-Induced Muscle Damage and Oxidative Stress. *Antioxidants* **2018**, *7*, 50. [CrossRef]
200. Cheng, A.J.; Jude, B.; Lanner, J.T. Intramuscular mechanisms of overtraining. *Redox Biol.* **2020**, *35*, 101480. [CrossRef]
201. Leal, D.V.; Standing, A.S.I.; Furmanski, A.L.; Hough, J. Polymorphonuclear leucocyte phagocytic function, γδ T-lymphocytes and testosterone as separate stress-responsive markers of prolonged, high-intensity training programs. *Brain Behav. Immun.—Health* **2021**, *13*, 100234. [CrossRef]
202. Turner, J.E.; Hodges, N.J.; Bosch, J.A.; Aldred, S. Prolonged depletion of antioxidant capacity after ultraendurance exercise. *Med. Sci. Sports Exerc.* **2011**, *43*, 1770–1776. [CrossRef] [PubMed]
203. Kajaia, T.; Maskhulia, L.; Chelidze, K.; Akhalkatsi, V.; McHedlidze, T. Implication of relationship between oxidative stress and antioxidant status in blood serum. *Georgian Med News* **2018**, *284*, 71–76.
204. Rossi, P.; Buonocore, D.; Altobelli, E.; Brandalise, F.; Cesaroni, V.; Iozzi, D.; Savino, E.; Marzatico, F. Improving Training Condition Assessment in Endurance Cyclists: Effects of Ganoderma lucidum and Ophiocordyceps sinensis Dietary Supplementation. *Evidence-Based Complement. Altern. Med.* **2014**, *2014*, 979613. [CrossRef] [PubMed]
205. Jun, M.; Venkataraman, V.; Razavian, M.; Cooper, B.; Zoungas, S.; Ninomiya, T.; Webster, A.C.; Perkovic, V. Antioxidants for chronic kidney disease. *Cochrane Database Syst. Rev.* **2012**, *10*, CD008176. [CrossRef]

206. Tarnopolsky, M.A. Mitochondrial DNA shifting in older adults following resistance exercise training. *Appl. Physiol. Nutr. Metab.* **2009**, *34*, 348–354. [CrossRef]
207. Bouzid, M.A.; Filaire, E.; Matran, R.; Robin, S.; Fabre, C. Lifelong Voluntary Exercise Modulates Age-Related Changes in Oxidative Stress. *Int. J. Sports Med.* **2018**, *39*, 21–28. [CrossRef]
208. Bejma, J.; Ji, L.L. Aging and acute exercise enhance free radical generation in rat skeletal muscle. *J. Appl. Physiol.* **1999**, *87*, 465–470. [CrossRef]
209. Sovatzidis, A.; Chatzinikolaou, A.; Fatouros, I.G.; Panagoutsos, S.; Draganidis, D.; Nikolaidou, E.; Avloniti, A.; Michailidis, Y.; Mantzouridis, I.; Batrakoulis, A.; et al. Intradialytic cardiovascular exercise training alters redox status, reduces inflammation and improves physical performance in patients with chronic kidney disease. *Antioxidants* **2020**, *9*, 868. [CrossRef]
210. Wilund, K.R.; Tomayko, E.J.; Wu, P.T.; Chung, H.R.; Vallurupalli, S.; Lakshminarayanan, B.; Fernhall, B. Intradialytic exercise training reduces oxidative stress and epicardial fat: A pilot study. *Nephrol. Dial. Transplant.* **2010**, *25*, 2695–2701. [CrossRef]
211. Pechter, U.; Maaroos, J.; Mesikepp, S.; Veraksits, A.; Ots, M. Regular low-intensity aquatic exercise improves cardio-respiratory functional capacity and reduces proteinuria in chronic renal failure patients. *Nephrol. Dial. Transplant.* **2003**, *18*, 624–625. [CrossRef]
212. Knap, B.; Marija, P.; Večerić-Haler, Ž. Effect of Exhausting Exercise on Oxidative Stress in Health, Hemodialysis and Professional Sport. *Nat. Sci.* **2019**, *11*, 307–314. [CrossRef]
213. Abreu, C.C.; Cardozo, L.; Stockler-Pinto, M.B.; Esgalhado, M.; Barboza, J.E.; Frauches, R.; Mafra, D. Does resistance exercise performed during dialysis modulate Nrf2 and NF-κB in patients with chronic kidney disease? *Life Sci.* **2017**, *188*, 192–197. [CrossRef] [PubMed]
214. Wang, C.J.; Johansen, K.L. Are dialysis patients too frail to exercise? *Semin. Dial.* **2019**, *32*, 291–296. [CrossRef] [PubMed]

Disclaimer/Publisher's Note: The statements, opinions and data contained in all publications are solely those of the individual author(s) and contributor(s) and not of MDPI and/or the editor(s). MDPI and/or the editor(s) disclaim responsibility for any injury to people or property resulting from any ideas, methods, instructions or products referred to in the content.

MDPI
St. Alban-Anlage 66
4052 Basel
Switzerland
Tel. +41 61 683 77 34
Fax +41 61 302 89 18
www.mdpi.com

International Journal of Molecular Sciences Editorial Office
E-mail: ijms@mdpi.com
www.mdpi.com/journal/ijms

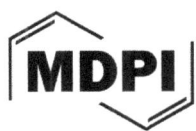

www.ingramcontent.com/pod-product-compliance
Lightning Source LLC
LaVergne TN
LVHW070748100526
838202LV00013B/1328